Clinical Calculations
With Applications to General and Specialty Areas

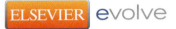

YOU'VE JUST PURCHASED
MORE THAN
A TEXTBOOK!

Evolve Student Resources for *Joyce Kee and Sally Marshall:*
Clinical Calculations With Applications to General
and Specialty Areas, eighth edition, **include the following:**

- **Drug Calculations Companion, Version 5**
  A completely updated, interactive
  student tutorial that includes an
  extensive menu of various topic
  areas within drug calculations such
  as oral, parenteral, pediatric, and
  intravenous calculations to name
  a few. It contains over 600 practice
  problems covering ratio and
  proportion, formula, and dimensional
  analysis methods.

Activate the complete learning experience that comes with each
textbook purchase by registering at

http://evolve.elsevier.com/KeeMarshall/clinical/

REGISTER TODAY!

Clinical Calculations

With Applications to General and Specialty Areas
Eighth Edition

Joyce LeFever Kee, RN, MS

Associate Professor Emerita
College of Health Sciences
Department of Nursing
University of Delaware
Newark, Delaware

Sally M. Marshall, RN, MSN

Formerly, Nursing Service
Department of Veterans Affairs
Regional Office of Medical Center
Wilmington, Delaware

Katy Woods, RN, BSN, DNP-C

Nurse Anesthesia Specialty
University of Maryland
Baltimore, Maryland

Mary Catherine (Katie) Forrester, RN, MSN, ACNP-BC

Vanderbilt University Hospital Trauma and Burn Center
Nashville, Tennessee

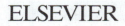

ELSEVIER

3251 Riverport Lane
St. Louis, Missouri 63043

CLINICAL CALCULATIONS WITH APPLICATIONS TO
GENERAL AND SPECIALTY AREAS, EIGHTH EDITION

ISBN: 978-0-323-39088-0

Notices

Knowledge and best practice in this field are constantly changing. As new research and experience broaden our understanding, changes in research methods, professional practices, or medical treatment may become necessary.

Practitioners and researchers must always rely on their own experience and knowledge in evaluating and using any information, methods, compounds, or experiments described herein. In using such information or methods they should be mindful of their own safety and the safety of others, including parties for whom they have a professional responsibility.

With respect to any drug or pharmaceutical products identified, readers are advised to check the most current information provided (i) on procedures featured or (ii) by the manufacturer of each product to be administered, to verify the recommended dose or formula, the method and duration of administration, and contraindications. It is the responsibility of practitioners, relying on their own experience and knowledge of their patients, to make diagnoses, to determine dosages and the best treatment for each individual patient, and to take all appropriate safety precautions.

To the fullest extent of the law, neither the Publisher nor the authors, contributors, or editors, assume any liability for any injury and/or damage to persons or property as a matter of products liability, negligence or otherwise, or from any use or operation of any methods, products, instructions, or ideas contained in the material herein.

Previous editions copyrighted 2013, 2009, 2004, 2000, 1996, 1992, 1988

Library of Congress Cataloging-in-Publication Data

Names: Kee, Joyce LeFever, author. | Marshall, Sally M., author. | Woods,
  Katy, author. | Forrester, Mary Catherine, author.
Title: Clinical calculations : with applications to general and specialty
  areas / Joyce LeFever Kee, Sally M. Marshall, Katy Woods, Mary Catherine
  (Katie) Forrester.
Description: Eighth edition. | St. Louis, Missouri : Elsevier Inc., [2016]
|
  Includes bibliographical references and index.
Identifiers: LCCN 2015046362 | ISBN 9780323390880
Subjects: | MESH: Drug Dosage Calculations | Pharmaceutical
  Preparations--administration & dosage | Nurses' Instruction
Classification: LCC RS57 | NLM QV 748 | DDC 615.1/4--dc23 LC record available
at http://lccn.loc.gov/2015046362

Senior Content Strategist: Yvonne Alexopoulos
Content Development Manager: Jean Sims Fornango
Senior Content Development Specialist: Danielle M. Frazier
Publishing Services Manager: Julie Eddy
Senior Project Manager: Mary G. Stueck
Design Direction: Brian Salisbury

Printed in Canada
Last digit is the print number: 9 8 7 6 5 4 3 2 1

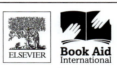

*To my granddaughter, Kimberly Cibroski, BSN, Nurse,
Emergency Room, ChristianaCare, Newark, Delaware*
Joyce Kee

In memory of my mother, Lois
Sally Marshall

To my parents, Bill and Rebecca, and my husband, Mark
Katie Forrester

To our nursing colleagues

Reviewers

Rose Mary Gee, PhD, RN
Assistant Professor
School of Nursing
Georgia Southern University
Statesboro, Georgia

Jessica Gonzales, ARNP, MSN, RN
Nursing Instructor
Lake Washington Institute of Technology
Redmond, Washington

Lori A. McGill, DNP, RN
Professor
College of Nursing
RN-to-BSN Program
St. Petersburg College
Pinellas Park, Florida

Bobbi Steelman, BSEd, MAEd, CPhT
Director of Education/Pharmacy Technician Program
Director
Daymar College
Bowling Green, Kentucky

Collene Thaxton, RN, MSN
Associate Professor
Mount Wachusett Community College
Gardner, Massachusetts

Preface to the Instructor

Clinical Calculations with Applications to General and Specialty Areas arose from the need to bridge the learning gap between education and practice. We believe that this bridge is needed for the student to understand the wide range of clinical calculations used in nursing practice. This book provides a comprehensive application of calculations in nursing practice.

Clinical Calculations has been expanded in this eighth edition on topics in several areas to show the interrelationship between calculation and drug administration. The use of the latest methods, techniques, and equipments are included: unit dose dispensing system, electronic medication administration record (eMAR), computerized prescriber order system (CPOS), various methods of calculating drug doses with the use of body mass index (BMI), ideal body weight (IBW) with adjusted body weight (ABW), insulin pump, patient-controlled analgesia pumps, multi-channel infusion pumps, IV filters, and many more. This text also provides the six (6) methods for calculating drug dosages—basic formula, ratio and proportion, fractional equation, dimensional analysis, body weight, and body surface area.

The chapter, "Prevention of Medication Errors," has been updated. It includes examples of the types of medication errors, ways to prevent medication errors, and the "10 Rights" in drug administration. A separate chapter, "Insulin Administration" has been added.

Clinical Calculations is unique in that it has problems not only for the general patient areas but also for the specialty units—pediatrics, critical care, pediatric critical care, labor and delivery, and community. This text is useful for nurses at all levels of nursing education who are learning for the first time how to calculate dosage problems and for beginning practitioners in specialty areas. It also can be used in nursing refresher courses, in-service programs, hospital units, home health care, and other settings of nursing practice.

This book is divided into five parts. Part I is the basic math review, written concisely for nursing students to review Roman numerals, fractions, decimals, percentages, and ratio and proportion. A post-math review test follows. The post-math test can be taken first and, if the student has a score of 90% of higher, the basic review section can be omitted. Part II covers metric and household measurement systems used in drug calculations; conversion of units; reading drug labels, drug orders, eMAR, computerized prescriber order systems, and abbreviations; and methods of calculations. We suggest that you assign Parts I and II, which cover delivery of medication, before the class. Part III covers calculation of drug and fluid dosages for oral, injectable, insulin administration, and intravenous administration. Clinical drug calculations for specialty areas are found in Part IV, which includes pediatrics, critical care for adults and children, labor and delivery, and community. Part V contains the post-test for students to test their competency in mastering oral, injectable, intravenous, and pediatric drug calculations. A passing grade is 88%.

Appendix A includes guidelines for administration of medications (oral, injectable, and intravenous), and Appendix B contains nomograms.

Each chapter has a content list, objectives, introduction, and numerous practice problems. The practice problems are related to clinical drug problems that are currently used in clinical settings. Illustrations of tablets, capsules, medicine cup, syringes, ampules, vials, intravenous bag and bottle, IV tubing, electronic IV devices, intramuscular injection sites, central venous sites, and many other related images are provided throughout the text.

Calculators may be used in solving dosage problems. Many institutions have calculators available. The student should work the problem without a calculator and then check the answer with a calculator.

FEATURES FOR THE EIGHTH EDITION

- The chapter on prevention of medication errors has been updated, and a new chapter on insulin administration has been added.
- Problems using the newest drug labels are provided in most chapters.
- Six methods for calculating drug dosages have been divided into two chapters. Chapter 6 gives four methods: basic formula, ratio and proportion, fractional equations, and dimensional analysis. Chapter 7 contains two individual methods for calculating drug doses: body weight and body surface area.
- Additional dimensional analysis has been added to the examples of drug dosing and to the answers to practice problems in most of the chapters.
- Additional drug problems have been added throughout.
- Emphasis is placed on the metric system along with the household system of measurement.
- Several chapters have nomograms for adults and children.
- Explanation on the unit dose dispensing system, computer-based drug administration, computerized prescriber order system, bar code medication administration, MAR, electronic medication administration record (eMAR), and automation of medication dispensing administration are provided.
- Incorporation of guidelines for safe practice and the medication administration set by the Joint Commission (TJC) and the Institute for Safe Medicine Practices (ISMP) are included.
- Explanation of the four groups of inhaled medications include: MDI inhalers with and without spacers, dry powder inhalers, and nebulizers.
- Calculations by BMI, IBW, and ABW for obese and debilitated persons are presented.
- Body Surface Area (BSA or m^2) using the square root method is included.
- Use of fingertip units for cream applications is illustrated.
- Explanations are provided for the use of the insulin pump, insulin pen injectors, and the patient-controlled analgesic pump.
- Illustrations of new types of syringes, safety needle shield, various insulin and tuberculin syringes, and needleless syringes are provided.
- Illustrations of pumps are provided, including insulin, enteral infusion, and various intravenous infusion pumps (single and multi-channel, patient-controlled analgesia, and syringe).
- Coverage of direct intravenous injection (IV push or IV bolus) is provided with practice problems in Chapter 11.
- Updated methods and information for critical care, pediatrics, and labor and delivery calculations are presented.

ANCILLARIES

Evolve resources for instructors and students can be found online at http://evolve.elsevier.com/KeeMarshall/clinical/

The Instructor Resources are designed to help you present the material in this text and include the following:
- Test Bank—now with over 500 questions.
- TEACH consists of customizable Lesson Plans and Lecture Outlines, and PowerPoint slides. It is an online resource designed to help you to reduce your lesson preparation time, give you new and creative ideas to promote student learning, and help you to make full use of the rich array of resources in the Clinical Calculations teaching package.
- Drug Label Glossary—includes all of the drug labels from the text. Instructors can search for labels by trade or generic name.
- *NEW VERSION!* ***Drug Calculations Comprehensive Test Bank,*** version 4. This generic test bank contains over 700 questions on general mathematics, converting within the same system of measurement, converting between different systems of measurement, oral dosages, parenteral dosages, flow rates, pediatric dosages, IV calculations, and more.

Student Resources provide students with additional tools for learning and include the following:
- *NEW VERSION!* **Drug Calculations Companion,** version 5. This is a completely updated, interactive student tutorial that includes an extensive menu of various topic areas within drug calculations, such as oral, parenteral, pediatric, and intravenous calculations. It contains over 600 practice problems covering ratio and proportion, formula, and dimensional analysis methods.

Preface to the Student

Clinical Calculations with Applications to General and Specialty Areas, eighth edition, can be used as a self-instructional mathematics and dosage calculation review tool.

Part I, *Basic Math Review,* is a review of math concepts usually taught in middle school. Some students may need to review Part I as a refresher of basic math and then take the comprehensive math test at the end of the chapter. Others may choose to take the math test first. If your score on this test is 90% or higher, you should proceed to Part II; if your score is less than 90%, you should review Part I.

Part II, *Systems, Conversion, and Methods of Drug Calculation,* should be studied before the class on oral, injectable, insulin administration, and intravenous calculations, which are covered in Part III. In Part II you will learn the various systems of drug administration, conversion within the various systems, charting (MAR and eMAR), drug orders, abbreviations, methods of drug calculation, how to prevent medication errors, and alternative methods for drug administration. You can study Part II on your own. Chapter 6, "Methods of Calculation," gives the four methods commonly used to calculate drug dosages. You or the instructor should select one of the four methods to calculate drug dosages. Use that method in all practice problems starting in Chapter 6. This approach will improve your proficiency in the calculation of drug dosages.

Part III, *Calculations for Oral, Injectable, and Intravenous Drugs,* is usually discussed in class and during a clinical practicum. Before class, you should review the four chapters in Part III. Questions may be addressed and answered during class time. During the class or clinical practicum, you may practice drug calculations and the drawing up of drug doses in a syringe.

Part IV, *Calculations for Specialty Areas,* is usually presented when the topics are discussed in class. You should review the content in these chapters—"Pediatrics," "Critical Care," "Pediatric Critical Care," "Labor and Delivery," and "Community"—before the scheduled class. According to the requirements of your specific nursing program, this content may or may not be covered.

Part V, *Post–Test,* has 65 post-test questions you should solve to determine your competency in mastering oral, injectable, intravenous, and pediatric drug calculations.

Take a look at the following features so that you may familiarize yourself with this text and maximize its value:

Caution boxes alert you to potential problems related to various medications and their administration.

Figure 8-3 A, Pill/tablet cutter. **B,** Silent Knight tablet crushing system. (**B,** Used with permission from Links Medical Products, Inc., Irvine, California.)

Pill/Tablet Cutter and Crusher

A pill or tablet cutter can be used to evenly split or divide a scored or unscored tablet. The pill cutter *cannot* be used to cut/divide enteric-coated tablets or capsules, time-released, sustained-released, or controlled-released capsules. Pill/tablet cutters can be purchased at a drug-store (Figure 8-3). If the patient cannot swallow pills or tablets, best practice is to consult with the prescriber or pharmacist to find if a liquid form of the drug is available. If the medication is not manufactured in liquid form, then a pill crusher (Figure 8-3, *B*) can be used to reduce tablets to a powdered form that can be mixed with water, juice, fruit sauce, or ice cream. Not all pills can be crushed; see Caution below.

> ⚠ **CAUTION**
> - Enteric-coated tablets have a special coating that allows them to move through the stomach and be dissolved in the small intestine so that the medication doesn't irritate the gastric mucosa.
> - Time-released, sustained-release, or controlled-release tablets slowly release drug over a period of time.
> - Layered tablets have medications that may be released at different times. The outer coating dissolves quickly, and the tablet core will dissolve slowly.

Calculation of Tablets and Capsules

The following steps should be taken to determine the drug dose:
1. Check the drug order.
2. Determine the drug available (generic name, brand name, and dosage per drug form).
3. Set up the method for drug calculation (basic formula, ratio and proportion, fraction equation, or dimensional analysis).
4. Convert to like units of measurement within the same system before solving the problem. Use the unit of measure on the drug container to calculate the drug dose.
5. Solve for the unknown (X).

Adding Drugs Used for Continuous Intravenous Administration

Nurses may need to prepare medications from vials and add the medication into the patient's IV solution bag for some continuous infusions. This process of mixing or compounding an IV solution should be completed before the IV bag or bottle is hung. The medication is prepared using sterile technique and is added through the injection port to the bag or bottle that is to be rotated, or gently agitated, to ensure that the drug is dispersed. Failure to adequately disperse the medication can result in a higher concentration of medication close to the bottom of the bag or bottle. This would deliver a higher concentration of the added medication, potentially causing harm to the patient. Medication labels must be placed on the IV bag or bottle, clearly stating the patient's name and any other identifiers as specified by policy, such as name of the drug, amount, concentration, and strength of all ingredients without abbreviation; also, date, nurse's initials, time, and the time the IV should be completed should be provided. It is important to follow institutional policies and procedures when adding medication to continuous IV fluid.

> **NOTE**
>
> **DO NOT** add the drug while the infusion is running unless the bag is rotated. A drug solution injected into an upright infusing IV solution causes the drug to concentrate into the lower portion of the IV bag and not be dispersed. The patient will receive a concentrated drug solution, and this can be harmful (e.g., if the drug is potassium chloride).

Types of Solutions

All IV solutions contain various solutes and electrolytes that are added for specific therapies. Common solutes include dextrose (D) and sodium chloride (NaCl). The strength of the solution is expressed in percent (%), such as 0.45%, which means 0.45 g in 100 mL. Common commercially prepared IV solutions are dextrose in water (D_5W), dextrose with one-half normal saline solution (D_5 0.45%), normal saline solution (0.9% NaCl), one-half normal saline solution (0.45% NaCl), and lactated Ringer's solution (LR). Lactated Ringer's solution contains sodium, chloride, potassium, calcium, and lactate.

Tonicity of IV Solutions

The terms *tonicity* and *osmolality* have been used interchangeably, but *tonicity* refers to the concentration of IV solution, whereas *osmolality* is the concentration of body fluids (e.g., blood, serum). IV solutions produce tonicity in the cells of the body; this is the movement of water molecules into and out of the cells because of their surrounding aqueous environment. IV solutions are divided into three categories: hypertonic, hypotonic, and isotonic. The range of tonicity is measured in milliosmoles, and the normal range is 240 to 340 mOsm: +50 mOsm and/or −50 mOsm of 290 mOsm. Hypertonic solutions cause water molecules to diffuse out of the cells and exert a hyperosmolar effect. For example, a hypertonic solution is D_5 0.9% normal saline (NaCl) because it has an osmolarity of 560 mOsm. Hypotonic solutions cause water molecules to diffuse into the cells and exert a hypo-osmolar effect. A solution of 0.45% normal saline (NaCl) is hypo-osmolar and has an osmolarity of 154 mOsm. D_5W is iso-osmolar with an osmolality of 250 mOsm; however, the dextrose is metabolized quickly, leaving only water, thus making the solution hypotonic. Isotonic solutions maintain the same concentration of water molecules on both sides of the cell, so no net movement occurs. The osmolarity of isotonic solutions is 240 to 340 mOsm, similar to blood, lactated Ringer's (LR), and 0.9% normal saline (NaCl) solution. Table 11-2 lists the names of selected IV solutions, their tonicity, and their osmolarity, as well as the abbreviations for these solutions.

Notes emphasize important points for students as they learn material in each chapter.

You Must Remember boxes identify pertinent concepts that students should commit to memory.

Health, www.Dailymed.nlm.nih.gov), and Lexicomp, on the unit for prompt information about the drug to be given, especially if it is a high-alert drug. Some examples of high-alert drugs are: potassium chloride, insulin, heparin, opiates, and anticancer agents. Refer to Chapter 13.

> **YOU MUST REMEMBER**
>
> The person who administers the medication, usually the nurse, is responsible if an ME occurs.

Here are some examples of the types of medication errors (MEs):

1. The physician or health care provider makes a prescribing error and/or the written drug order is **NOT** legible.
2. Transcription errors occur because the medications have similar names; the decimals and zeros are not correctly written; or numbers are transposed.
3. Telephone and verbal orders are misinterpreted.
4. Interruptions occur when preparing medications.
5. Drug labels look similar (names and color), and packing obscures print on the label.
6. Trade names and generic names for drugs are used interchangeably, which causes confusion.
7. Oral dosages and intravenous dosages are different for the same drug.
8. Subcutaneous insulin is given in a tuberculin syringe and **NOT** in an insulin syringe.
9. The pharmacy delivers the wrong drug.
10. Intravenous medication is given too fast or too concentrated.
11. The amount of the drug is incorrectly calculated.
12. The drug is given intramuscularly or subcutaneously and should be given intravenously OR the drug is given intravenously and should be given intramuscularly.
13. Two incompatible drugs are given intravenously, which can cause crystallization of the drugs.
14. Two or three patients with the same names are on the same unit and their identification wristbands are hard to read. One patient receives another's medication.
15. Medication is given and not monitored, and an overdose occurs.
16. An infusion pump malfunctions or is incorrectly programmed.

Ways to prevent medication errors (MEs):

1. Ask the physician or health care provider to rewrite or clarify medication order.
2. Use only approved abbreviations from The Joint Commission (TJC) list for medication dosages. Do not use "u" for unit; it should be spelled out. Avoid use of a slash mark (/), which could be interpreted as a one (1).
3. Do not use abbreviations for medication names (e.g., MSO_4 for morphine sulfate).
4. Use leading zeros for doses less than a unit (e.g., **0.1** mg; **NOT .1** mg). Do not use a zero following a whole number (e.g., 5 mg; **NOT** 5.0 mg). The decimal point after 5 may not be noticed and would look like 50 mg.
5. Check medication orders with written order and MAR/eMAR.
6. Check the drug dose sent from the pharmacy with the MAR/eMAR.
7. Prepare medications in a clean, distraction-free environment.
8. Never administer a medication that has been prepared by another nurse.
9. Have another nurse check the dosage preparation, especially if in doubt. Recalculate drug dosage as needed.
10. Check if the patient is allergic to any specific drugs. If an allergy exists, report the type of reaction the patient experiences.
11. Check the patient's identification band with the eMAR and bar code.
12. Do not leave medication at the bedside. Stay with the patient until the medications are swallowed.

*NEW VERSION! **Drug Calculations Companion,*** version 4. This is a completely updated, interactive student tutorial that includes an extensive menu of various topic areas within drug calculations, such as oral, parenteral, pediatric, and intravenous calculations. It contains over 600 practice problems covering ratio and proportion, formula, and dimensional analysis methods.

evolve Look for this icon at the end of the chapters. It will refer you to ***Drug Calculations Companion,*** version 5 for additional practice problems and content information.

ACKNOWLEDGMENTS

We wish to extend our sincere appreciation to the individuals who have helped with this eighth edition: Sara Ahmed, PharmD, BCPS, ChristianaCare Health Care System, Wilmington, Delaware; Sarah Marshall Pragg, for her graphic design and editing; and to our husbands, Edward Kee and Robert Marshall, for their support.

Joyce LeFever Kee
Sally M. Marshall

Contents

PART I

BASIC MATH REVIEW

Objectives
- Convert Roman numerals to Arabic numerals.
- Multiply and divide fractions and decimals.
- Solve ratio and proportion problems.
- Change percentages to decimals, fractions, and ratio and proportion.
- Demonstrate an understanding of Roman numerals, fractions, decimals, ratio and proportion, and percentage by passing the math test.

The basic math review assists nurses in converting Roman and Arabic numerals, multiplying and dividing fractions and decimals, and solving ratio and proportion problems and percentage problems. Nurses need to master basic math skills to solve drug dosage problems for the administration of medication.

A math test, found on pages 11 to 14, follows the basic math review. The test may be taken first, and, if a score of 90% or greater is achieved, the math review, or Part I, can be omitted. If the test score is less than 90%, the student should do the basic math review section. Some students may choose to start with Part I and then take the test.

Answers to the Practice Problems are at the end of Part I, before the Post-Math Test.

NUMBER SYSTEMS

Two systems of numbers currently used are Arabic and Roman. Both systems are used in drug administration.

Arabic System

The Arabic system is expressed in the numbers 0, 1, 2, 3, 4, 5, 6, 7, 8, and 9. These can be written as whole numbers or with fractions and decimals. This system is commonly used today.

Roman System

Numbers used in the Roman system are designated by selected capital letters, e.g., I, V, X. Roman numbers can be changed to Arabic numbers.

Conversion of Systems

Roman Number	Arabic Number
I	1
V	5
X	10
L	50
C	100

The apothecary system of measurement uses Roman numerals for writing drug dosages. The Roman numerals are written in lowercase letters, e.g., i, v, x, xii. The lowercase letters can be topped by a horizontal line, e.g., ī, v̄, x̄, x̄ii. These can be written with or without a horizontal line over the numerals.

Roman numerals can appear together, such as xv and ix. Reading multiple Roman numerals requires the use of addition and subtraction.

Method A

If the first Roman numeral is greater than the following numeral(s), then **ADD.**

EXAMPLES   v̄iii = 5 + 3 = 8
            x̄v = 10 + 5 = 15

Method B

If the first Roman numeral is less than the following numeral(s), then **SUBTRACT.** Subtract the first numeral from the second (i.e., the smaller from the larger).

EXAMPLES   īv = 5 − 1 = 4
            īx = 10 − 1 = 9

Some Roman numerals require both addition and subtraction to ascertain their value. Read from left to right.

EXAMPLES $\overline{xix}$ = 10 + 9(10 − 1) = 19
          $\overline{xxxiv}$ = 30(10 + 10 + 10) + 4(5 − 1) = 34

PRACTICE PROBLEMS ▶ I ROMAN NUMERALS

Answers can be found on page 9.

1. $\overline{xvi}$

10 5 1 =
16

2. $\overline{xii}$

10 +1 +1 = 12

3. $\overline{xxiv}$

10+ 10 + 11 = 5   26
20 + 4 = 24

4. $\overline{xxxix}$

$\dfrac{10+10+10-1+10}{9}$ = 39

5. XLV

10 − 50 + 5 = 45
10 − 55

6. XC

10 − 100 = 90

FRACTIONS

Fractions are expressed as part(s) of a whole or part(s) of a unit. A fraction is composed of two basic numbers: a *numerator* (the top number) and a *denominator* (the bottom number). The denominator indicates the total number of parts.

EXAMPLES   Fraction: $\dfrac{3}{4}$ numerator (3 of 4 parts)
                 denominator (4 of 4 parts, or 4 total parts)

The value of a fraction depends mainly on the denominator. When the denominator increases, for example, from $\frac{1}{10}$ to $\frac{1}{20}$, the value of the fraction decreases, because it takes more parts to make a whole.

EXAMPLES   Which fraction has the greater value: $\frac{1}{4}$ or $\frac{1}{6}$? The denominators are 4 and 6.

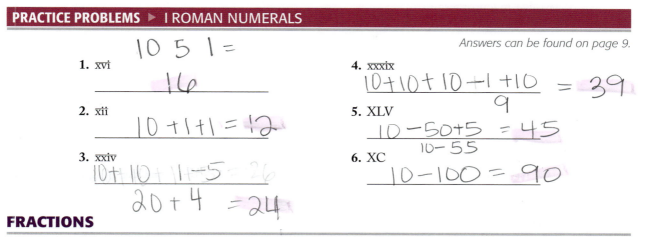

Pie $\frac{1}{4}$ $\frac{1}{6}$ ← too many parts to make whole

A   B

The larger value is $\frac{1}{4}$, because four parts make the whole, whereas for $\frac{1}{6}$, it takes six parts to make a whole. Therefore $\frac{1}{6}$ has the smaller value.

Proper, Improper, and Mixed Fractions

In a *proper fraction* (simple fraction), the numerator is less than the denominator, e.g., $\frac{1}{2}$, $\frac{2}{3}$, $\frac{3}{4}$, $\frac{2}{6}$. (When possible, the fraction should be reduced to its lowest terms, e.g., $\frac{2}{6}$ = $\frac{1}{3}$ [2 goes into 2 and 6].)

In an *improper fraction*, the numerator is greater than the denominator, e.g., $\frac{4}{2}$, $\frac{8}{5}$, $\frac{14}{4}$. (Reduce improper fractions to whole numbers or mixed numbers, e.g., $\frac{4}{2}$ = 2 [$\frac{4}{2}$ means the same as 4 ÷ 2]; $\frac{8}{5}$ = $1\frac{3}{5}$ [8 ÷ 5, 5 goes into 8 one time with 3 left over, or $\frac{3}{5}$]; and $\frac{14}{4}$ = $3\frac{2}{4}$ = $3\frac{1}{2}$ [14 ÷ 4, 4 goes into 14 three times with 2 left over, or $\frac{2}{4}$, which can then be reduced to $\frac{1}{2}$].)

A *mixed number* is a whole number and a fraction, e.g., $1\frac{3}{5}$, $3\frac{1}{2}$. Mixed numbers can be changed to improper fractions by multiplying the denominator by the whole number, then adding the numerator, e.g., $1\frac{3}{5}$ = $\frac{8}{5}$ (5 × 1 = 5 + 3 = 8).

Fractions may be added, subtracted, multiplied, or divided. Multiplying fractions and dividing fractions are the two common methods used in solving dosage problems.

Multiplying Fractions

To multiply fractions, multiply the numerators and then the denominators. Reduce the fraction, if possible, to lowest terms.

EXAMPLES   **PROBLEM 1:** $\dfrac{1}{3} \times \dfrac{3}{5} = \dfrac{\overset{1}{3}}{\underset{5}{15}} = \dfrac{1}{5}$

The answer is $\frac{3}{15}$, which can be reduced to $\frac{1}{5}$. The number that goes into both 3 and 15 is 3. Therefore 3 goes into 3 one time, and 3 goes into 15 five times.

PROBLEM 2: $\dfrac{1}{3} \times 6 = \dfrac{6}{3} = 2$

A whole number can also be written as that number over one ($\frac{6}{1}$). Six is divided by 3 ($6 \div 3$); 3 goes into 6 two times.

PROBLEM 3: $\dfrac{4}{5} \times 12 = \dfrac{48}{5} = 9\dfrac{3}{5}$

Dividing Fractions

To divide fractions, invert the *second fraction*, or divisor, and then multiply.

EXAMPLES   **PROBLEM 1:** $\dfrac{3}{4} \div \dfrac{3}{8} \text{ (divisor)} = \dfrac{\overset{1}{3}}{\underset{1}{4}} \times \dfrac{\overset{2}{8}}{\underset{1}{3}} = \dfrac{2}{1} = 2$

When dividing, invert the divisor $\frac{3}{8}$ to $\frac{8}{3}$ and multiply. To reduce the fraction to lowest terms, 3 goes into both 3s one time, and 4 goes into 4 and 8 one time and two times, respectively.

PROBLEM 2: $\dfrac{1}{6} \div \dfrac{4}{18} = \dfrac{1}{\underset{1}{6}} \times \dfrac{\overset{3}{18}}{4} = \dfrac{3}{4}$

Six and 18 are reduced, or canceled, to 1 and 3.

PROBLEM 3: $3\dfrac{2}{3} \div \dfrac{5}{6} = \dfrac{11}{\underset{1}{3}} \times \dfrac{\overset{2}{6}}{5} = \dfrac{22}{5} = 4\dfrac{2}{5}$

Change $3\frac{2}{3}$ to an improper fraction and invert $\frac{5}{6}$ to $\frac{6}{5}$ and then multiply. Reduce 3 and 6 to 1 and 2.

Decimal Fractions

Change fraction to decimal. Divide the numerator by the denominator.

EXAMPLES   **PROBLEM 1:** $\dfrac{3}{4} = 4\overline{)3.00}^{\,0.75}$ or 0.75

Therefore $\frac{3}{4}$ is the same as 0.75.

PROBLEM 2: $\quad \dfrac{12}{8} = 8\overline{)12.0}^{\,1.5}$ or 1.5

$$\begin{array}{r} 8 \\ \hline 4\,0 \\ 4\,0 \\ \hline \end{array}$$

PRACTICE PROBLEMS ▶ II FRACTIONS

Answers can be found on pages 9 and 10.

Round off to the nearest <u>tenth unless otherwise indicated.</u>

1. a. Which has the greatest value: $\frac{1}{50}$, $\frac{1}{100}$, or $\frac{1}{150}$? _____ $\frac{1}{50}$ _____

    b. Which has the lowest value: $\frac{1}{50}$, $\frac{1}{100}$, or $\frac{1}{150}$? _____ $\frac{1}{150}$ _____

2. Reduce improper fractions to whole or mixed numbers.

    a. $\frac{12}{4} =$ 3

    b. $\frac{20}{5} =$ 4

    c. $\frac{22}{3} =$ $7\frac{1}{3}$

    d. $\frac{32}{6} =$ $5\frac{2}{6} = 5\frac{1}{3}$ $6 \times 5 = 30$ $\frac{32}{30}\,_2$

3. Multiply fractions to whole number(s) or lowest fraction or decimal.

    a. $\frac{2}{3} \times \frac{1}{8} =$ $\frac{2}{24}\, \frac{2}{2} = \frac{1}{12}$

    $\frac{12}{5} \times \frac{15}{4}$ **b.** $2\frac{2}{5} \times 3\frac{3}{4} =$ $\frac{180}{20} = 9$

    c. $\frac{500}{350} \times 5 =$ $\frac{2500}{350}$ $5\frac{5}{7}$

    d. $\frac{400,000}{200,000} \times 3 =$

4. Divide fractions to whole number(s) or lowest fraction or decimal.

    a. $\frac{2}{3} \div 6 =$

    b. $\frac{1}{4} \div \frac{1}{5} =$

    c. $\frac{1}{6} \div \frac{1}{8} =$

    d. $\frac{1}{150} / \frac{1}{100} = (\frac{1}{150} \div \frac{1}{100}) =$

    e. $\frac{1}{200} \div \frac{1}{300} =$

    f. $9\frac{3}{5} \div 4 =$

        $\frac{48}{5} \div \frac{4}{1} =$

5. Change each fraction to a decimal.

    a. $\frac{1}{4} =$ **b.** $\frac{1}{10} =$ **c.** $\frac{2}{5} =$

    d. $\frac{35}{4} =$ **e.** $\frac{78}{5} =$

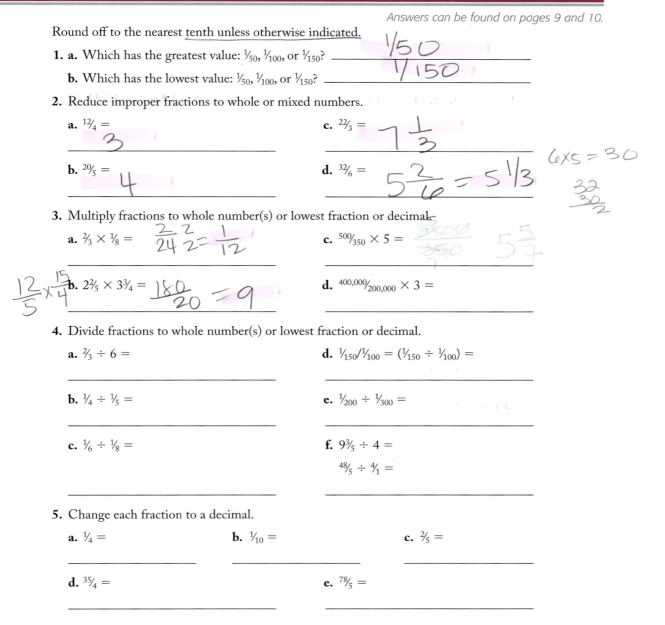

DECIMALS

Decimals consist of (1) whole numbers (numbers to the left of decimal point) and (2) decimal fractions (numbers to the right of decimal point). The number 2468.8642 is an example of the division of units for a whole number with a decimal fraction.

Whole Numbers					Decimal Fractions			
2	4	6	8	•	8	6	4	2
Thousands	Hundreds	Tens	Units		Tenths	Hundredths	Thousandths	Ten Thousandths

Decimal fractions are written in tenths, hundredths, thousandths, and ten-thousandths. Frequently, decimal fractions are used in drug dosing. The metric system is referred to as the *decimal system*. After decimal problems are solved, decimal fractions are generally rounded off to tenths. *If the hundredth column is 5 or greater, the tenth is increased by 1, e.g., 0.67 is rounded up to 0.7 (tenths).*

Decimal fractions are an integral part of the metric system. Tenths mean 0.1 or $\frac{1}{10}$, hundredths mean 0.01 or $\frac{1}{100}$, and thousandths mean 0.001 or $\frac{1}{1000}$. When a decimal is changed to a fraction, the denominator is based on the number of digits to the right of the decimal point (0.8 is $\frac{8}{10}$, 0.86 is $\frac{86}{100}$).

EXAMPLES **PROBLEM 1:** 0.5 is $\frac{5}{10}$, or 5 tenths.
PROBLEM 2: 0.55 is $\frac{55}{100}$, or 55 hundredths.
PROBLEM 3: 0.555 is $\frac{555}{1000}$, or 555 thousandths.

Multiplying Decimals

To multiply decimal numbers, multiply the multiplicand by the multiplier. Count how many numbers (spaces) are to the right of the decimals in the problem. Mark off the number of decimal spaces in the answer (right to left) according to the number of decimal spaces in the problem. Answers are rounded off to the nearest **tenths.**

EXAMPLES
```
 1.34    multiplicand
×2.3     multiplier
 402
268
3.082    or   3.1 (rounded off in tenths)
```

Answer: 3.1. Because 8 is greater than 5, the "tenth" number is increased by 1.

Dividing Decimals

To divide decimal numbers, move the decimal point in the divisor to the right to make a whole number. The decimal point in the dividend is also moved to the right according to the number of decimal spaces in the divisor. Answers are rounded off to the nearest **tenths.**

EXAMPLES Dividend ÷ Divisor

$$2.46 \div 1.2 \text{ or } \frac{2.46}{1.2} =$$

$$\text{(divisor)} \quad 1.2\overline{)2.4\,60} \text{ (dividend)} \quad \frac{2.05 = 2.1}{}$$

$$\underline{2\,4}$$

$$60$$

$$\underline{60}$$

$$0$$

PRACTICE PROBLEMS ▶ III DECIMALS

Answers can be found on page 10.

Round off to the nearest tenths.

1. Multiply decimals.

a. 6.8 × 0.123 =   **b.** 52.4 × 9.345 =

_____   _____

2. Divide decimals.

a. 69 ÷ 3.2 =   **c.** 100 ÷ 4.5 =

_____   _____

b. 6.63 ÷ 0.23 =   **d.** 125 ÷ 0.75 =

_____   _____

3. Change decimals to fractions.

a. 0.46 =   **b.** 0.05 =   **c.** 0.012 =

_____   _____   _____

4. Which has the greatest value: 0.46, 0.05, or 0.012? Which has the smallest value? _____

RATIO AND PROPORTION

A *ratio* is the relation between two numbers and is separated by a colon, e.g., 1:2 (1 is to 2). It is another way of expressing a fraction, e.g., 1:2 = ½.

Proportion is the relation between two ratios separated by a double colon (::) or equals sign (=).

To solve a ratio and proportion problem, the inside numbers *(means)* are multiplied and the outside numbers *(extremes)* are multiplied. To solve for the unknown, which is X, the X goes to the left side and is followed by an equals sign.

EXAMPLES **PROBLEM 1:** 1:2::2:X (1 is to 2, as 2 is to X)

means

extremes

Multiply the extremes and the means, and solve for X.

X = 4 (1 X is the same as X)

Answer: 4 (1:2::2:4)

PROBLEM 2: 4:8 :: X:12

8 X = 48

$X = {}^{48}\!/_8 = 6$

Answer: 6 (4:8::6:12)

PROBLEM 3: A ratio and proportion problem may be set up as a fraction.

Ratio and Proportion	*Fraction*
2:3::4:X	$\dfrac{2}{3} = \dfrac{4}{X}$ (cross-multiply)
2 X = 12	2 X = 12
$X = {}^{12}\!/_2 = 6$	X = 6

Answer: 6. Remember to cross-multiply when the problem is set up as a fraction.

PRACTICE PROBLEMS ▶ IV RATIO AND PROPORTION

Answers can be found on page 10.

Solve for X.

1. 2:10::5:X

_____

2. 0.9:100 = X:1000

_____

3. Change the ratio and proportion to a fraction and solve for X.
3:5::X:10

_____

4. It is 500 miles from Washington, DC, to Boston, MA. Your car averages 22 miles per 1 gallon of gasoline. How many gallons of gasoline will be needed for the trip?

_____

PERCENTAGE

Percent (%) means 100. Two percent (2%) means 2 parts of 100, and 0.9% means 0.9 part (less than 1) of 100. A percent can be expressed as a fraction, a decimal, or a ratio.

EXAMPLES

Percent		Fraction	Decimal	Ratio
60%	=	$^{60}/_{100}$	0.6	60:100
0.45%	=	$^{0.45}/_{100}$ or $^{45}/_{10,000}$	0.0045	0.45:100 or 45:10,000

Note: *To change a percent to a decimal, move the decimal point two places to the left.*

PRACTICE PROBLEMS ▶ V PERCENTAGE

Answers can be found on page 10.

Change percent to fraction, decimal, and ratio.

Percent	Fraction	Decimal	Ratio
1. 2%			
2. 0.33%			
3. 150%			
4. ½% (0.5%)			
5. 0.9%			

ANSWERS

I Roman Numerals

1. $10 + 5 + 1 = 16$
2. $10 + 2 = 12$
3. $20 (10 + 10) + 4 (5 - 1) = 24$
4. $30 (10 + 10 + 10) + 9 (10 - 1) = 39$
5. $40 (50 - 10) + 5 = 45$
6. $100 - 10 = 90$

II Fractions (Round off to the nearest tenths unless otherwise indicated.)

1. a. $^{1}/_{50}$ has the greatest value.
  b. $^{1}/_{150}$ has the lowest value.
2. a. 3
  b. 4
  c. $7\frac{1}{3}$
  d. $5^{2}/_{6}$ or $5\frac{1}{3}$
3. a. $^{2}/_{24} = ^{1}/_{12}$

  b. $^{12}/_{5} \times ^{15}/_{4} = \dfrac{180}{20} = 9$

  c. $\dfrac{\overset{10}{\cancel{500}}}{\underset{7}{\cancel{350}}} \times 5 = \dfrac{50}{7} = 7.1$

  d. $\dfrac{\overset{2}{\cancel{400{,}000}}}{\underset{1}{\cancel{200{,}000}}} \times 3 = 6$

4. a. $^{2}/_{3} \div 6 = ^{2}/_{3} \times ^{1}/_{6}$
    $= ^{2}/_{18} = ^{1}/_{9} = 0.11$
  b. $^{1}/_{4} \div ^{1}/_{5} =$
    $^{1}/_{4} \times ^{5}/_{1} = ^{5}/_{4} =$
    $1\frac{1}{4}$, or 1.25 or 1.3

  c. $\dfrac{1}{6} \div \dfrac{1}{8} = \dfrac{1}{\underset{3}{\cancel{6}}} \times \dfrac{\overset{4}{\cancel{8}}}{1} = \dfrac{4}{3} = 1.33,\ \text{or}\ 1.3$

  d. $^{1}/_{150} \div ^{1}/_{100} = \dfrac{1}{\underset{3}{\cancel{150}}} \times \dfrac{\overset{2}{\cancel{100}}}{1}$

    $= ^{2}/_{3}$, or 0.666, or 0.67 or 0.7
  e. $^{1}/_{200} \div ^{1}/_{300} = ^{1}/_{200} \times ^{300}/_{1} = ^{300}/_{200} = 1\frac{1}{2}$, or 1.5

  f. $\dfrac{48}{5} \div \dfrac{4}{1} = \dfrac{48}{5} \times \dfrac{1}{4} = \dfrac{48}{20} = 2.4$

5. a. $\dfrac{1}{4} = 4\overline{)1.00}$ $\dfrac{0.25}{}$ or 0.3 rounded off

b. $\dfrac{1}{10} = 10\overline{)1.00}$ $\dfrac{0.10}{}$ or 0.1

c. $\dfrac{2}{5} = 5\overline{)2.00}$ $\dfrac{0.40}{}$ or 0.4

d. $\dfrac{35}{4} = 4\overline{)35.00}$ $\dfrac{8.75}{}$ or 8.8 rounded off

e. $\dfrac{78}{5} = 5\overline{)78.00}$ $\dfrac{15.60}{}$ or 15.6

III Decimals

1. a. 0.8364, or 0.8

$$\begin{array}{r} \times 0.123 \\ \hline 6.8 \\ 984 \\ 738 \\ \hline \end{array}$$

  0.8364, or 0.8 (round off to tenths: 3 hundredths is less than 5)
   b. 489.6780, or 489.7 (7 hundredths is greater than 5)
2. a. 21.56, or 21.6 (6 hundredths is greater than 5, so the tenth is increased by one)
   b. 28.826, or 28.8 (2 hundredths is less than 5, so the tenth is not changed)
   c. $100 \div 4.5 = 4.5\overline{)100.0} = 22.2$, or 22 (rounded off to whole number)
   d. $125 \div 0.75 = 0.75\overline{)125.00} = 166.6$, or 167 (rounded off to whole number)
3. a. $^{46}\!/_{100} = ^{23}\!/_{50}$ **b.** $^{5}\!/_{100} = ^{1}\!/_{20}$ **c.** $^{12}\!/_{1000} = ^{3}\!/_{250}$
4. 0.46 has the greatest value; 0.012 has the lowest value. Forty-six hundredths is greater than 12 thousandths.

IV Ratio and Proportion

1. $2X = 50$
    $X = 25$
2. $100X = 900$
    $X = 9$
3. $^3\!/_5 = {}^x\!/_{10} = 5X = 30$
            $X = 6$

4. 1 gal : 22 miles :: X gal : 500
        $22X = 500$
        $X = 22.7$ gal
  22.7 gallons of gasoline are needed.

V Percentage

Percent	Fraction	Decimal	Ratio
1. 2	$^2\!/_{100}$	0.02	2 : 100
2. 0.33 or 0.3	$^{0.33}\!/_{100}$ or $^{33}\!/_{10,000}$	0.0033	0.33 : 100 or 33 : 10,000
3. 150	$^{150}\!/_{100}$	1.50	150 : 100
4. 0.5	$^{0.5}\!/_{100}$ or $^{5}\!/_{1000}$	0.005	0.5 : 100 or 5 : 1000
5. 0.9	$^{0.9}\!/_{100}$ or $^{9}\!/_{1000}$	0.009	0.9 : 100 or 9 : 1000

POST-MATH TEST

Answers can be found on pages 13 and 14.

The math test is composed of five sections: Roman and Arabic numerals, fractions, decimals, ratios and proportions, and percentages. There are 60 questions. A passing score is 54 or more correct answers (90%). A nonpassing score is 7 or more incorrect answers. Answers to the Post-Math Test can be found on pages 13 and 14.

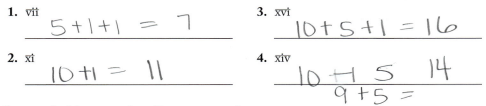

M D C L X V I
1000 500 100 50 10 5 1

Roman and Arabic Numerals

Convert Roman numerals to Arabic numerals.

1. vii

5 + 1 + 1 = 7

3. xvi

10 + 5 + 1 = 16

2. xi

10 + 1 = 11

4. xiv

10 + 5   14
9 + 5 =

Convert Arabic numerals to Roman numerals.

5. 4

IV

7. 29

XXIX

6. 18

XVIII
10 5

8. 37

XXXVII

Fractions

Which fraction has the larger value?

9. $\frac{1}{100}$ or $\frac{1}{150}$?

1/100

10. $\frac{1}{3}$ or $\frac{1}{2}$?

1/2

Reduce improper fractions to whole or mixed numbers.

11. $\frac{45}{9}$ =

5

12. $\frac{74}{3}$ =

$24\frac{2}{3}$

Change a mixed number to an improper fraction.

13. $5\frac{2}{3}$ =

17/3

Change fractions to decimals.

14. $\frac{2}{3} =$ (reduce to tenths)

15. $\frac{1}{12} =$ (reduce to tenths)

_____

_____

Multiply fractions (reduce to lowest terms or to tenths).

16. $\frac{7}{8} \times \frac{4}{6} =$

17. $2\frac{3}{5} \times \frac{5}{8} =$

_____

_____

18. $21\frac{3}{4} \times \frac{7}{8} =$

19. $4\frac{4}{5} \times 3\frac{2}{3} =$

_____

_____

Divide fractions.

20. $\frac{1}{2} \div \frac{1}{3} =$

22. $\frac{1}{8} \div \frac{1}{12} =$

_____

_____

21. $6\frac{3}{4} \div 3 =$

23. $20\frac{3}{4} \div \frac{1}{6} =$

_____

_____

Decimals

Round off decimal numbers to tenths.

24. $0.87 =$

26. $0.42 =$

_____

_____

25. $2.56 =$

_____

Change decimals to fractions.

27. $0.68 =$

29. $0.012 =$

_____

_____

28. $0.9 =$

30. $0.33 =$

_____

_____

Multiply decimals (round off to tenths or whole numbers).

31. $0.34 \times 0.6 =$

32. $2.123 \times 0.45 =$

_____

_____

Divide decimals.

33. $3.24 \div 0.3 =$

34. $69.4 \div 0.23 =$

_____

_____

Ratio and Proportion

Change ratios to fractions.

35. $3:4 =$

37. $65:90 =$

36. $1:175 =$

38. $0.9:100 =$

Solve ratio and proportion problems.

39. $2:3::8:X$

41. $3:100 = X:1000$

40. $0.5:20::X:100$

42. $5:25 = 10:X$

Change ratios and proportions to fractions and solve.

43. $1:2::4:X$

45. $0.9:10 = X:100$

44. $5:50::X:300$

Percentage

Change percents to fractions.

46. $3\% =$ **47.** $27\% =$ **48.** $1.2\% =$ **49.** $5.75\% =$

Change percents to decimals (round off to tenths, hundredths, or thousandths).

50. $8\% =$ **52.** $0.9\% =$ **54.** $0.25\% =$

51. $15\% =$ **53.** $3.5\% =$ **55.** $0.45\% =$

Change percents to ratios.

56. $35\% =$ **58.** $4\% =$ **60.** $0.45\% =$

57. $12.5\% =$ **59.** $0.9\% =$

ANSWERS   POST-MATH TEST

Roman and Arabic Numerals

1. 7   **3.** 16   **5.** iv   **7.** xxix
2. 11   **4.** 14   **6.** xviii   **8.** xxxvii

Fractions

9. $\frac{1}{100}$

10. $\frac{1}{2}$

11. 5

12. $24\frac{2}{3}$

13. $\frac{17}{3}$

14. 0.66 or 0.7

15. 0.08 or 0.1

16. $\frac{28}{48}$ or $\frac{7}{12}$ or 0.58 or 0.6

17. $\frac{13}{\cancel{5}} \times \frac{\cancel{5}^{1}}{8} = \frac{13}{8} = 1\frac{5}{8}$

18. $\frac{87}{4} \times \frac{7}{8} = \frac{609}{32} = $ 19.03 or 19.0 or 19 (rounded off)

19. $\frac{24}{5} \times \frac{11}{3} = \frac{264}{15} = 17.6$

20. $\frac{1}{2} \times \frac{3}{1} = \frac{3}{2} = 1\frac{1}{2}$

21. $\frac{\cancel{27}^{9}}{4} \times \frac{1}{\cancel{3}_{1}} = \frac{9}{4} = 2\frac{1}{4}$

22. $\frac{1}{\cancel{8}_{2}} \times \frac{\cancel{12}^{3}}{1} = \frac{3}{2} = 1\frac{1}{2}$

23. $\frac{83}{\cancel{4}_{2}} \times \frac{\cancel{6}^{3}}{1} = \frac{249}{2} = $ 124.5 or 125 whole number

Decimals

24. 0.9

25. 2.6

26. 0.4

27. $\frac{68}{100}$

28. $\frac{9}{10}$

29. $\frac{12}{1000}$

30. $\frac{33}{100}$

31. 0.204 or 0.2

32. 0.95535, or 0.96 or 1

33. 10.8

34. 301.739 or 301.7

Ratio and Proportion

35. $\frac{3}{4}$

36. $\frac{1}{175}$

37. $\frac{65}{90}$

38. $\frac{9}{1000}$

39. 12

40. 2.5

41. 30

42. 50

43. $\frac{1}{2} \times \frac{4}{X} =$
(cross-multiply)
X = 8

44. $\frac{\cancel{5}^{1}}{\cancel{50}_{10}} = \frac{X}{300}$

10 X = 300

X = 30

45. $\frac{0.9}{10} = \frac{9}{100}$

10 X = 90

X = 9

Percentage

46. $\frac{3}{100}$

47. $\frac{27}{100}$

48. $\frac{12}{1000}$

49. $\frac{575}{10,000}$

50. 0.08 or 0.1

51. 0.15

52. 0.009

53. 0.035

54. 0.0025

55. 0.0045

56. 35:100

57. 12.5:100 or 125:1000

58. 4:100

59. 0.9:100 or 9:1000

60. 0.45:100 or 45:10,000

---

evolve   Additional practice problems are available in the Mathematics Review section of Drug Calculations Companion, version 5, on Evolve.

PART II

SYSTEMS, CONVERSION, AND METHODS OF DRUG CALCULATION

CHAPTER 1

Systems Used for Drug Administration and Temperature Conversion

Objectives
- Identify the system of measurement accepted worldwide and the system of measurement used in home settings.
- List the basic units and subunits of weight, volume, and length of the metric system.
- Explain the rules for changing grams to milligrams and milliliters to liters.
- Give abbreviations for the frequently used metric units and subunits.
- List the basic units of measurement for volume in the household system.
- Convert units of measurement within the metric system and within the household system.
- Convert Fahrenheit to Celsius and Celsius to Fahrenheit

Outline
METRIC SYSTEM
 Conversion Within the Metric System
APOTHECARY SYSTEM
HOUSEHOLD SYSTEM
 Conversion Within the Household System
 Temperature Conversion

The three systems used for measuring drugs and solutions are the metric, apothecary, and household systems. The metric system, developed in 1799 in France, is the chosen system for measurements in the majority of European countries. The metric system, also referred to as *the decimal system,* is based on units of 10. Since the enactment of the Metric Conversion Act of 1975, the United States has been moving toward the use of this system. The intention of the act is to adopt the International Metric System worldwide. The metric system is known as the *International System of Units,* abbreviated as SI units. Eventually, it will be the only system used in drug dosing.

The apothecary system dates back to the Middle Ages and has been the system of weights and measurements used in England since the seventeenth century. It was brought to the United States from England. The system is also referred to as *the fractional system* because anything less than one is expressed in fractions. In the United States, the apothecary system is rapidly being phased out and is being replaced by the metric system. You may omit the apothecary system if you desire.

Standard household measurements are used primarily in home settings. With the trend toward home care, conversions to household measurements may gain importance.

METRIC SYSTEM

The metric system is a decimal system based on multiples of 10 and decimal fractions of 10. There are three basic units of measurement. These basic units are as follows:

Gram (g, gm, G, Gm): unit for weight
Liter (l, L): unit for volume or capacity
Meter (m, M): unit for linear measurement or length

Prefixes are used with the basic units to describe whether the units are larger or smaller than the basic unit. The prefixes indicate the size of the unit in multiples of 10. The prefixes for basic units are as follows:

Prefix for Larger Unit		Prefix for Smaller Unit	
Kilo	1000 (one thousand)	Deci	0.1 (one-tenth)
Hecto	100 (one hundred)	Centi	0.01 (one-hundredth)
Deka	10 (ten)	Milli	0.001 (one-thousandth)
		Micro	0.000001 (one-millionth)
		Nano	0.000000001 (one-billionth)

Abbreviations of metric units that are frequently written in drug orders are listed in Table 1-1. Lowercase letters are usually used for abbreviations rather than capital letters.

The metric units of weight, volume, and length are given in Table 1-2. Meanings of the prefixes are stated next to the units of weight. Note that the larger units are 1000, 100, and 10 times the basic units (in bold type) and the smaller units differ by factors of 0.1, 0.01, 0.001, 0.000001, and 0.000000001. The size of a basic unit can be changed by multiplying or dividing by 10. Micrograms and nanograms are the exceptions: one (1) milligram = 1000 micrograms, and one (1) microgram = 1000 nanograms. Micrograms and nanograms are changed by 1000 instead of by 10.

Conversion Within the Metric System

Drug administration often requires conversion within the metric system to prepare the correct dosage. Two basic methods are given for changing larger to smaller units and smaller to larger units.

TABLE 1-1 Metric Units and Abbreviations

	Names	Abbreviations
Weight	Kilogram	kg, Kg
	Gram	g, gm, G, Gm
	Milligram	mg, mgm
	Microgram	mcg
	Nanogram	ng
Volume	Kiloliter	kl, kL
	Liter	l, L
	Deciliter	dl, dL
	Milliliter	ml, mL
	Microliter	mcL
Length	Kilometer	km, Km
	Meter	m, M
	Centimeter	cm
	Millimeter	mm

TABLE 1-2 Units of Measurement in the Metric System With Their Prefixes

Weight per Gram	Meaning
*1 kilogram (kg) = 1000 grams	One thousand
1 hectogram (hg) = 100 grams	One hundred
1 dekagram (dag) = 10 grams	Ten
*1 gram (g) = 1 gram	**One**
1 decigram (dg) = 0.1 gram ($\frac{1}{10}$)	One-tenth
1 centigram (cg) = 0.01 gram ($\frac{1}{100}$)	One-hundredth
*1 milligram (mg) = 0.001 gram ($\frac{1}{1000}$)	One-thousandth
*1 microgram (mcg) = 0.000001 gram ($\frac{1}{1,000,000}$)	One-millionth
*1 nanogram (ng) = 0.000000001 gram ($\frac{1}{1,000,000,000}$)	One-billionth

Volume per Liter	Length per Meter
*1 kiloliter (kL) = 1000 liters	1 kilometer (km) = 1000 meters
1 hectoliter (hL) = 100 liters	1 hectometer (hm) = 100 meters
1 dekaliter (daL) = 10 liters	1 dekameter (dam) = 10 meters
*1 liter (l, L) = 1 liter	**1 metric (m) = 1 meter**
*1 deciliter (dL) = 0.1 liter	1 decimeter (dm) = 0.1 meter
1 centiliter (cL) = 0.01 liter	1 centimeter (cm) = 0.01 meter
*1 milliliter (mL) = 0.001 liter	1 millimeter (mm) = 0.001 meter
1 microliter (mcL) = 0.000001 liter	

*Commonly used units of measurements.

Method A (Larger to Smaller)

To change from a *larger* unit to a *smaller* unit, multiply by 10 for each unit decreased, or move the decimal point one space to the right for each unit changed.

When changing three units from larger to smaller, such as from gram to milligram (a change of three units), multiply by 10 three times (or by 1000), or move the decimal point three spaces to the right.

Change 1 gram (g) to milligrams (mg):

a. $1 \times 10 \times 10 \times 10 = 1000$ mg

b. $1 \text{ g} \times 1000 = 1000$ mg

or

c. $1 \text{ g} = 1.000$ mg (1000 mg)

When changing two units, such as kilogram to dekagram (a change of two units from larger to smaller), multiply by 10 twice (or by 100), or move the decimal point two spaces to the right.

Change 2 kilograms (kg) to dekagrams (dag):

a. $2 \times 10 \times 10 = 200$ dag

b. $2 \text{ kg} \times 100 = 200$ dag

or

c. $2 \text{ kg} = 2.00$ dag (200 dag)

When changing one unit, such as liter to deciliter (a change of one unit from larger to smaller), multiply by 10, or move the decimal point one space to the right.

Change 3 liters (L) to deciliters (dL):

a. $3 \times 10 = 30$ dL

b. $3 \text{ L} \times 10 = 30$ dL

or

c. $3 \text{ L} = 3.0$ dL (30 dL)

A micro unit is one thousandth of a milli unit, and a nano unit is one thousandth of a micro unit. To change from a milli unit to a micro unit, multiply by 1000, or move the decimal place three spaces to the right. Changing micro units to nano units involves the same procedure, multiplying by 1000 or moving the decimal place three spaces to the right.

EXAMPLES **PROBLEM 1:** Change 2 grams (g) to milligrams (mg).

$$2 \text{ g} \times 1000 = 2000 \text{ mg}$$

or

$$2 \text{ g} = 2.000 \text{ mg } (2000 \text{ mg})$$

PROBLEM 2: Change 10 milligrams (mg) to micrograms (mcg).

$$10 \text{ mg} \times 1000 = 10{,}000 \text{ mcg}$$

or

$$10 \text{ mg} = 10.000 \text{ mcg } (10{,}000 \text{ mcg})$$

PROBLEM 3: Change 4 liters (L) to milliliters (mL).

$$4 \text{ L} \times 1000 = 4000 \text{ mL}$$

or

$$4 \text{ L} = 4.000 \text{ mL } (4000 \text{ mL})$$

PROBLEM 4: Change 2 kilometers (km) to hectometers (hm).

$$2 \text{ km} \times 10 = 20 \text{ hm}$$

or

$$2 \text{ km} = 2.0 \text{ hm } (20 \text{ hm})$$

Method B (Smaller to Larger)

To change from a *smaller* unit to a *larger* unit, divide by 10 for each unit increased, or move the decimal point one space to the left for each unit changed.

When changing three units from smaller to larger, divide by 1000, or move the decimal point three spaces to the left.
Change 1500 milliliters (mL) to liters (L):
a. $1500 \text{ mL} \div 1000 = 1.5 \text{ L}$
        or
b. $1500 \text{ mL} = 1\,500. \text{ L } (1.5 \text{ L})$

When changing two units from smaller to larger, divide by 100, or move the decimal point two spaces to the left.
Change 400 centimeters (cm) to meters (m):
a. $400 \text{ cm} \div 100 = 4 \text{ m}$
        or
b. $400 \text{ cm} = 4\,00. \text{ m } (4 \text{ m})$

When changing one unit from smaller to larger, divide by 10, or move the decimal point one space to the left.

Change 150 decigrams (dg) to grams (g):

a. 150 dg ÷ 10 = 15 g

or

b. 150 dg = 15 0. g (15 g)

EXAMPLES **PROBLEM 1:** Change 8 grams (g) to kilograms (kg).

8 g ÷ 1000 = 0.008 kg

or

8 g = 008. kg (0.008 kg)

PROBLEM 2: Change 1500 milligrams (mg) to decigrams (dg).

1500 mg ÷ 100 = 15 dg

or

1500 mg = 15 00. dg (15 dg)

PROBLEM 3: Change 750 micrograms (mcg) to milligrams (mg).

750 mcg ÷ 1000 = 0.75 mg

or

750 mcg = 750. mg (0.75 mg)

PROBLEM 4: Change 2400 milliliters (mL) to liters (L).

2400 mL ÷ 1000 = 2.4 L

or

2400 mL = 2 400. L (2.4 L)

PRACTICE PROBLEMS ▶ I METRIC SYSTEM (CONVERSION WITHIN THE METRIC SYSTEM)

Answers can be found on page 24.

1. Conversion from larger units to smaller units: *Multiply* by 10 for each unit changed (multiply by 10, 100, 1000), or move the decimal point one space to the *right* for each unit changed (move one, two, or three spaces), Method A.

[handwritten: 7.5]

a. 7.5 grams to milligrams

[handwritten: 7500 mg]

[handwritten in left margin: 1 milligram = 1,000 micrograms]

b. 10 milligrams to micrograms

[handwritten: 10.000 = 10,000 micrograms]

c. 35 kilograms to grams

[handwritten: 35,000 g]

d. 2.5 liters to milliliters

[handwritten: 2500 mL]

e. 1.25 liters to milliliters

_1250mL_

f. 20 centiliters to milliliters

_200mL_

g. 18 decigrams to milligrams

_1800 mL_

h. 0.5 kilograms to grams

500grams

2. Conversion from smaller units to larger units: *Divide* by 10 for each unit changed (divide by 10, 100, 1000), or move the decimal point one space to the *left* for each unit changed (move one, two, or three spaces), Method B.

a. 500 milligrams to grams

_500, =0.5g_

b. 7500 micrograms to milligrams

_7500, 7.5mg_

c. 250 grams to kilograms

_250 0.25kg_

d. 4000 milliliters to liters

_4000mL 4L_

e. 325 milligrams to grams

_325 mg .325g_

f. 100 milliliters to deciliters

_100mL 1dl_

g. 2800 milliliters to liters

_2800ml 2.8L_

h. 75 millimeters to centimeters

_75mm 7.5cm_

APOTHECARY SYSTEM

The apothecary system was started in England in the early seventeenth century. It was a system of measurement commonly used before the universal acceptance of the International Metric System. Now, all pharmaceuticals are manufactured using the metric system, and the apothecary system is no longer included on most drug labels. All medication should be prescribed and calculated using metric measures.

Occasionally the drug may be prescribed in grains or fluid ounces (apothecary system). Examples of those drugs include aspirin grain (gr) v or x (325 or 650 mg), nitroglycerin tablets gr 1/150 (0.4 mg), codeine gr 1/2 or 1 (30 or 60 mg), and morphine gr 1/6 (10 mg). Table 2-1 (page 28) is the conversion table for the Approximate Metric, Apothecary, and Household Equivalents. The table can be used if a drug is ordered in the apothecary system but needs to be converted into the metric system. With the apothecary system, Roman numerals are written in lowercase letters, e.g., gr x (10 grains).

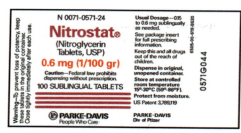

Figure 1-1 This label for nitroglycerin tablets shows the strength of the drug using both the metric system (0.6 mg) and apothecary system (1/100 gr).

An example of a drug that includes both metric and apothecary measurements on the label is nitroglycerin, 0.6 mg (metric) and 1/100 (apothecary) (see Figure 1-1).

HOUSEHOLD SYSTEM

The use of household measurements is on the increase because more patients/clients are being cared for in the home. The household system of measurement is less accurate than the metric system because of a lack of standardization of spoons, cups, and glasses. A teaspoon (t) is considered 5 mL, although it could represent anywhere from 4 to 6 mL. Three household teaspoons are equal to one tablespoon (T). A drop size can vary with the size of the lumen of the dropper. Basically, a drop and a minim are considered equal. Again, household measurements must be considered approximate measurements. Some of the household units are the same as the apothecary units because there is a blend of these two systems.

The community health nurse may use and teach the household units of measurements to patients/clients.

Table 1-3 gives the commonly used units of measurement in the household system. You might want to memorize the equivalents in Table 1-3 or refer to the table as needed.

Conversion Within the Household System

For changing larger units to smaller units and smaller units to larger units within the household system, the same methods that applied to the apothecary system can be used. With household measurements, a fluid ounce is usually indicated as an ounce.

Method C

To change a *larger* unit to a *smaller* unit, multiply the constant value found in Table 1-3 by the number of the larger unit.

EXAMPLES **PROBLEM 1:** 2 medium-size glasses = _____ 16 _____ ounces (oz).

1 medium glass = 8 fl oz (8 is the constant value)

2 × 8 = 16 oz

1 medium glass= 8oz

1oz = 30mL

TABLE 1-3 Units of Measurement in the Household System

1 drop (gt) (gtt) = 1 minim (m)	1 coffee cup (c) = 6 to 8 ounces (oz)
1 teaspoon (t) = 60 drops (gtt) = 5 mL	1 medium-size glass = 8 ounces (oz)
1 tablespoon (T) = 3 teaspoons (t)	1 measuring cup = 8 ounces (oz)
1 ounce (oz) = 2 tablespoons (T)	

1000mL = 1qt lat = 32oz

PROBLEM 2: 3 tablespoons (T) = _____9_____ teaspoons (t).   *3 × 3*
1 T = 3 t (3 is the constant value)
$3 \times 3 = 9$ t

PROBLEM 3: 5 ounces (oz) = _____10_____ tablespoons (T).   *1 ounce = 2 Table*
1 oz = 2 T (2 is the constant value)   *5 × 2*
$5 \times 2 = 10$ T

PROBLEM 4: 2 teaspoons (t) = _____120_____ drops (gtt).   *1 tea = 60 drops*
1 t = 60 gtt (60 is the constant value)
$2 \times 60 = 120$ gtt

Method D

To change a *smaller* unit to a *larger* unit, divide the constant value found in Table 1-3 into the number of the larger unit.

> ✎ **NOTE**
>
> The constant values are the numbers of the smaller units in Table 1-3.

EXAMPLES **PROBLEM 1:**

120 drops (gtt) = _____ teaspoons (t).
1 t = 60 gtt (60 is the constant value)
$120 \div 60 = 2$ t

PROBLEM 3:

18 ounces (oz) = _____ coffee cups (c).
1 c = 6 oz (6 is the constant value)
$18 \div 6 = 3$ c
If it is a large coffee cup, use 8 oz.

PROBLEM 2:

6 teaspoons (t) = _____ tablespoons (T).
1 T = 3 t (3 is the constant value)
$6 \div 3 = 2$ T

PROBLEM 4:

4 tablespoons (T) = _____ ounces (oz).
1 oz = 2 T (2 is the constant value)
$4 \div 2 = 2$ oz

PRACTICE PROBLEMS ▶ II HOUSEHOLD SYSTEM (CONVERSION WITHIN THE HOUSEHOLD)

Answers can be found on page 25.

1. Give the equivalents using Method C, changing larger units to smaller units.

   a. 2 glasses = _____ oz

   b. 3 ounces = _____ T

   c. 4 tablespoons = _____ t

   d. 1½ coffee c (cups) = _____ oz

   e. ½ teaspoon = _____ gtt

2. Give the equivalents using Method D, changing smaller units to larger units.

a. 9 teaspoons = _____ T

b. 6 tablespoons = _____ oz

c. 90 drops = _____ t

d. 12 ounces = _____ coffee c (cups)

e. 24 ounces = _____ medium-size glasses

Temperature Conversion

Temperature is commonly measured by two scales, Celsius and Fahrenheit. Celsius (C), or centigrade, describes temperature with 0° C as the freezing point of water and 100°C as the boiling point of water. The Celsius scale is widely used around the world. Medical devices and scientific equipment often use the Celsius scale because it is a base-10 system like the metric system. The Fahrenheit (F) scale describes temperature with the freezing point of water as 32° F and the boiling point of water as 212° F. The Fahrenheit scale is primarily used in the United States and its territories.

To convert from Fahrenheit to Celsius the formula is:

$$[C] = ([°F] - 32) \times 5/9$$

To convert from Celsius to Fahrenheit the formula is:

$$[F] = ([°C] \times 9/5) + 32$$

PRACTICE PROBLEMS ▶ IIII TEMPERATURE CONVERSION

Answers can be found on page 25.

a. Change 98.6° F to Celsius _37°C_

b. Change 101° F to Celsius _38.3°C_

c. Change 104° F to Celsius _40°C_

d. Change 22° C to Fahrenheit _71.6°F_

e. Change 30° C to Fahrenheit _86°F_

ANSWERS

I Metric System

1. a. 7.5 g to mg
   7.5 g × 1000 = 7500 mg
         or
   7.500 mg (7500 mg)

b. 10,000 mcg
c. 35,000 g
d. 2500 mL
e. 1250 mL
f. 200 mL
g. 1800 mg
h. 500 g

2. a. 500 mg to g
   500 ÷ 1000 = 0.5 g
         or
   500 mg = 500. g (0.5 g)

b. 7.5 mg
c. 0.25 kg
d. 4 L
e. 0.325 g
f. 1 dL
g. 2.8 L
h. 7.5 cm

II Household System

1. a. 2 glasses = _____ oz
   2 × 8 = 16 oz
  b. 6 T
  c. 12 t
  d. 9 or 12 oz
  e. 30 gtt

2. a. 9 teaspoons = _____ T
   9 ÷ 3 = 3 T
  b. 3 oz
  c. 1½ t
  d. 1½ or 2 c
  e. 3 medium-size glasses

III Temperature Conversion

a. $°C = ([98.6° F] - 32) × 5/9$
   $°C = 66.6 × 5/9$
      $= 333/9$
   $°C = 37$

b. $°C = ([101° F] - 32) × 5/9$
      $= 69 × 5/9$
      $= 345/9$
   $°C = 38.3$

c. $°C = ([104° F] - 32) × 5/9$
      $= 72 × 5/9$
      $= 360/9$
   $°C = 40$

d. $°F = ([22° C] × 9/5) + 32$
      $= 198/5 + 32$
      $= 39.6 + 32$
   $°F = 71.6$

e. $°F = ([30° C] × 9/5) + 32$
      $= 270/5 + 32$
      $= 54 + 32$
   $°F = 86$

SUMMARY PRACTICE PROBLEMS

Answers can be found on page 26.

Make conversions within the two systems.

1. Metric system

  a. 30 mg = _30,000_ mcg

  b. 3 g = _3000_ mg

  c. 6 L = _6000_ mL

  d. 1.5 kg = _1500_ g

  e. 10,000 mcg = _10,000_ mg

  f. 500 mg = _0.5_ g

  g. 2500 mL = _2.5_ L

  h. 125 g = _0.125_ kg

  i. 120 mm = _12_ cm

  j. 5 m = _500_ cm

2. Household system

  a. 12 t = _4_ T

  b. 5 medium-size glasses = _40_ oz

  c. 3 T = _9_ t

  d. 2 coffee c (cups) = _12 or 16_ oz

  e. 24 oz = _3 or 4_ coffee c (cups)

  f. 4 oz = _____ T

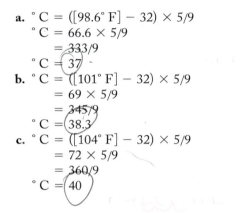

1 T = 3 t

5 × 8

1 oz = 2 T

ANSWERS   SUMMARY PRACTICE PROBLEMS

1. a. 30,000 mcg
   b. 3000 mg
   c. 6000 mL
   d. 1500 g
   e. 10 mg
   f. 0.5 g
   g. 2.5 L
   h. 0.125 kg
   i. 12 cm
   j. 500 cm

2. a. 4 T
   b. 40 oz
   c. 9 t
   d. 12 oz or 16 oz
   e. 3-4 coffee c (cups)
   f. 8 T

---

evolve   Additional information is available in the Introducing Drug Measures section of Drug Calculations Companion, version 5, on Evolve.

CHAPTER 2

Conversion Within the Metric, Apothecary, and Household Systems

Objectives   • Convert grams to milligrams and milligrams to grams.
                • Convert drug dosage by weight from one system to another system by using the ratio method.
                • Utilize the conversion table for metric, apothecary, and household systems.
                • Convert liters/milliliters to ounces and milliliters to tablespoons and teaspoons.

Outline   **UNITS, MILLIEQUIVALENTS, AND PERCENTS**
              METRIC, APOTHECARY, AND HOUSEHOLD EQUIVALENTS
              CONVERSION IN METRIC AND HOUSEHOLD SYSTEMS BY LIQUID VOLUME
              CONVERSION IN METRIC AND HOUSEHOLD SYSTEMS BY LENGTH

Today, conversion within the metric system is more common than conversion within the metric-apothecary systems. Although the apothecary system is being phased out, some physicians still order drug dosages by apothecary units. If the faculty find that the apothecary system is not being used in their institutions, they may wish to omit the apothecary equivalents and conversion shown in Table 2-1.

Drug doses are usually ordered in metric units (grams, milligrams, liters, and milliliters). To calculate a drug dosage, **the same unit of measurement must be used.** Therefore, you must memorize the metric equivalents. After the conversion is made, the dosage problem can be solved. Some authorities state that it is easier to *convert to the unit used on the container (bottle).*

Dosage conversion tables are available in many institutions; however, when you need a conversion table, one might not be available. Nurses should memorize metric equivalents or should be able to convert within the system.

UNITS, MILLIEQUIVALENTS, AND PERCENTS

Units, milliequivalents, and percents are measurements and are used to indicate the strength or potency of certain drugs. When a drug is developed, its strength is based on chemical assay or biological assay. Chemical assay denotes strength by weight, e.g., milligrams or grains. Biological assays are used for drugs in which the chemical composition is difficult to determine. Biological assays assess potency by determining the effect that one unit of the drug can have on a laboratory animal. Units mainly measure the potency of hormones, vitamins, anticoagulants, and some antibiotics. Drugs that were once standardized by units and were later synthesized to their chemical composition may still retain units as an indication of potency, e.g., insulin.

Milliequivalents measure the strength of an ion concentration. Ions are given primarily for electrolyte replacement. They are measured in milliequivalents (mEq), one of which is $\frac{1}{1000}$ of the equivalent weight of an ion. Potassium chloride (KCl) is a common electrolyte replacement and is ordered in milliequivalents.

Percents, the concentrations of weight dissolved in a volume, are always expressed as units of mass per units of volume. Common concentrations are g/mL, g/L, and mg/mL. These concentrations, expressed as percentages, are based on the definition of a 1% solution as 1 g of a drug in 100 mL of solution. Dextrose 50% in a 50-mL pre-filled syringe is a concentration of 50 g of dextrose in 100 mL of water. Calcium gluconate 10% in a 30-mL bottle is a concentration of 10 g of calcium gluconate in 100 mL of solution. Proportions can also express concentrations. A solution that is 1:100 has the same concentration as a 1% solution. Epinephrine 1:1000 means that 1 g of epinephrine was dissolved in a 1000-mL solution.

Units, milliequivalents, and percents cannot be directly converted into the metric, apothecary, or household system.

METRIC, APOTHECARY, AND HOUSEHOLD EQUIVALENTS

Knowing how to convert drug doses among the systems of measurement is essential in the clinical setting. In discharge teaching for individuals receiving liquid medication, converting metric to household measurement may be important.

Table 2-1 gives the metric and apothecary equivalents by weight and the metric, apothecary, and household equivalents by volume.

TABLE 2-1   Approximate Metric, Apothecary, and Household Equivalents

	Metric System	Apothecary System	Household System
Weight	1 kg; 1000 g	2.2 lb	2.2 lb
	30 g	1 oz	
	15 g	4 dr	
	1 g; 1000 mg*	15 (16) gr	
	0.5 g; 500 mg	7½ gr	
	0.3 g; 300 mg	5 gr	
	0.1 g; 100 mg	1½ gr	
	0.06 g; 60 (65) mg*	1 gr	
	0.03 g; 30 (32) mg	½ gr	
	0.01 g; 10 mg	⅙ gr	
	0.6 mg	$\frac{1}{100}$ gr	
	0.4 mg	$\frac{1}{150}$ gr	
	0.3 mg	$\frac{1}{200}$ gr	
	1 mg = 1000 mcg		
Volume	1 L; 1000 mL	1 qt; 32 fl oz	1 qt; 32 fl oz
	0.5 L; 500 mL	1 pt; 16 fl oz	1 pt; 16 fl oz
	0.24 L; 240 mL	8 fl oz	1 glass or 8 oz
	0.18 L; 180 mL	6 fl oz	1 c or 6 oz
	30 mL	1 oz or 8 dr	2 T or 6 t or 1 oz
	15 mL	½ oz or 4 dr	1 T or ½ oz
	4-5 mL		1 t
	4 mL	1 dr or 60 minims (♏)	1 t
	1 mL	15 (16) ♏	15-16 gtt (drops)
Height	2.54 cm	1 inch	1 inch
Length	0.0254 m	1 inch	—
Distance	25.4 mm	1 inch	1 inch

*Equivalents commonly used for computing conversion problems by ratio.
Note: ½ may be written as ss.

Remember, conversion from one system to another is an approximation. Though the apothecary system is not or infrequently used, the table is included as a reference for approximate metric, apothecary, and household equivalents.

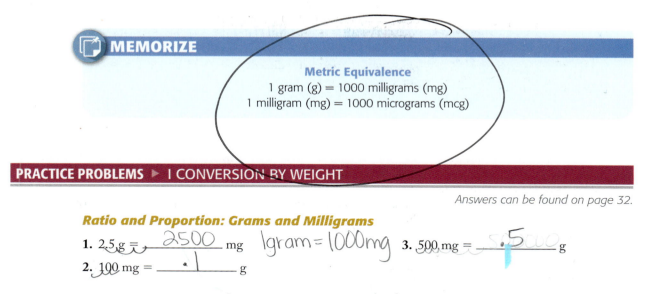

MEMORIZE

Metric Equivalence
1 gram (g) = 1000 milligrams (mg)
1 milligram (mg) = 1000 micrograms (mcg)

PRACTICE PROBLEMS ▶ I CONVERSION BY WEIGHT

Answers can be found on page 32.

Ratio and Proportion: Grams and Milligrams

1. 2.5 g = ___2500___ mg   1 gram = 1000 mg   3. 500 mg = ___.5.500___ g

2. 100 mg = ___.1___ g

CONVERSION IN METRIC AND HOUSEHOLD SYSTEMS BY LIQUID VOLUME

MEMORIZE

Metric and Household Equivalents
1000 mL = 1 L = 1 qt = 32 oz
1 ounce (oz) = 30 mL

Liters and Ounces: 1 L = 32 oz

a. To convert liters and quarts to ounces, *multiply* the number of liters by 32, the constant value.
b. To convert ounces to liters or quarts, *divide* the number of ounces by 32, the constant value.

EXAMPLES   PROBLEM 1: Change 3 liters to ounces.

$$3 \text{ L} \times 32 = 96 \text{ oz}$$

PROBLEM 2: Change 64 ounces to liters.

$$64 \text{ oz} \div 32 = 2 \text{ L (liters)}$$

Ounces and Milliliters: 1 oz = 30 mL

a. To convert ounces to milliliters, *multiply* the number of ounces by 30, the constant value.
b. To convert milliliters to ounces, *divide* the number of milliliters by 30, the constant value.

EXAMPLES   **PROBLEM 1:**   Change 5 ounces to milliliters (mL).

$$5 \text{ oz} \times 30 = 150 \text{ mL}$$

PROBLEM 2:   Change 120 milliliters to ounces.

$$120 \text{ mL} \div 30 = 4 \text{ oz}$$

Ratio and Proportion

The ratio method is useful when smaller units are converted within the two systems.

If it is difficult for you to recall these methods, then use the ratio and proportion method to convert from one system to the other.

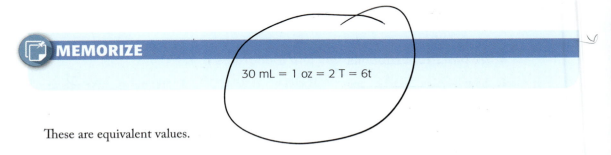

MEMORIZE

30 mL = 1 oz = 2 T = 6t

These are equivalent values.

EXAMPLES   **PROBLEM 1:**   Change 20 mL to teaspoons.

$$
\begin{array}{cc}
\textit{Known} & \textit{Desired} \\
\text{mL:t} & :: \text{mL:t} \\
30:6 & :: 20:X \\
\end{array}
$$

$$30 \, X = 120$$
$$X = 4 \, t \text{ (teaspoons)}$$

PROBLEM 2:   Change 15 mL to tablespoons.

$$
\begin{array}{cc}
\textit{Known} & \textit{Desired} \\
\text{mL:T} & :: \text{mL:T} \\
30:2 & :: 15:X \\
\end{array}
$$

$$30 \, X = 30$$
$$X = 1 \, T \text{ (tablespoon)}$$

PROBLEM 3:   Change 5 oz to tablespoons.

$$
\begin{array}{cc}
\textit{Known} & \textit{Desired} \\
\text{oz:T} & :: \text{oz:T} \\
1:2 & :: 5:X \\
\end{array}
$$

$$X = 10 \, T \text{ (tablespoons)}$$

PRACTICE PROBLEMS ▶ II CONVERSION BY LIQUID VOLUME

Answers can be found on page 32.

Constant = 32

Liters and Ounces (Round to the nearest tenths.)

1. 2.5 L = __80__ oz

2. 0.25 L = __8__ oz

3. 40 oz = __1.25__ L → 1.3 L

4. 24 oz = __.75__ L → 0.8 L

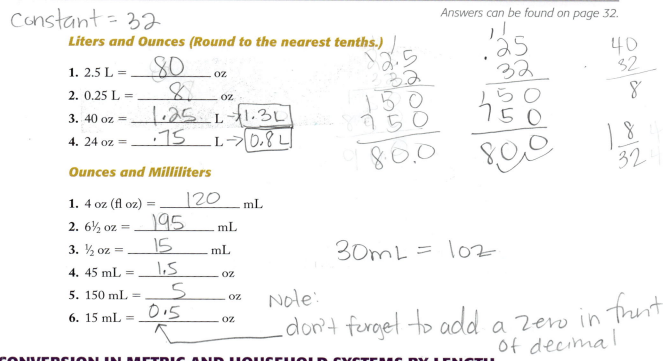

Ounces and Milliliters

1. 4 oz (fl oz) = __120__ mL

2. 6½ oz = __195__ mL

3. ½ oz = __15__ mL

4. 45 mL = __1.5__ oz

5. 150 mL = __5__ oz

6. 15 mL = __0.5__ oz

30 mL = 1 oz

Note:
don't forget to add a zero in frnt of decimal

CONVERSION IN METRIC AND HOUSEHOLD SYSTEMS BY LENGTH

Inches and Meters: 1 inch = 0.0254 meter (constant value)

a. To convert inches to meters, **multiply** the number of inches by 0.0254, the constant value.

b. To convert meters to inches, **divide** the number of meters by 0.0254, the constant value.

EXAMPLES **PROBLEM 1:** Change 12 inches to meters (m).

12 inches × 0.0254 = 0.3048 or 0.305 meter or 0.3 meter

PROBLEM 2: Change 0.6 meter to inches.

0.6 meter ÷ 0.0254 = 23.6 inches

Inches and Centimeters: 1 inch = 2.54 centimeters (constant value)

a. To convert inches to centimeters, multiply the number of inches by 2.54, the constant value.

b. To convert centimeters to inches, divide the numbers of centimeters by 2.54, the constant value.

EXAMPLES **PROBLEM 1:** Change 12 inches to centimeters (cm).

12 inches × 2.54 = 30.48 cm (centimeters) or 30.5 cm

PROBLEM 2: Change 60 cm to inches.

60 cm ÷ 2.54 = 23.6 inches

Answers can be found on pages 32 and 33.

Inches to Meters (Change feet to inches [e.g., 6 ft 2 inches = 74 inches])

1. 6 ft 2 inches = _____ m

2. 5 ft 2 inches = _____ m

3. 6 ft 5 inches = _____ m

4. 2 ft 10 inches = _____ m

5. 4 ft 7 inches = _____ m

Inches to Centimeters

1. 2 inches = _____ cm

2. 3 inches = _____ cm

3. ½ inch = _____ cm

4. 6 inches = _____ cm

5. 8 inches = _____ cm

ANSWERS

I Conversion by Weight

Ratio and Proportion: Grams and Milligrams

1. g:mg ∷ g:mg
    1:1000∷2.5:X
         X = 2500 mg
            or
Move decimal point three spaces to the right
(conversion within the metric system).
2.5 g = 2.500 mg

2. mg:g∷ mg:g
    1000:1∷100:X
    1000 X = 100
         X = 0.1 g

3. mg:g∷ mg:g
    1000:1∷500:X
    1000 X = 500
         X = 0.5 g

II Conversion by Liquid Volume

Liters and Ounces

1. 2.5 L × 32 = 80 oz
2. 0.25 L × 32 = 8 oz

3. 40 oz ÷ 32 = 1.25 L or 1.3 L
4. 24 oz ÷ 32 = 0.75 L or 0.8 L

Ounces and Milliliters

1. 4 oz × 30 = 120 mL
2. 6.5 oz × 30 = 195 mL
3. 0.5 oz × 30 = 15 mL

4. 45 mL ÷ 30 = 1½ oz or 1.5 oz
5. 150 mL ÷ 30 = 5 oz
6. 15 mL ÷ 30 = ½ oz or 0.5 oz

III Conversion by Length

Inches to Meters

1. 74 inches × 0.0254 = 1.879 or 1.880 m
2. 62 inches × 0.0254 = 1.575 m
3. 77 inches × 0.0254 = 1.956 m

4. 34 inches × 0.0254 = 0.864 m
5. 55 inches × 0.0254 = 1.397 m

Inches to Centimeters

1. 2 inches × 2.54 = 5.08 cm
2. 3 inches × 2.54 = 7.62 cm
3. ½ inch × 2.54 = 1.27 cm

4. 6 inches × 2.54 = 15.24 cm
5. 8 inches × 2.54 = 20.32 cm

SUMMARY PRACTICE PROBLEMS

Answers can be found on page 35.

Metric Conversion

Before the drug dosage problems can be solved, the nurse must convert to one drug unit, either from grams to milligrams **or** milligrams to grams. This will be explained in more detail in Chapter 8.

> **YOU MUST REMEMBER**
>
> *Multiply* when converting from larger to smaller units, and *divide* when converting from smaller to larger units.

Weight: Metric System: Conversion Within

1. To convert grams to milligrams, move the decimal point three spaces to the *right*.

    a. 1.0 g = _____ mg

    b. 0.8 g = _____ mg

    c. 0.3 g = _____ mg

    d. 0.1 g = _____ mg

2. To convert milligrams to grams, move the decimal point three spaces to the *left*.

    a. 750 mg = _____ g

    b. 250 mg = _____ g

    c. 1200 mg = _____ g

    d. 400 mg = _____ g

Volume: Metric and Household Conversion

3. To convert liters and quarts to ounces, (multiply/divide) _____ the number of liters by _____; to convert ounces to liters and quarts, (multiply/divide) _____ the number of ounces by _____.

    a. 3 L = _____ oz

    b. 1½ qt = _____ oz

    c. 64 fl oz = _____ qt

    d. ½ L = _____ oz

    e. 8 oz = _____ L or qt

    f. 24 oz = _____ qt

4. To convert ounces to milliliters, (multiply/divide) _____ the number of ounces by _____; to convert milliliters to ounces, (multiply/divide) _____ the number of milliliters by _____.

    a. 1½ oz = _____ mL

    b. 15 mL = _____ oz

    c. 60 mL = _____ oz

    d. 75 mL = _____ oz

    e. 3 fl oz = _____ mL

    f. 8 oz = _____ mL

5. To convert milliliters to drops, (multiply/divide) _____ the number of milliliters by _____ ; to convert drops to milliliters (multiply/divide) _____ the number of drops by _____.

   a. 15 mL = _____ gtt

   b. 10 gtt = _____ mL

   c. 18 gtt = _____ mL

   d. 4 mL = _____ gtt

   e. 30 gtt = _____ mL

   f. ½ mL = _____ gtt

6. Ratio and proportion.

> **YOU MUST REMEMBER**
>
> 30 mL = 1 oz = 2 T = 6 t (fl oz and oz have been used interchangeably with liquids)

   a. Change 16 oz to L or qt

   _____

   b. Change 1½ oz to T

   _____

   c. Change 1 T to t

   _____

   d. Change 20 mL to t

   _____

   e. Change 2½ oz to mL

   _____

   f. Change 4 oz to mL

   _____

7. Patient intake for lunch included a carton of milk (8 oz), cup of coffee (6 oz), small glass of apple juice (4 oz), and gelatin (4 oz). How many milliliters (mL) did the patient consume for lunch?

   _____

8. Add 8-hour intake: IV: 30 mL/hr, 230 mL in IV medications. PO intake: juice 4 oz, tea 6 oz, water 3 oz, gelatin 4 oz, ginger ale 5 oz, and milk 8 oz. What was the patient's intake (IV and PO) in

   8 hours? _____ mL

9. Add 8-hour intake: IV: 60 mL/hr; 250 mL in IV medications. PO intake: juice 4 oz; water 3 oz; gelatin 2 oz; and broth 4 oz. What was the patient's intake (IV and PO) in 8 hours?

   _____ mL

ANSWERS   SUMMARY PRACTICE PROBLEMS

Weight

1. a. 1000 mg
   b. 800 mg

   c. 300 mg
   d. 100 mg

2. a. 0.750 or 0.75 g
   b. 0.250 or 0.25 g

   c. 1.200 or 1.2 g
   d. 0.400 or 0.4 g

Volume

3. multiply, 32; divide, 32
   a. 3 L × 32 = 96 oz
   b. 1.5 qt × 32 = 48 oz
   c. 64 oz ÷ 32 = 2 qt

   d. 0.5 L × 32 = 16 oz
   e. 8 oz ÷ 32 = $\frac{8}{32}$ = ¼ L or ¼ qt or 0.25 or 0.3 qt
   f. 24 oz ÷ 32 = $\frac{24}{32}$ = ¾ qt or 0.75 or 0.8 qt

4. multiply, 30; divide, 30
   a. 1½ oz × 30 = 45 mL
   b. 15 mL ÷ 30 = $\frac{15}{30}$ = ½ oz or 0.5 oz
   c. 60 mL ÷ 30 = 2 oz

   d. 75 mL ÷ 30 = 2½ oz or 2.5 oz
   e. 3 oz × 30 = 90 mL
   f. 8 oz × 30 = 240 mL

5. multiply, 15; divide, 15
   a. 15 mL × 15 = 225 gtt
   b. 10 gtt ÷ 15 = $\frac{10}{15}$ = ⅔ ml or 0.67 or 0.7 mL
   c. 18 gtt ÷ 15 = 1⅕ ml or 1.2 mL

   d. 4 mL × 15 = 60 gtt
   e. 30 gtt ÷ 15 = 2 mL
   f. ½ mL × 15 = 7.5 gtt or 8 gtt

6. Ratio and proportion
   Known   Desired
   a. L:oz::L:oz
      1:32::X:16
      32 X = 16
      X = ½ L
   b. oz:T::oz:T
      1:2::1½:X
      X = 3 T
   c. T:t::T:t
      2:6::1:X
      2 X = 6
      X = 3 t
   d. mL:t::mL:t
      30:6::20:X
      30 X = 120
      X = 4 t
   e. oz:mL::oz:mL
      1:30::2½:X
      X = 75 mL
   f. oz:mL::oz:mL
      1:30::4:X
      X = 120 mL

7.   (1 ounce = 30 mL)
      Milk = 240 mL
      Coffee = 180 mL
   Apple juice = 120 mL
      Gelatin = <u>120 mL</u>
                660 mL
   The patient's intake for lunch is 660 mL.

8. IV:30 mL × 8 hr = 240 mL
      IV medications = 230 mL
   Juice (4 oz × 30 mL) = 120 mL
      Tea = 180 mL
      Water = 90 mL
      Gelatin = 120 mL
      Ginger ale = 150 mL
      Milk = <u>240 mL</u>
             1370 mL
   The patient's intake in 8 hours (IV and PO) is 1370 mL.

9. IV:60 mL/hr × 8 hr = 480 mL
      IV medications = 250 mL
      Juice = 120 mL
      Water = 90 mL
      Gelatin = 60 mL
      Broth = <u>120 mL</u>
              1120 mL
   The patient's intake in 8 hours (IV and PO) is 1120 mL.

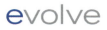 Additional information is available in the Introducing Drug Measures section of Drug Calculations Companion, version 5, on Evolve.

CHAPTER 3

Interpretation of Drug Labels, Drug Orders, Bar Codes, MAR and eMAR, Automation of Medication Dispensing Administration, and Abbreviations

Objectives
- Identify brand names, generic names, drug forms, dosages, expiration dates, and lot numbers on drug labels.
- Explain difference between military and traditional time.
- Give examples of drugs with "look-alike" drug names.
- Name the components of a drug order.
- Explain the computer-based medication administration system.
- Explain the use of the bar code for unit dose drug.
- Identify drug information for charting.
- Provide meanings of abbreviations: drug form, drug measurement, and routes and times of drug administration.

INTERPRETATION OF DRUG LABELS

Pharmaceutical companies label drugs with their brand name of the drug in large letters and the generic name in smaller letters. The form of the drug (tablet, capsule, liquid, or powder) and dosage are printed on the drug label.

Many of the calculation problems in this book use drug labels. By using drug labels, the student can practice solving drug problems that are applicable to clinical practice. The student should know what information is on a drug label and how this information is used in drug calculations. All drug labels provide eight basic items of data: (1) brand (trade) name, (2) generic name, (3) dosage, (4) form of the drug, (5) expiration date, (6) lot number, (7) name of the manufacturer, and (8) drug information and directions.

EXAMPLE   DRUG LABEL

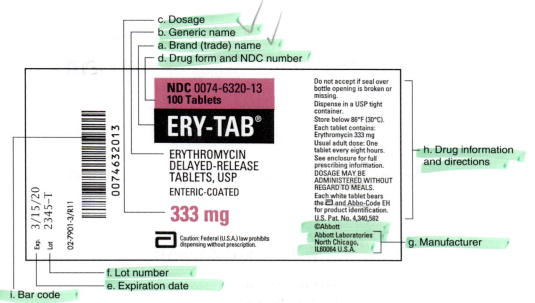

a. **The brand (trade) name** is the commercial name given by the pharmaceutical company (manufacturer of the drug). It is printed in large, bold letters.

b. **The generic name** is the chemical name given to the drug, regardless of the drug manufacturer. It is printed in smaller letters, usually under the brand name. Drugs are usually referred to by their generic name.

c. **The dosage strength** is the drug dose per drug form (tablet, capsule, liquid) as stated on the label.

d. **The National Drug Code number (NDC)** is the universal product identifier required by the U.S. Food and Drug Administration. The numbers identify the manufacturer, distributor, strength, dosage, formulation (tablets, capsules, liquids), and package size.

e. **The expiration date** refers to the length of time the drug can be used before it loses its potency. Drugs should not be administered after the expiration date. The nurse must check the expiration date of all drugs that he or she administers.

f. **The lot number** identifies the drug batch in which the medication was produced. Occasionally, a drug is recalled according to the lot number.

g. **The manufacturer** is the pharmaceutical company that produces the brand-name drug.

h. **Specific drug-related information and directions.** This information along with more detail can be found in the package insert.

i. **The bar code** contains all drug identifiers, such as control lot, batch number, NDC number, and expiration date. This is on all prescription and nonprescription medications.

Examples of drug labels are given, and practice problems for reading drug labels follow the examples.

EXAMPLE **ORAL DRUG (SOLID FORM)**

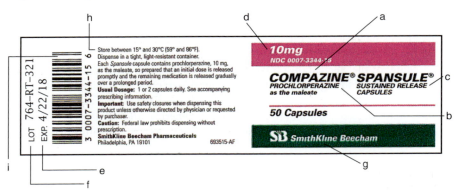

a. Brand (trade) name is Compazine.
b. Generic name is prochlorperazine.
c. Drug form is a sustained-release capsule (SR capsule).
d. Dosage is 10 mg per capsule.
e. Expiration date is 4/22/18 (after this date, the drug should be discarded).
f. Lot number is 764-RT-321.
g. Manufacturer name is SmithKline Beecham Pharmaceuticals.
h. Drug information includes dosages, storage, and safety measures.
i. Bar code.

EXAMPLE **ORAL DRUG (LIQUID FORM)**

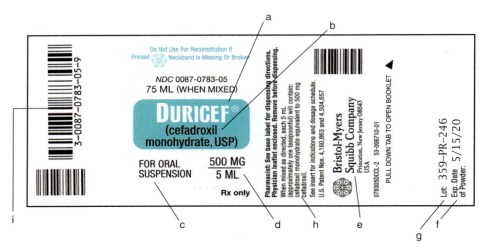

a. Brand (trade) name is Duricef.
b. Generic name is cefadroxil monohydrate.
c. Drug form is oral suspension.
d. Dosage is 500 mg per 5 mL.
e. Manufacturer is Bristol-Myers Squibb Company.
f. Expiration date is 5/15/20.
g. Lot number is 359-PR-246.
h. See package insert for more information.
i. Bar code.

EXAMPLE INJECTABLE DRUG

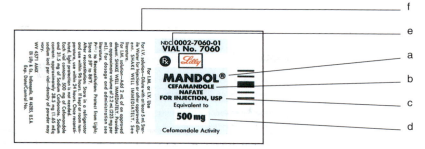

a. Brand name is Mandol.

b. Generic name is cefamandole nafate.

c. Drug form is drug powder that must be reconstituted in sterile water for use.

d. Dosage is 500 mg drug powder.

e. Drug container is vial.

f. Directions for drug reconstitution. For IV use: Add 5 mL of sterile water into the vial. Shake the vial well to completely dissolve the drug powder. For IM use: Add 2 mL of sterile water into the vial and shake thoroughly. The total volume of sterile water in the vial will equal 2.2 mL. The powder will increase the total volume by 0.2 mL.

Refer to Chapter 9 for more information on medication reconstitution.

PRACTICE PROBLEMS ▶ I INTERPRETATION OF DRUG LABELS

Answers can be found on page 55.

1.

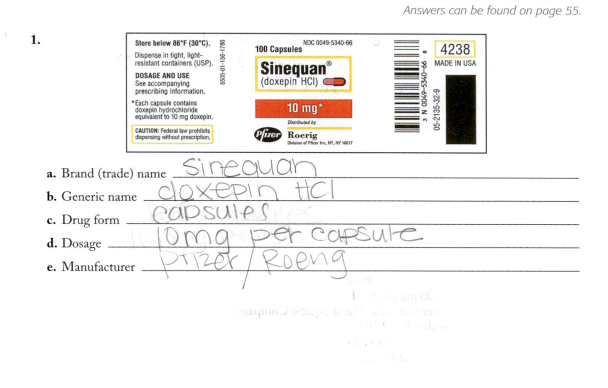

a. Brand (trade) name ___Sinequan___

b. Generic name ___doxepin HCl___

c. Drug form ___capsules___

d. Dosage ___10mg per capsule___

e. Manufacturer ___Pfizer/Roerig___

2.

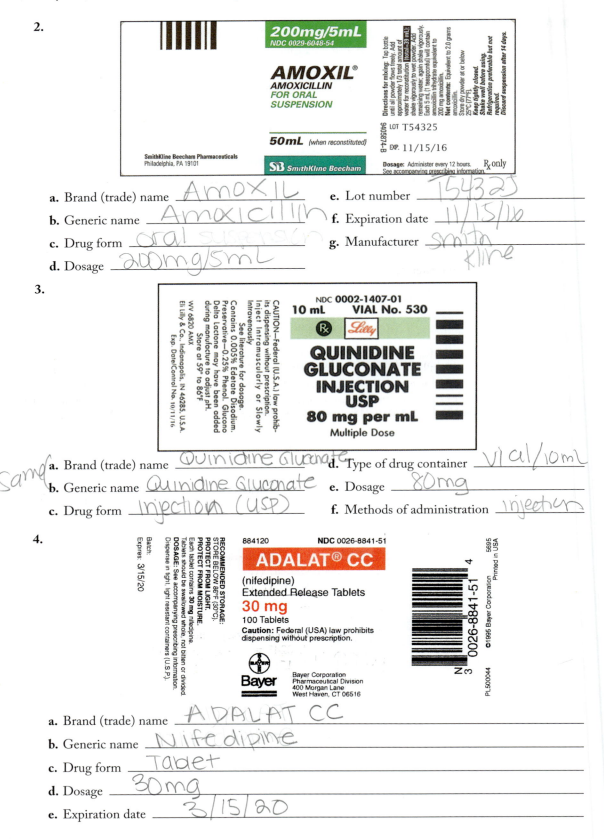

200mg/5mL
NDC 0029-6048-54

AMOXIL®
AMOXICILLIN
FOR ORAL
SUSPENSION

50mL *(when reconstituted)*

SmithKline Beecham Pharmaceuticals
Philadelphia, PA 19101

SB *SmithKline Beecham*

LOT T54325
EXP. 11/15/16

Dosage: Administer every 12 hours.
See accompanying prescribing information.   R̠only

a. Brand (trade) name   *Amoxil*
b. Generic name   *Amoxicillin*
c. Drug form   *oral suspension*
d. Dosage   *200mg/5mL*

e. Lot number   *T54325*
f. Expiration date   *11/15/16*
g. Manufacturer   *Smith Kline*

3.

NDC 0002-1407-01
10 mL   VIAL No. 530

Lilly

**QUINIDINE
GLUCONATE
INJECTION
USP
80 mg per mL**
Multiple Dose

Same

a. Brand (trade) name   *Quinidine Gluconate*
b. Generic name   *Quinidine Gluconate*
c. Drug form   *Injection (USP)*

d. Type of drug container   *vial/10mL*
e. Dosage   *80mg*
f. Methods of administration   *injection*

4.

Batch:
Expires: 3/15/20

RECOMMENDED STORAGE:
STORE BELOW 86°F (30°C).
PROTECT FROM LIGHT.
PROTECT FROM MOISTURE.
Each tablet contains **30 mg** nifedipine.
Tablets should be swallowed whole, not bitten or divided.
DOSAGE: See accompanying prescribing information.
Dispense in tight, light resistant containers (U.S.P.).

884120   NDC 0026-8841-51

ADALAT® CC

(nifedipine)
Extended Release Tablets
30 mg
100 Tablets
Caution: Federal (USA) law prohibits
dispensing without prescription.

Bayer

Bayer Corporation
Pharmaceutical Division
400 Morgan Lane
West Haven, CT 06516

0026-8841-51   4

N 3

©1995 Bayer Corporation   5695
Printed in USA
PL500044

a. Brand (trade) name   *ADALAT CC*
b. Generic name   *Nifedipine*
c. Drug form   *Tablet*
d. Dosage   *30mg*
e. Expiration date   *3/15/20*

5.

NDC 0006-7782-30
2.5 mL INJECTION
AquaMEPHYTON®
(PHYTONADIONE)
Aqueous Colloidal Solution
10 mg per mL
Dist. by:
MERCK & CO., INC.
West Point, PA 19486, USA

MULTIPLE DOSE VIAL
FOR ROUTE OF
ADMINISTRATION AND DOSAGE:
SEE ACCOMPANYING CIRCULAR
Store in a dark place.
CAUTION: Federal (USA)
law prohibits dispensing
without prescription.

2.5 mL | No. 7782   9073108

a. Brand name ___AquaMEPHYTON___

b. Generic name ___Phytonadione___

c. Drug form ___Injection (Aqueous colloidal solution)___

d. How many mL in vial ___2.5mL___

e. Dosage 1 mL = ___10mg___ mg

f. Manufacturer ___MERCK & CO INC___

g. Drug label suggests storing ___in dark place___

Military (International) Time versus Traditional Time

Understanding the difference between military time and traditional time is essential in the health care field because almost all nursing settings use military time for documentation, medication administration, and for scheduling routine care and treatments. Military time uses a 24-hour clock, preventing potential documentation and medication errors as each time occurs only once a day. Military time requires 4 digits, the first two representing the hour and the second two digits representing the minutes. Unlike traditional time, military time does not separate the hours and minutes with a colon. Also, AM and PM are omitted because a 12-hour clock is not used in military time. Example: 5:43 AM = 0543. Example: 11:07 PM = 2307.

Use Figure 3-1 to solve conversion problems.

PRACTICE PROBLEMS ▶ II MILITARY TIME AND TRADITIONAL TIME CONVERSIONS

Answers can be found on page 55.

Outer # = AM
Inner # = PM

Convert traditional times to military time.
1. 9:30 AM = ___0930 am___
2. 10:05 PM = ___2205 pm___
3. 4:55 PM = ___1655 pm___

Convert military times to traditional time.
4. 0245 = ___2:45am___
5. 1515 = ___3:15pm___
6. 0001 = ___12:01am___

___0000 = midnight in medical field___

Figure 3-1 24-hour clock. In military time, midnight is considered 2400; however, midnight is referred to and written as 0000 in the medical field.

DRUG DIFFERENTIATION

Some drugs with similar names, such as quinine and quinidine, have different chemical drug structures. Extreme care must be exercised when administering drugs that "look alike" or have similar spellings.

EXAMPLES **PERCOCET**

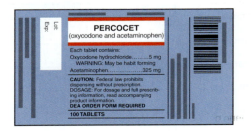

PERCODAN

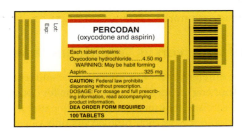

Percocet contains oxycodone and acetaminophen, whereas Percodan contains oxycodone and aspirin. A patient may be allergic to aspirin or should not take aspirin; therefore it is important that the patient be given Percocet. *Read the drug labels carefully and check patient for an allergy band.*

EXAMPLES **HYDROXYZINE AND HYDRALAZINE**

Hydroxyzine is an antianxiety drug, and hydralazine is an antihypertensive drug.

EXAMPLES **QUINIDINE AND QUININE**

Quinidine sulfate is an antidysrhythmic drug, and quinine sulfate is an antimalarial drug.

Drug Orders

Medication orders may be prescribed and written by a licensed health care provider (HCP) with prescriptive authority, which includes physicians (MD), osteopathic physicians (DO), dentists (DDS), podiatrists (DPM), nurse practitioners (NP), and physician assistants (PA). Drug prescriptions in private practice or in clinics are written on a small prescription pad and are filled by a pharmacist at a drugstore or hospital (Figure 3-2). Some facilities have moved to computerized prescriptions. The physician enters the patient's drug order into a prescription template on a computer. The prescription then can be printed out for the patient or sent electronically over a secure network directly to the patient's chosen pharmacy. For hospitalized patients, the drug orders may be written on a doctor's order sheet and signed by the prescribing licensed HCP (Figure 3-3), or a computerized drug order system may be used. If the order is given by telephone (TO), the order must be cosigned by the physician within 24 hours. Most health care institutions have policies concerning verbal or telephone drug orders. The nurse must know and follow the institution's policy.

Roger J. Smith, Jr., M.D.
678 Apple Street
Wilmington, Delaware 19810

(123) 456-7891

_____

Name _____ Age _____

Address _____ Date _____

R$_x$ ~~ADULT MEDICATION~~
         ~~PHYTONADIONE~~
         ~~Injection CAPM~~
         ~~2.5mL~~

Generic permitted _____

Label _____   _____ M.D.

Safety cap _____

Refill _____ times

Figure 3-2 Prescription pad medication order.

CITY HOSPITAL Dover, Delaware		PATIENT'S NAME Room #
Date	**Time**	**Patient's Orders**
12/2/16	0900	Zoloft 75mg po daily

Figure 3-3 Patient's order sheet.

The basic components of a drug order are (1) date and time the order was written, (2) drug name, (3) drug dosage, (4) route of administration, (5) frequency of administration, and (6) physician's or HCP's signature. It is the nurse's responsibility to follow the physician's or HCP's order, but if any one of these components is missing, the drug order is incomplete and cannot be carried out. If the order is illegible, is missing a component, or calls for an inappropriate drug or dosage, clarification from the provider who wrote the order must be obtained before the order is carried out. It is the nurse's responsibility to know what medication he or she is giving and why the patient is receiving it.

Examples of drug orders and their interpretations are as follows:

6/3/16	0900	Digoxin 0.25 mg, po, daily
		(give 0.25 mg of digoxin by mouth daily)

Ibuprofen 400 mg, po, q4h, PRN
(give 400 mg of ibuprofen by mouth every 4 hours as needed)

Cefadyl 500 mg, IM, q6h
(give 500 mg of Cefadyl intramuscularly every 6 hours)

Prednisone 5 mg, po, q8h × 5 days
(give 5 mg of prednisone by mouth every 8 hours for 5 days)

PRACTICE PROBLEMS ▶ III INTERPRETATION OF DRUG ORDERS

Answers can be found on page 55.

Interpret these drug orders. For abbreviations that you do not know, see the section on abbreviations later in this chapter.

1. Procrit 40,000 units, SC, weekly

_____

2. Furosemide 40 mg, IV, bid

_____

3. Meperidine 50 mg, IM, q3-4h, PRN

_____

4. Prednisone 10 mg, po, tid × 5 days

_____

List what is missing in the following drug orders.

5. Codeine 30 mg, po, PRN for pain _____

6. Digoxin 0.25 mg, daily _____

7. TheoDur 200 mg _____

8. Penicillin V K 200,000 units, for days _____

_____

TABLE 3-1 Types of Drug Orders

Types/Description	Examples
Standing orders: A standing order may be typed or written on the patient's order sheet. It may be an order that is given for a number of days, or it may be a routine order that is part of an order set that applies to all patients who have had the same type of procedure. Standing orders may include PRN orders.	Erythromycin 250 mg, po, q6h, 5 days Demerol 50 mg, IM, q3-4h, PRN, pain Colace 100 mg, po, hs, PRN
One-time (single) orders: One-time orders are given once, usually at a specified time. One-time orders can include STAT orders.	Preoperative orders: Meperidine 75 mg, IM, 0730 Atropine SO_4 0.4 mg, IM, 0730
PRN orders: PRN orders are given at the patient's request and at the nurse's discretion concerning safety and need. Narcotics are time-framed and renewed every 48-72 hours.	Acetaminophen 1000 mg IV q6h PRN × 24 hr for fevers > 38° C Ondansetron HCl (Zofran), 4 mg, q4-8h, PRN for nausea
STAT orders: A STAT order is for a one-time dose of drug to be given immediately.	Regular insulin 10 units, subQ, STAT

There are four types of drug orders: (1) standing order, (2) one-time (single) order, (3) PRN (whenever necessary) order, and (4) STAT (immediate) order (Table 3-1). Many of the drugs ordered for nonhospitalized patients are normally standing orders that can be renewed (refilled) for 6 to 12 months. Narcotic orders are *not* automatically refilled; if the narcotic use is extended, the physician writes another prescription or calls the pharmacy.

UNIT-DOSE DISPENSING SYSTEM (UDDS)

The unit-dose drug dispensing system (UDDS) was developed to decrease medication errors, reduce the waste of medication, and improve the efficiency of the nurse when administering medication. The UDDS has almost replaced the ward stock system (Table 3-2). In the ward stock system, bulk drug supplies were delivered to the medication room in each patient area. In the medication room, the nurse would prepare the patient's dose from the large multidose containers or multiple-dose vials; the correct dosage of medication must be taken from the container each time and labeled. In unit-dose dispensing, the pharmacy can provide individual doses in packets or containers for each patient. The pharmacy buys the drugs in bulk and repackages the medication in individual dose packets labeled with the drug name, dosage, and usually a bar code. Many variations are seen in how drugs are stored and delivered to patient care areas. Unit-dose cart cabinets (Figure 3-4) with individualized drawers labeled with the patient's name, room number, and bed number are most common. Each drawer is filled with 24 hours of medication as prescribed by the physician and filled and verified by the pharmacist. The drawers may be refilled or exchanged every 24 hours. When the nurse administers medication, the patient's drawer is accessed, and the appropriate drug is withdrawn.

TABLE 3-2 Methods of Drug Distribution

	Stock Drug Method	Unit-Dose Method
Description	Drug is stored in a large container on the floor and is dispensed from the container for all patients.	Drug is packaged in single doses by the pharmacy for 24-hour dosing.
Advantages	Drug is always available, which eliminates time spent waiting for drug to arrive from the pharmacy. Cost efficiency is enhanced by having large quantities of the drug.	Fewer drug errors are made. Packaging saves the nurse time otherwise spent in preparing the drug dose. Correct dose is provided with *no* calculation needed. Drug is billed for specific number of doses.
Disadvantages	Drug error is more prevalent because the drug is "poured" by many persons. More drugs are available to choose from; this may cause errors. Drug expiration date on the container may be missed.	Time delay is seen in receipt of drug from the pharmacy. If doses are contaminated or damaged, they are not immediately replaceable.

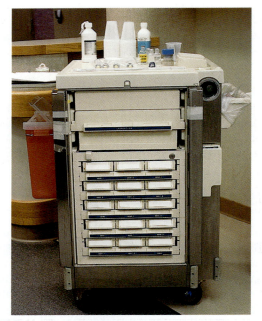

Figure 3-4 Unit-dose cabinet. (From Clayton, B. D., Willihnganz, M. J. [2013]. *Basic pharmacology for nurses.* 16th ed. St. Louis: Mosby.)

Unit-dose dispensing has eliminated the need for many drug calculations that were essential with the ward stock system. Drug manufacturers are working to develop single doses for all medications but extra packaging is costly. In addition, not all medications that are prescribed for a patient are dosed in the exact amount manufactured. Therefore the nurse must master manual calculations and must have working knowledge of the process and formulas needed for medications to be given safely.

COMPUTER-BASED DRUG ADMINISTRATION (CBDA)

Computer-based drug administration (CBDA) is a technological software system that is designed to prevent medication errors. The concept began when the Centers for Disease Control and Prevention (CDC) reported a rise in the number of medication-related deaths between 1983 and 1993. Since that time, the National Coordinating Council for Medication Error Reporting and Prevention has made several recommendations regarding the causes of medication errors; one example of its changes is the bar coding of medications. The federal government through the Department of Veterans Affairs hospitals has developed a software program that automates the medication administration process to improve accuracy and efficiency in documentation. Currently, this system is composed of the computerized prescriber order system (CPOS), the bar-code medication administration (BCMA) system, the electronic medication administration record (eMAR), and the pharmacy information system (PIS). Future software will be expanded to track medications in all forms and to include the whole process of prescribing, administering, monitoring, and documenting.

COMPUTERIZED PRESCRIBER ORDER SYSTEM (CPOS)

The process begins with the computerized prescriber order (entry) system (CPOS), by which the physician or HCP can search for and select medications from a scrolling list (Figure 3-5). Once the medication is selected, the next screen displays all the possible doses, routes, and schedules (Figure 3-6). Once the physician selects those components of the order, he or she can view the screen and make changes. If the screen information is correct, the physician signs the order with his or her personal electronic code, and the order is sent through the PIS, where the order is processed.

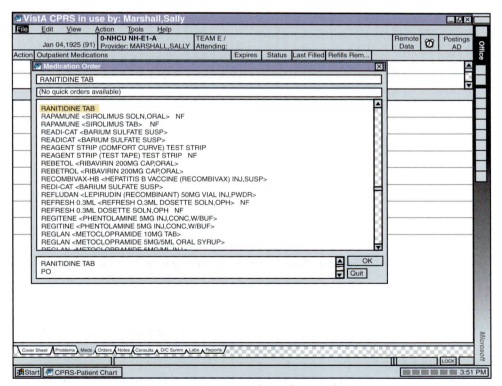

Figure 3-5 CPOS screen for medication selection.

VistA CPRS in use by: Marshall,Sally						
File Edit View Action Tools Help						

0-NHCU NH-E1-A	TEAM E /	Remote	Postings
Jan 04,1925 (91) Provider: MARSHALL,SALLY	Attending	Data	AD

Action	Outpatient Medications	Expires	Status	Last Filled	Refills Rem...
	RANITIDINE HCL 150MG TAV (CMOP) Qty: 11 for 6 days SIG: TAKE ONE TABLET BY MOUTH TWO TIMES DAILY	Nov 27,16	Expired	Nov 21,16	0
	METFORMIN HCL 500MG TAB Qty: 6 for 6 days SIG: TAKE ONE TABLET BY MOUTH EVERY EVENING WITH DINNER FOR	Nov 27,16	Expired	Nov 21,16	0

Action	Inpatient Medications	Stop Date	Status
	*ACETAMINOPHEN TAB Give: 1000MG PO Q6H PRN	Mar 12,16	Active
	TRAZODONE TAB Give: 100MG PO At Bedtime	Mar 09,16	Active
	FOSINOPRIL TAB Give: 20MG PO Daily	Feb 21,16	Active
	PAROXETINE TAB Give: 20MG PO Daily	Feb 13,16	Active
	FELODIPINE TAB, SA Give: 10MG PO Daily	Feb 06,16	Active
	METFORMIN TAB,ORAL Give: 1000MG PO QAM GLY/MET	Jan 10,16	Active
	*METFORMIN TAB,ORAL Give: 500MG PO QPM GLY/MET	Jan 09,16	Active
	RANITIDINE TAB Give: 150MG PO BID	Jan 02,16	Active

Cover Sheet / Problems \ Meds / Orders \ Notes / Consults / D/C Summ \ Labs / Reports /

Figure 3-6 CPOS medication selection screen.

Bar Code Medication Administration

Bar codes are mandatory on medication packaging produced by drug suppliers. Pharmacies can buy drugs in bulk and repackage the medication individually in cellophane envelopes or packets for the unit dose, with each drug and dose having a specific bar-code number. The pharmacy delivers bar-coded drugs to hospital units at specified times, and drugs are kept in special carts within designated areas in patient care locations.

When the nurse is ready to administer the medications, she or he accesses the BCMA system, which displays the medication record screen, and uses the bar-code reader to scan the patient's wristband and the bar code on the drug (Figures 3-7 and 3-8).

The software validates the correct patient, drug, and dosage, along with the right route and time. The software is intended to enhance patient safety by clarifying orders, improving communication, and augmenting clinical judgment.

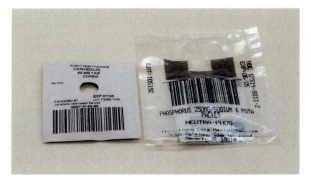

Figure 3-7 Bar code for unit drug dose.

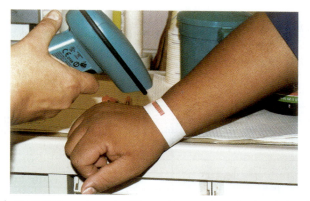

Figure 3-8 Bar-code reader. It is used to scan the patient's wristband.

Automation of Medication Dispensing Administration

Automated dispensing cabinets (ADCs) are medication cabinets that store, dispense, and track drugs in patient areas. They were developed to reduce medication errors, increase pharmacy and nursing efficiency, increase security, support efforts to maintain The Joint Commission and regulatory compliance, and control costs. ADCs permit nurses to access the system with a user ID, personal password, or biometric fingerprint scan to obtain medication in the patient area without having to wait for medication to come from a centralized pharmacy. The three most common dispensing systems are the Pyxis MedStation system (Figure 3-9), Omnicell OmniRx, and the AcuDose-Rx. These systems support storage of vials, ampules, unit-dose packages, prefilled syringes, liquid cups, pre-mixed IVs, large-volume IVs, and other forms of packing. Now almost 90% of all ADCs are linked to the pharmacy information system's patient medication profile; this ensures that the nurse accesses only medication for a specific patient.

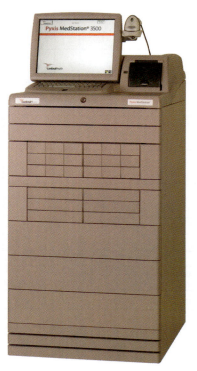

Figure 3-9 Pyxis MedStation system. (From Cardinal Health, San Diego, Calif.)

HOPE HOSPITAL			Patient's Name	John Smith				
				123-24-8449				
Medication Administration Record (MAR)			Age: 78					
			Room#					
Nurse's signature/Title		Initial	6033					
Joyce L. Kee, RN		JK						
Sally Marshall, RN		SM						
Jane Jones, LPN		JJ	Allergies:					
			Penicillin					

DATE ORDER	STOP DATE	Medication Dose – Route – Frequency	TIME	Date, Initial, HT Rate, BP														
				5/16		5/17		5/18		5/19								
5/16		Digoxin 0.25 mg po daily Hold if HR < 60	0800	JK	92	JK	86	JK	88	SM	84							
5/16	5/20 @0000	Prednisone 5 mg po q8h × 5 days	0800	JK		JK		JK		SM								
			1600	SM		JJ		SM		JK								
			0000	JJ		SM		JJ		JJ								
5/16		Atenolol 50 mg po daily Hold if SBP < 100	0800	JK	152/110	JK	146/90	JK	148/72	SM	145/75							

One-Time/PRN/STAT Medications				
Date	Medication/Dose Route/Frequency	Time/ Initial	Reason	Result
5/18	Ibuprofen 400 mg po q4h PRN	0930 SM	Left knee pain 5 of 10	1030 knee pain has improved 1 of 10

Figure 3-10 Medication administration record (MAR).

Medication Administration Record (MAR and eMAR)

Documentation for the MAR should be completed immediately after medications are given. Failing to do so may result in (1) forgetting to chart/document, or (2) administration of drugs by another nurse who thought that the drugs were not given. Although the MAR may vary among health care facilities, all include basic information, such as the patient's name, identification number, date of birth, location, weight, allergies, sex, and date of admission. Drug information on the MAR that is common to all records includes the following: (1) date the drug was ordered, (2) drug name, (3) dosage, (4) route of administration, (5) frequency of administration, (6) date and time the drug was given, and (7) the nurse's signature and initials. Handwritten MARs (Figure 3-10) should be avoided because of the high risk of transcription error.

The electronic medication administration record (eMAR) (Figure 3-11) is the counterpart to BCMA. It is a paperless system that displays on the computer screen the medications to be administered and the appropriate times for each. The nurse uses his or her own specific code to log on to the system, and when the drug is scanned, it is documented as given.

FRIDAY 10/12/16 - 0700 thru SATURDAY 10/13/16 - 0659

Meyer, Lois M.
WESOF W303-2
Age: 87   Sex: F
Primary Dx: Chest pain

Unit#:
Admitted: 10/12/16
Ht: 152.40 cm   Wt: 49.8 kg

ST ANNE HOSPITAL
MEDICATION ADMINISTRATION RECORD
Acct#:   Page: 1
Attending Dr: Benjamin Simmons, MD
Run Date/Time: 10/12/16 - 2237
                              DOB: 12/28/1928

ALLERGIES: Drug: PCN, ERYTHROMYCIN, IV DYE
Other: NO ALLERGIES RECORDED
Pharmacy: IODINE (INCLUDES RADIOPAQUE AGENTS W/IODINE). MACROLIDE ANTIBIOTICS, PENICILLINS

Init	IV Flushes: Routine		0700-1459	1500-2259	2300-0659
	Sodium Chloride 0.9% **IV** Flush peripheral IV lines with 5 mls 0.9 NS q 8 hours and central lines per protocol.		Time _____ Init _____ # Flushed_____	Time _____ Init _____ # Flushed_____	Time _____ Init _____ # Flushed_____

Init	SCHED MEDS	DOSE		0700-1459	1500-2259	2300-0659
	DOCUSATE SODIUM (DOCUSATE SODIUM) START: 10/12 D/C: 11/11/16 AT 2244	**100 MG**	PO Q12 RX 002306792			
	PRAVACHOL (PRAVASTATIN SODIUM) Give at: BEDTIME START: 10/12 D/C: 11/11/16 AT 2244	**80 MG**	PO RX 002306793			
	METOPROLOL TARTRATE (METOPROLOL TARTRATE) HOLD FOR SBP<110 OR HR<55 Check apical rate and BP before drug admin. START: 10/12 D/C: 11/11/16 AT 2244	**50 MG**	PO Q12 RX 002306794			
	ACCUPRIL (QUINAPRIL HCL) HOLD FOR SBP<120 START: 10/12 D/C: 11/11/16 AT 2244	**40 MG**	PO Q12 RX 002306795			
	NITROGLYCERIN 2% (NITROGLYCERIN 2%) HOLD FOR SBP<100 START: 10/12 D/C: 11/11/16 AT 2244	**1 INCH**	TP Q6 RX 002306796			0000 0600
	ALPRAZOLAM (ALPRAZOLAM) START: 10/12 D/C: 10/14/16 AT 1601	**0.25 MG**	PO Q8 RX 002306791			0000

Init	PRN MEDS	DOSE		0700-1459	1500-2259	2300-0659
	NITROSTAT 25 TABS/BOTTLE (NITROGLYCERIN) Chest discomfort. May repeat q 5 min x 3. If no relief after 3 doses. Stat ECG & call Physician. START: 10/12 D/C: 11/11/16 at 1833	**0.4 MG**	SL STAT RX 002306718 PRN			

Figure 3-11 Electronic medication administration record (eMAR).

Note all medication hold parameters before administering any medication.

ABBREVIATIONS

Drug Measurements and Drug Forms

Many abbreviations, symbols, acronyms, and dose designations in health care developed over time from the need to communicate and document care. The nurse must learn these and properly interpret them when administering drug therapy. Here are lists of acceptable abbreviations used in three categories: (1) drug measurements and drug forms, (2) routes of drug administration, and (3) times of administration. Not all abbreviations are used in every institution. The nurse should follow the institution's policies for documentation and communication.

Abbreviation	Meaning
cap	capsule
elix	elixir
g, gm, G, GM	gram
gtt	drops
kg	kilogram
l, L	liter
m^2	square meter
mcg	microgram
mEq	milliequivalent
mg	milligram
mL, ml	milliliter
m, min	minim
oz	ounce
pt	pint
qt	quart
SR	sustained release
supp	suppository
susp	suspension
T.O.	telephone order
T, tbsp	tablespoon
t, tsp	teaspoon
V.O.	verbal order

Routes of Drug Administration

Abbreviation	Meaning
ID	intradermal
IM	intramuscular
IV	intravenous
IVPB	intravenous piggyback
KVO	keep vein open
Ⓛ	left
NGT	nasogastric tube
PO, po, os	by mouth
R, Ⓡ	right
SC, subc, sc, SQ, subQ	subcutaneous
SL, sl, subl	sublingual
TKO	to keep open
Vag	vaginal

Times of Administration

Abbreviation	Meaning
AC, ac	before meals
ad lib	as desired
B.i.d., b.i.d., bid	twice a day
c̄	with
NPO	nothing by mouth
PC, pc	after meals
PRN, p.r.n.	whenever necessary, as needed
q	every
qAM	every morning
qh	every hour
q2h	every 2 hours
q4h	every 4 hours
q6h	every 6 hours
q8h	every 8 hours
Q.i.d., q.i.d., qid	four times a day
s̄	without
SOS	once if necessary; if there is a need
STAT	immediately
T.i.d., t.i.d., tid	three times a day

"Do Not Use" Abbreviations

Misconstrued and misinterpreted abbreviations can result in harmful outcomes. Two organizations, The Joint Commission (TJC), formerly known as The Joint Commission on Accreditation of Healthcare Organizations, and the Institute for Safe Medication Practices (ISMP), whose purpose is to improve quality of care and promote patient safety, have issued "Do Not Use" lists of error-prone abbreviations, symbols, acronyms, and dose designations with suggestions for alternatives to avoid mistakes and patient harm. The nurse must be alert and recognize drug orders with abbreviations or symbols that could cause potential problems.

The following is a combined list from TJC and ISMP of abbreviations and symbols that have been frequently misinterpreted and that have caused harmful errors.

The "Do Not Use" Abbreviation List

Abbreviation	Meaning	Use Instead
A.D., ad	Right ear	Right ear
&	and	and
A.S., as	Left ear	Left ear
@	at	at
A.U., au	Both ears	Both ears
cc	cubic centimeter	mL (milliliter)
D/C	Discharge or discontinue	Discharge or discontinue
Drug name abbreviations		Write out the full name of the drug
hs	At bedtime	Bedtime
HS	Half-strength	Half-strength or at bedtime
i/d	One daily	1 daily
IJ	Injection	Injection
IN	Intranasal	Intranasal or NAS
IU	International unit	International unit
< and >	Less than and greater than	Less than and greater than

Abbreviation	Meaning	Use Instead
o.d. or OD	Once daily	Daily
O.D., od	Right eye	Right eye
OJ	Orange juice	Orange juice
O.S., os	Left eye	Left eye
O.U., ou	Both eyes	Both eyes
Per os	By mouth, orally	PO, by mouth, or orally
q.d. or QD	Every day	Daily
qhs or qHS	Nightly at bedtime	Nightly
qn	Nightly or at bedtime	Nightly or at bedtime
q.o.d. or QOD	Every other day	Every other day
q1d	Daily	Daily
q6PM	Every evening at 6 PM	6 PM daily
/ (slash mark)	Separates doses or means per	per
ss	Sliding scale or 1/2	Sliding scale
SSI	Sliding scale insulin	Sliding scale insulin
SSRI	Sliding scale regular insulin	Sliding scale insulin
tiw or TIW	Three times a week	Three times weekly
U or u	Unit	Unit
UD	ut dictum or as directed	As directed
Ug	microgram	mcg (microgram)

Please refer to TJC website at *www.jointcommission.org* and to the Institute for Safe Medication Practices at *www.ismp.org* for more detailed safety information.

PRACTICE PROBLEMS ▶ IV ABBREVIATIONS

Answers can be found on page 55.

If you have more than three incorrect answers, review the abbreviations and meanings. Then quiz yourself again.

1. cap _____
2. SR _____
3. fl oz _____
4. g, G, gm, GM _____
5. gtt _____
6. L _____
7. mL _____
8. mcg _____
9. mg _____
10. oz _____
11. T, tbsp _____
12. t, tsp _____
13. IM _____

14. IV _____
15. KVO or TKO _____
16. subcut _____
17. c̄ _____
18. A.C., ac _____
19. NPO _____
20. PC, pc _____
21. q4h _____
22. Q.i.d., q.i.d., qid _____
23. T.i.d., t.i.d., tid _____
24. B.i.d., b.i.d., bid _____
25. STAT _____

ANSWERS

I Interpretation of Drug Labels

1. a. Sinequan
b. doxepin
c. capsule
d. 10 mg per capsule
e. Pfizer/Roerig

2. a. Amoxil
b. amoxicillin
c. liquid for oral suspension when reconstituted
d. 200 mg/5 mL
e. Lot #T54325
f. Expiration date: 11/15/20
g. SmithKline Beecham

3. a. quinidine gluconate
b. quinidine gluconate (same as brand name)
c. liquid for injection
d. vial (multiple-dose vial), total amount is 10 mL per vial
e. 80 mg per mL
f. IM or IV

4. a. Adalat
b. nifedipine
c. tablet
d. 30 mg
e. 3/15/20

5. a. Aquamephyton
b. phytonadione
c. Aqueous colloidal solution, injectable
d. 2.5 mL
e. 10 mg
f. Merck & Co.
g. In a dark place

II Military Time and Traditional Time Conversions

1. 0930
2. 2205

3. 1655
4. 2:45 AM

5. 3:15 PM
6. 12:01 AM

III Interpretation of Drug Orders

1. Give 40,000 units of Procrit subcutaneously, once a week
2. Give 40 mg of furosemide intravenously, two times per day
3. Give 50 mg of meperidine intramuscularly every 3 to 4 hours whenever necessary
4. Give 10 mg of prednisone by mouth three times a day for 5 days
5. frequency of administration
6. route of administration
7. route and frequency of administration
8. route and frequency of administration and stop date

IV Abbreviations

1. capsule
2. sustained release
3. fluid ounce
4. gram
5. drop
6. liter
7. milliliter
8. microgram
9. milligram

10. ounce
11. tablespoon
12. teaspoon
13. intramuscular
14. intravenous
15. keep vein open
16. subcutaneous
17. with

18. before meals
19. nothing by mouth
20. after meals
21. every 4 hours
22. four times a day
23. three times a day
24. two times a day
25. immediately

evolve   Additional information is available in the Safety in Medication Administration section of Drug Calculations Companion, version 5.

CHAPTER 4

Prevention of Medication Errors

Objectives
- Know the organizations that are monitoring medication errors.
- Identify high-alert drugs.
- Discuss some of the causes of medication errors (MEs).
- Explain ways that medication errors can be prevented.
- Describe the Rights in drug administration.

Outline **PREVENTING MEDICATION ERRORS**
THE RIGHTS IN DRUG ADMINISTRATION

PREVENTING MEDICATION ERRORS

The purpose of drug therapy is to improve the patient's quality of life while minimizing the risk. There are risks, some known and some unknown, associated with every medication. An adverse drug event/reaction (ADE/ADR) is an incident that causes physical, mental, or functional harm associated with a medication or the delivery of that medication. One type of adverse drug event/reaction is a medication error (ME), which is a mistake made in prescribing, dispensing, administering, and/or patient monitoring. Although medication errors are considered preventable, over 100,000 MEs were reported by hospitals nationwide in 2001, according to a study conducted by the Institute for Safe Medication Practices (ISMP). As a result of these medication errors, at least 7,000 deaths occurred per year at a cost of $2 billion. However, the reporting of MEs is voluntary, not mandatory. So the actual figures of MEs are probably much higher.

Currently there are 40 health care groups—private, governmental, and professional—that are working together to report, understand, and prevent medication errors. These stakeholders include: the ISMP, National Coordinating Council for Medication Error Reporting and Prevention (NCC-MERP), Food and Drug Administration (FDA), American Hospital Association, American Medical Association, American Nurses Association, United States Pharmacopeia (USP), the National Academy of Medicine (formerly Institute of Medicine, IOM), American Society of Health-System Pharmacists, The Joint Commission (TJC), and AARP. The NC-MERP has developed tools for reporting and categorizing medication errors. The FDA rules state that a bar code and the national drug code, which identifies the drug strength and its dosage form, are required for human drug products and blood. The ISMP has identified lists of high-alert drugs that should be carefully monitored to prevent adverse drug reactions. Nurse educators have resources through the Quality and Safety Education for Nurses (QSEN) Institute to assist students to learn the complexities of safe practice in drug administration.

Of the MEs reported in 2001, about half are intercepted, and of those, 86% were intercepted by nurses. With so many drugs in use today, the nurse should have access to drug reference books and online resources, such as Micromedex, DailyMed (can be obtained from the National Institutes of

Health, www.Dailymed.nlm.nih.gov), and Lexicomp, on the unit for prompt information about the drug to be given, especially if it is a high-alert drug. Some examples of high-alert drugs are: potassium chloride, insulin, heparin, opiates, and anticancer agents. Refer to Chapter 13.

> ## YOU MUST REMEMBER
>
> The person who administers the medication, usually the nurse, is responsible if an ME occurs.

Here are some examples of the types of medication errors (MEs):

1. The physician or health care provider makes a prescribing error and/or the written drug order is **NOT** legible.
2. Transcription errors occur because the medications have similar names; the decimals and zeros are not correctly written; or numbers are transposed.
3. Telephone and verbal orders are misinterpreted.
4. Interruptions occur when preparing medications.
5. Drug labels look similar (names and color), and packing obscures print on the label.
6. Trade names and generic names for drugs are used interchangeably, which causes confusion.
7. Oral dosages and intravenous dosages are different for the same drug.
8. Subcutaneous insulin is given in a tuberculin syringe and **NOT** in an insulin syringe.
9. The pharmacy delivers the wrong drug.
10. Intravenous medication is given too fast or too concentrated.
11. The amount of the drug is incorrectly calculated.
12. The drug is given intramuscularly or subcutaneously and should be given intravenously OR the drug is given intravenously and should be given intramuscularly.
13. Two incompatible drugs are given intravenously, which can cause crystallization of the drugs.
14. Two or three patients with the same names are on the same unit and their identification wristbands are hard to read. One patient receives another's medication.
15. Medication is given and not monitored, and an overdose occurs.
16. An infusion pump malfunctions or is incorrectly programmed.

Ways to prevent medication errors (MEs):

1. Ask the physician or health care provider to rewrite or clarify medication order.
2. Use only approved abbreviations from The Joint Commission (TJC) list for medication dosages. Do not use "u" for unit; it should be spelled out. Avoid use of a slash mark (/), which could be interpreted as a one (1).
3. Do not use abbreviations for medication names (e.g., MSO_4 for morphine sulfate).
4. Use leading zeros for doses less than a unit (e.g., **0.1** mg; **NOT .1** mg). Do not use a zero following a whole number (e.g., 5 mg; **NOT** 5.0 mg). The decimal point after 5 may not be noticed and would look like 50 mg.
5. Check medication orders with written order and MAR/eMAR.
6. Check the drug dose sent from the pharmacy with the MAR/eMAR.
7. Prepare medications in a clean, distraction-free environment.
8. Never administer a medication that has been prepared by another nurse.
9. Have another nurse check the dosage preparation, especially if in doubt. Recalculate drug dosage as needed.
10. Check if the patient is allergic to any specific drugs. If an allergy exists, report the type of reaction the patient experiences.
11. Check the patient's identification band with the eMAR and bar code.
12. Do not leave medication at the bedside. Stay with the patient until the medications are swallowed.

13. Know whether the medication the patient is to receive would be contraindicated because of the patient's health (liver disease and Tylenol [acetaminophen]) or because of a possible drug interaction with another drug the patient is taking.
14. Assess physical parameters (e.g., apical pulse, respiration, BP, INR, and electrolyte values) before administering the medication that could affect these parameters.
15. Monitor the effects of the administered drug, the rate of IV flow, and the patient's response to the medication.
16. Check when to administer medication for a patient whose status is nothing by mouth (NPO). When in doubt, check with the health care provider (HCP) or nurse manager.
17. Record medications that are given immediately after their administration.
18. Report MEs immediately to the HCP.
19. Educate the patient and family about the drug and its action.
20. Know the compatibility of drugs that are being given. Report any contraindications.

Nurses often work in busy environments with constant distractions. When giving medications, it is important to concentrate fully on the task and know the usual drug dosage of the medication you are giving. If your facility does not have a current drug reference book that is easily accessible, then a drug reference text should be obtained. If a nurse is unsure about a drug order or dosage, then consultation is required with the pharmacy, physician, HCP, or nurse manager before administering the medication. Keeping the patient safe is the nurse's responsibility. The nurse is the licensed practitioner who administers the medication and monitors the medication's response. Nurses are the final line of defense. Be a patient advocate, and always ask if you are unsure.

THE RIGHTS IN DRUG ADMINISTRATION

To provide safe drug administration, the nurse should practice the "10 Rights": the right patient, the right drug, the right dose, the right time, the right route, the right documentation, the right to refuse the medication, the right assessment, the right education (patient), and the right evaluation (see Box 4-1).

Right Patient

The patient's identification band should always be checked before a medication is given. The nurse should do the following:
- Verify the patient's identity by checking his or her identification bracelet/wristband.
- Ask the patient his or her name and birth date. Do not call the patient by name. Some individuals answer to any name. The patient may have difficulty in hearing.
- Check the name on the patient's medication label.
- Check if the patient has allergies (check chart and ask the patient).

Right Drug

To avoid error, the nurse should do the following:
- Check the drug label three times: (1) first contact with the drug bottle or drug pack, (2) before pouring/preparing the drug, and (3) after preparation of the drug.
- Check that the drug order is complete and legible. If it is not, contact the physician, HCP, or charge nurse.
- Know the drug action.
- Check the expiration date. Discard an outdated drug or return the drug to the pharmacy.
- If the patient questions the drug, recheck the drug and drug dose. If in doubt, seek another HCP's advice, i.e., pharmacist, physician, licensed HCP. Some generic drugs differ in shape or color.

Right Dose

Stock drugs and unit doses are the two methods frequently used for drug distribution. Not all health care institutions use the unit-dose method (drugs prepared by dose in the pharmacy or by the pharmaceutical company). If the institution uses the unit-dose method, drugs in bottles should *not* be administered without the consent of the physician or pharmacist. The nurse should:

- Be able to calculate drug dose using the ratio and proportion, basic formula, fractional equation, or dimensional analysis methods.
- Know how to calculate drug dose by body weight (kg) or by body surface (BSA; m²). Doses of potent drugs (e.g., anticancer agents) and doses for children are frequently determined by body weight or BSA.
- Know the recommended dosage range for the drug. Check the *Physicians' Desk Reference*, the *American Hospital Formulary Service (AHFS) Drug Information*, nursing drug reference books, computerized drug reference programs, or other drug references. If the nurse believes that the dose is incorrect or is not within the therapeutic drug range, he or she should notify the charge nurse, physician, or pharmacist and should document all communications.
- Recalculate the drug dose if in doubt, or have a colleague recheck the dose and calculation.
- Question drug doses that appear incorrect.
- Have a colleague check the drug dose of potent or specified drugs, such as insulin, digoxin, narcotics, and anticancer agents. This procedure is required by some facilities.

Right Time

The drug dose should be given at a specified time to maintain a therapeutic drug serum level. Too-frequent dosing can cause drug toxicity, and missed doses can nullify the drug action and its effect. The nurse should:

- Administer the drug at the specified time(s). Usually, drugs can be given 30 minutes before or after the time prescribed.
- Omit or delay a drug dose according to specific circumstance, e.g., laboratory or diagnostic tests may be necessary. Notify the appropriate personnel of the reason.
- Administer drugs that are affected by food (e.g., tetracycline) 1 hour before or 2 hours after meals.
- Administer drugs that can irritate the gastric mucosa (e.g., potassium or aspirin) with food.
- Give some medications promptly or at a specified time (e.g., STAT drugs for pain or nausea drugs).
- Know that drugs with a long half-life ($t_{1/2}$) (e.g., 20 to 36 hours) are usually given once per day. Drugs with a short half-life, e.g., 1 to 6 hours, are given several times a day.
- Administer antibiotics at even intervals (e.g., q8h: 8 AM, 4 PM, midnight), rather than tid (8 AM, noon, 4 PM); q6h (6, 12, 6, 12), rather than qid (8-12-4-8) to maintain therapeutic drug serum level. If the patient is to receive a diuretic twice a day, q12h, 8 AM and 8 PM, the evening dose may be given at 4 PM (e.g., bid) because of the diuretic effect. If dose is given in the evening, it could cause urination late at night.

Right Route

The right route is necessary for the appropriate absorption of the medication. The more common routes of absorption are: (1) oral (by mouth, po) tablet, capsule, pill, liquid, or suspension; (2) sublingual (under the tongue for venous absorption, *not* to be swallowed); (3) buccal (between gum and cheek, *not* to be swallowed); (4) topical (applied to the skin); (5) inhalation (aerosol sprays); (6) instillation (in nose, eye, ear, rectum, or vagina); and (7) four parenteral routes: intradermal, subcutaneous, intramuscular, and intravenous. The nurse should:

- Know the drug route. If in doubt, check with the pharmacy. Ointment for the eye should have "ophthalmic" written on the tube. Drugs given sublingually (e.g., nitroglycerin tablet) should *not* be swallowed, because the effect of the drug would be lost.

- Administer injectables (subcutaneous and intramuscular) at appropriate sites (see Chapter 9).
- Use aseptic technique when administering drugs. Sterile technique is required with parenteral routes.
- Document the injection site used on the patient's paper chart (MAR) or eMAR.

Right Documentation

Document on the MAR or eMAR (computer), the time the drug was administered and the nurse's initials. To avoid overdosing or underdosing of drug, administration of medication should be recorded immediately.

- Put your initials on the MAR sheet or eMAR at the proper space immediately after administering the drug. With eMAR, click the mark as given, and the system will automatically sign the medication off with your initials.
- Refused drug: Circle your initials and document on the nurse's notes or on the MAR or eMAR.
- Omitted drug: Circle your initials and document on the nurse's notes or the MAR/eMAR. Document why the drug was omitted, such as the patient was NPO because of a laboratory or diagnostic test. The charge nurse or HCP should be notified.
- Delay in administering drug should be documented on the nurse's notes, MAR sheet, or eMAR. If the drug is to be administered once a day and is delayed, document the time the drug is given. Medications can be retimed on eMAR.
- High-alert medications must be cosigned whenever a dose changes or a new IV bag is hung. Check with your institution.

Right to Refuse Medication

The patient has a right to refuse medication. However,

- Explain to the patient the therapeutic effect of the drug. This will often diminish the patient's refusal.
- Document the medication and time the patient refused the drug and the reason for the patient's refusal.
- Notify the physician, HCP, and/or charge nurse that the patient refused the drug and why.
- If the refusal is due to the mental status of the patient, it should be reported.

Right Assessment

- Assess whether the ordered medication is safe to administer.
- Assess the patient's vital signs (VS) to determine medication safety. For example, a patient may be ordered Dilaudid 0.5 mg, IV. The patient's VS are BP 95/60, pulse 60, and respirations 8. After assessing VS, the Dilaudid IV would be determined to be unsafe to administer.
- Know that opioids can decrease blood pressure, pulse, and respirations.
- Assess the effects of the medication being administered.

Right Education

- Educate the patient about the purpose(s) for the ordered medications.
- Answer patient's questions about the medication he or she is taking. The patient will most likely comply in taking the medication if the patient understands the purpose and effects of the drug(s).
- Educate the patient about the possible effects of the medication, including side effects, especially with potent drugs.

Right Evaluation

- Evaluate the effects of the medication, particularly whether it was effective or not.
- Record on the MAR or eMAR the positive or negative effects of the medication(s).
- Report to the health care provider (HCP) if the medication was ineffective.
- Evaluate whether the medication is causing adverse reactions. Report immediately any adverse reactions.

BOX 4-1 CHECKLIST FOR THE "10 RIGHTS" IN DRUG ADMINISTRATION

Right Patient

- Check patient's identification bracelet.
- Ask the patient his or her name and birth date.
- Check the name on the patient's medication label.

Right Drug

- Check that the drug order is complete and legible.
- Check the drug label three times.
- Check the expiration date.
- Know the drug action.

Right Dose

- Calculate the drug dosage.
- Know the recommended dosage range for the drug.
- Recalculate the drug dosage with another nurse if in doubt.

Right Time

- Administer drug at the specified time(s).
- Document any delay or omitted drug dose.
- Administer drugs that irritate gastric mucosa with food.
- Administer drugs that cannot be administered with food 1 hour before or 2 hours after meals.
- Administer antibiotics at even intervals (q6h or q8h).

Right Route

- Know the route for administration of the drug.
- Use aseptic techniques when administering a drug.
- Document the injection site on the MAR/eMAR.

Right Documentation

- Place nurse's initials on the MAR sheet or eMAR.
- Document the reason for a patient **not** taking the drug.
- Indicate on the MAR sheet or eMAR whether the drug dose was delayed and the time it was given.

Right to Refuse Medication

- Document the time and date the patient refused the drug and the refusal reason.
- Notify the charge nurse and physician that the patient refused the drug.
- Explain the purpose and therapeutic effect of the drug to the patient.
- Record if the refusal could be due to the patient's mental status.

Continued

BOX 4-1 CHECKLIST FOR THE "10 RIGHTS" IN DRUG ADMINISTRATION—cont'd

Right Assessment

- Assess if the ordered medication is safe to administer.
- Assess the patient's vital signs and determine whether they are safe for the drug.
- Know that opioids can decrease vital signs.
- Assess the effects of the medication(s) being administered.

Right Education

- Educate the patient about the purpose(s) for the medication.
- Answer the patient's questions about the medication he or she is receiving.
- Educate the patient about possible side effects of the medication.

Right Evaluation

- Evaluate the effects of the medication.
- Record on the MAR or eMAR the effects of the medication(s).
- Report to the HCP if the medication was ineffective.
- Evaluate whether the medication caused adverse reactions.

evolve   Additional information is available in the Safety in Medication Administration section of Drug Calculations Companion, version 5.

CHAPTER 5

Alternative Methods for Drug Administration

Objectives
- Explain the correct method of applying a transdermal patch.
- Describe the administration nasal and ophthalmic medications.
- Explain the techniques for administering ear drops to adults and children.
- Recognize when intraosseous or intraspinal access should be utilized in the clinical setting.

Outline

The properties of a medication significantly influence its route of administration, which determines how it will be absorbed into the body. The two major routes of administration are enteral and parenteral. Drugs taken orally or sublingually are using an enteral route of administration. The parenteral route directly delivers the medication into the patient's systemic circulation (i.e., intravenous, intramuscular, intraosseous, and subcutaneous). Other methods of administration may be less common but are still important alternatives for medication delivery. Some other forms of medication administration include transdermal, inhalation, pharyngeal, topical, rectal, vaginal, nasal, eye, or ear drops, and intraspinal. The general nursing procedure for any drug administration is to wash hands, apply clean gloves, then proceed to administer the medication.

TRANSDERMAL PATCH

Purpose

The transdermal patch contains medication (Figure 5-1); the patch is applied to the skin for slow, systemic absorption, usually over 24 hours. Use of the transdermal route avoids the gastrointestinal problems associated with some oral medications and provides a more consistent drug level in the patient's blood.

Method

Transdermal Patch
1. Wear gloves to remove existing patch if present, then cleanse and dry the area of skin where the new patch will be applied. Commonly used areas are the chest, abdomen, arms, or thighs. Avoid areas that have hair.
2. Label the patch with date, time, and nurse's initials.
3. Remove the transparent cover (inside) of the patch. Do not touch the inside of the patch.
4. Apply the patch to the chosen area with the dull plastic side up.
5. Document location of transdermal patch on medication administration record or chart.

Note: There are some transdermal patches that absorb over 3 days (e.g., durgesic), some over 7 days (e.g., Catapres), and some over 1 month (e.g., contraceptive agents).

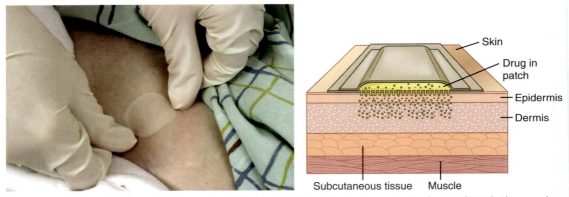

Figure 5-1 A, Transdermal nitroglycerin patch. (In Lilley, L. L., Collins, S. R., Harrington, S., Snyder, J. S. [2011]. *Pharmacology and the nursing process,* 6th ed., St. Louis: Mosby. From Rick Brady, Riva, MD.) **B,** Interior of the transdermal patch.

TYPES OF INHALERS AND NEBULIZERS

Purpose

The drug inhaler delivers a prescribed dose to be absorbed rapidly by the mucosal lining of the respiratory tract (Figure 5-2). The drug categories for respiratory inhalation are bronchodilators, which dilate bronchial tubes; glucocorticoids, which are anti-inflammatory agents; and mucolytics, which liquefy bronchial secretions.

Types

Inhalers can be divided into four groups: metered-dose inhalers (MDIs), MDI inhalers with spacers, dry powder inhalers, and nebulizers. Standard MDIs use a pressurized gas that expels the medication. The user must press the canister and inhale fully at the same time. Breath-activated MDIs are another type, in which the dose is triggered by inhaling through the mouthpiece; they require less coordination.

Spacer devices are used with MDIs and act as a reservoir to hold the medication until it is inhaled. These devices have a one-way valve that prevents the aerosol from escaping. Good coordination is not needed to use a spacer device.

Dry powder inhalers contain small amounts of medications that have to be strongly inhaled if the powder is to get into the lungs. This method is difficult for children younger than 6 years.

Nebulizers are devices that convert medication into a fine mist. The medication is usually prescribed in a prefilled dosette, which is placed in a nebulizer connected to a small compressor that aerosolizes the medication. The medication is inhaled via mouthpiece or face mask. Nebulizers are the choice for the weak, elderly, and small children and infants because no coordination is needed for this type of delivery.

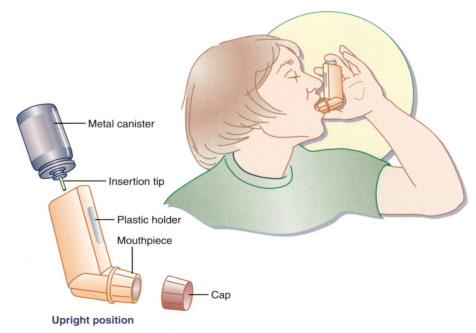

Metal canister

Insertion tip

Plastic holder

Mouthpiece

Cap

Upright position

Figure 5-2 Technique for using the aerosol inhaler. (From Kee, J. L., Hayes, E. R., & McCuistion, L. E. [2012]. *Pharmacology: a nursing process approach,* 7th ed., Philadelphia: Saunders.)

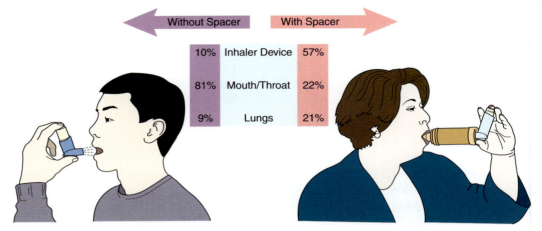

Without Spacer		With Spacer
10%	Inhaler Device	57%
81%	Mouth/Throat	22%
9%	Lungs	21%

Figure 5-3 Distribution of medication with and without a spacer.

Method

Metered–Dose Inhaler
1. Insert the medication canister into the plastic holder. If the inhaler has not been used recently or if it is being used for the first time, test spray before administering the metered dose.
2. Shake the inhaler well before using. Remove the cap from the mouthpiece.
3. Instruct the patient to breathe out through the mouth, expelling air. Place the mouthpiece into the patient's mouth, holding the inhaler upright (see Figure 5-2).
4. Instruct the patient to keep his or her lips securely around the mouthpiece and inhale. While the patient is inhaling, push the top of the medication canister once.
5. Instruct the patient to hold his or her breath for a few seconds. Remove the mouthpiece and take your finger off the canister. Tell the patient to exhale slowly.
6. If a second dose is required, wait 1 to 2 minutes, and repeat steps 3 to 5.
7. Cleanse the mouthpiece.

Method

Metered-Dose Inhaler with Spacer
This method is similar to an MDI with the following additions; see Figure 5-3.
1. Start to inhale as soon as the canister is depressed.
2. Check that the valve opens and closes with each breath.
3. Wash spacer as directed by manufacturer.
Note: For steroid inhalers, rinsing and gargling are necessary to remove residual steroid medication, thus preventing a sore throat or fungal overgrowth and infection.

NASAL SPRAY AND DROPS

Purpose

Most drugs in nasal spray and drop containers are intended to relieve nasal congestion typically caused by upper respiratory tract infections by shrinking swollen nasal membranes. Types of drugs given by this method are vasoconstrictors and glucocorticoids.

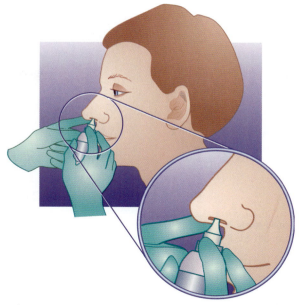

Figure 5-4 Administering nasal spray. (From Kee, J. L., Hayes, E. R., & McCuistion, L. E. [2015]. *Pharmacology: a nursing process approach,* 8th ed., Philadelphia: Saunders.)

Method

Nasal Spray
1. Instruct the patient to sit with his or her head tilted slightly back or slightly forward, according to the directions on the spray container.
2. Insert the tip of the container into one nostril and occlude the other nostril (Figure 5-4).
3. Instruct the patient to inhale as you squeeze the drug spray container. Repeat with the same nostril or other nostril if ordered.
4. Encourage the patient to keep his or her head tilted back for several minutes to promote absorption of the medication. The nose should not be blown until the head is upright.
5. Drink plenty of fluids after using a steroid nasal spray to avoid microbial overgrowth.

Method

Nasal Drops
1. Instruct the patient to sit with his or her head tilted back.
2. Insert the dropper into the nostril without touching the nasal membranes (Figure 5-5).
3. Instill the number of drops prescribed.
4. Instruct the patient to keep his or her head tilted back for 5 minutes and to breathe through the mouth.
5. Cleanse the dropper.
6. For the medication to reach the frontal and maxillary sinuses, the patient should slowly alternate turning his or her head from side to side while in the supine position. For the medication to reach the ethmoidal and sphenoidal sinuses, the patient will need to lean forward, bringing his or her head toward the knees.

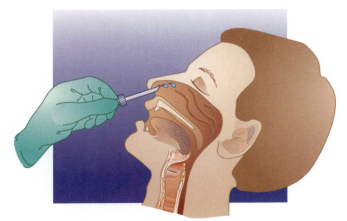

Figure 5-5 Administering nasal drops. (From Kee, J. L., Hayes, E. R., & McCuistion, L. E. [2015]. *Pharmacology: a nursing process approach,* 8th ed., Philadelphia: Saunders.)

EYE DROPS AND OINTMENT

Purpose

Eye medications are prescribed for various eye disorders, such as glaucoma, infection, and allergies, and for eye examination and eye surgery.

Method

Eye Drops
1. Instruct the patient to lie or sit with his or her head tilted back.
2. Instruct the patient to look up toward the ceiling and away from the dropper. Pull down the lower lid of the affected eye (Figure 5-6). Place the number of drops prescribed into the lower conjunctival sac. This prevents the drug from dropping onto the cornea. To prevent contamination DO NOT touch the end of the dropper on the eye or eyelashes.
3. Press gently on the medial nasolacrimal canthus (side closer to the nose) with a tissue to prevent systemic drug absorption.
4. If the other eye is affected, repeat the procedure in the other eye.
5. Instruct patient to blink once or twice and then to keep his or her eyes closed for several minutes. Use a tissue to blot away excess drug fluid.
6. When administering two or more different types of eye drops, wait 5 minutes between medications.

Method

Eye Ointment
1. Instruct the patient to lie or sit with his or her head tilted back.
2. Pull down the lower lid to expose the conjunctival sac of the affected eye (Figure 5-7).

3. Squeeze a strip of ointment about ¼-inch long (unless otherwise indicated) onto the conjunctival sac. Medication placed directly onto the cornea can cause discomfort or damage.
4. If the other eye is affected, repeat the procedure.
5. Instruct the patient to close his or her eyes for 2 to 3 minutes. Teach the patient to expect blurred vision for a short time after the application of the ointment.

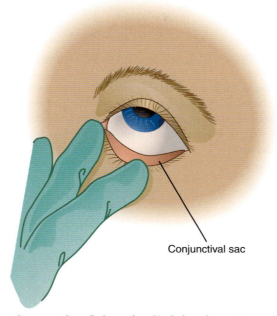

Figure 5-6 To administer eye drops, gently pull down the skin below the eye to expose the conjunctival sac. (From Kee, J. L., Hayes, E. R., & McCuistion, L. E. [2015]. *Pharmacology: a nursing process approach,* 8th ed., Philadelphia: Saunders.)

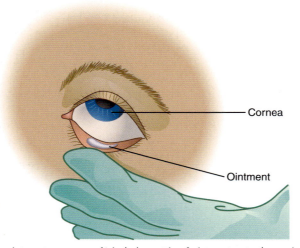

Figure 5-7 To administer eye ointment, squeeze a ¼-inch–long strip of ointment onto the conjunctival sac. (From Kee, J. L., Hayes, E. R., & McCuistion, L. E. [2015]. *Pharmacology: a nursing process approach,* 8th ed., Philadelphia: Saunders.)

EAR DROPS

Purpose

Ear medication is frequently prescribed to soften and loosen the cerumen (wax) in the ear canal, for anesthetic effect, to immobilize insects in the ear canal, and to treat infection such as fungal infections.

Method

Ear Drops
1. Instruct the patient to lie on the unaffected side or to sit upright with his or her head tilted toward the unaffected side.
2. Straighten the external ear canal (Figure 5-8) as follows: *Adult:* Pull the auricle of the ear up and back. *Child:* Pull the auricle of the ear down and back until age 3.
3. Instill the prescribed number of drops. Avoid contaminating the dropper.
4. Instruct the patient to remain in this position for 2 to 5 minutes to prevent the medication from leaking out of the ear.

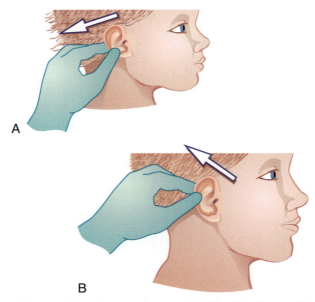

Figure 5-8 To administer ear drops, straighten the external ear canal by **(A)** pulling down and back on the auricle in children until age 3, and **(B)** pulling up and back on the auricle in adults. (From Kee, J. L., Hayes, E. R., & McCuistion, L. E. [2015]. *Pharmacology: a nursing process approach,* 8th ed., Philadelphia: Saunders.)

PHARYNGEAL SPRAY, MOUTHWASH, AND LOZENGE

Purpose

Sprays, mouthwashes, and lozenges can be prescribed to reduce throat irritation and for antiseptic and anesthetic effects. These methods are prescribed for a local effect on the throat and *not* for systemic use.

Method

Pharyngeal Spray
1. Instruct the patient to sit upright.
2. Place a tongue blade over the patient's tongue to improve visualization of the mouth and to prevent the tongue from becoming numb if an anesthetic is being administered.
3. Hold the spray pump nozzle outside the patient's mouth, and direct the spray to the back of the throat.

Method

Pharyngeal Mouthwash
1. Instruct the patient to sit upright.
2. Instruct the patient to swish the solution around the mouth, but *not* to swallow the solution, and then to spit it into an emesis basin or sink.

Method

Pharyngeal Lozenge
1. Instruct the patient to sit upright.
2. Instruct the patient to place the lozenge into his or her mouth and suck until it is fully dissolved. The lozenge should *not* be chewed or swallowed whole.

TOPICAL PREPARATIONS: LOTION, CREAM, AND OINTMENT

Purpose

Topical lotions, creams, and ointments are used to protect skin areas, prevent skin dryness, treat itching of skin areas, and relieve pain.

Method

Topical Lotion
1. Cleanse skin area with soap and water. Allow time for the area to air-dry, or gently pat it dry.
2. Shake the lotion container. Rub the lotion thoroughly into the skin unless otherwise indicated.

Method A

Topical Cream or Ointment
1. Cleanse the skin area. Allow time for the area to air-dry, or gently pat it dry.
2. Use a sterile tongue blade or gauze to apply the cream or ointment to the affected skin area. Use long, smooth strokes. A piece of sterile gauze may be placed over the medicated area after application to prevent soiling of clothing.

Method B

Topical Cream or Ointment
1. Cleanse the skin area. Allow time for the area to air-dry, or gently pat it dry.
2. Squeeze a line of ointment from the tube onto your gloved finger from the tip to the first skin crease; this is known as a fingertip unit (FTU) (Figure 5-9).
   One FTU weighs about 0.5 g.
3. Use the guidelines shown in Figure 5-10 to determine the number of FTUs to apply to various body areas.
4. Apply the medication to the affected area.

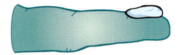

Figure 5-9 Fingertip unit: ointment squeezed from the tip of the finger to the first skin crease.

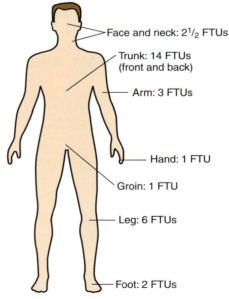

Face and neck: 2½ FTUs

Trunk: 14 FTUs (front and back)

Arm: 3 FTUs

Hand: 1 FTU

Groin: 1 FTU

Leg: 6 FTUs

Foot: 2 FTUs

Figure 5-10 Number of fingertip units for various body areas.

RECTAL SUPPOSITORY

Purpose

Rectal medications are used to relieve vomiting when the client is unable to take oral medication, to relieve pain or anxiety, to promote defecation, and to administer drugs that could be destroyed by digestive enzymes.

Method

Rectal Suppository
1. Place the patient on his or her left side in the Sims position.
2. Expose the anus by lifting the upper portion of the buttock. Check that the anus/rectum is not full of stool.
3. Lightly lubricate the suppository with water-soluble lubricant, and insert the narrow (pointed) end of the suppository into the anus, past the anal sphincter and into the rectum, approximately 3 inches or 7 to 8 centimeters (Figure 5-11).
4. Instruct the patient to remain in a supine or left lateral Sims position for 5 to 10 minutes.

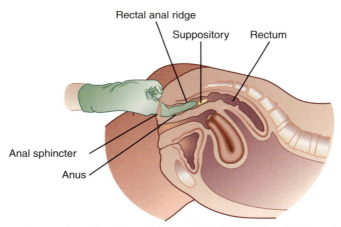

Figure 5-11 Inserting a rectal suppository. (From Kee, J. L., Hayes, E. R., & McCuistion, L. E. [2015]. *Pharmacology: a nursing process approach*, 8th ed., Philadelphia: Saunders.)

VAGINAL SUPPOSITORY, CREAM, AND OINTMENT

Purpose

Vaginal medications are used to treat vaginal infection or inflammation.

Method

Vaginal Suppository, Cream, and Ointment

1. Place the patient in the lithotomy position (knees bent with feet on the table or bed).
2. Place the vaginal suppository at the tip of the applicator.
   or
   Connect the top of the vaginal cream or ointment tube with the tip of the applicator. Squeeze the tube to fill the applicator.
3. Lubricate the applicator with water-soluble lubricant if necessary.
4. Insert applicator downward first, then upward and backward 3 to 4 inches or 8 to 10 centimeters (Figure 5-12).
5. Instruct patient to remain lying down for at least 5 to 15 minutes after the application. The patient may use a light pad in her underwear to prevent soiling of clothing. Bedtime is the suggested time for vaginal drug administration.
6. Instruct the patient to avoid using tampons after insertion of the vaginal medication.

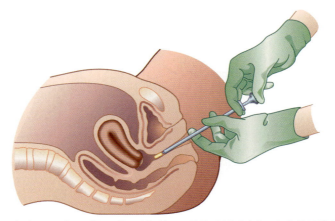

Figure 5-12 Inserting a vaginal suppository. (From Kee, J. L., Hayes, E. R., & McCuistion, L. E. [2015]. *Pharmacology: a nursing process approach,* 8th ed., Philadelphia: Saunders.)

INTRAOSSEOUS ACCESS

Purpose

Intraosseous (IO) infusions are used for patients in emergent, urgent, and medically necessary situations when intravenous access is difficult or unobtainable (Figure 5-13). The IO catheters are injected directly through the bone cortex into the soft marrow interior, either manually or with a driver/drill device. Once the IO catheter is placed, there is immediate access to the venous system for fluid and medication infusion. Common sites for IO catheter placement are the proximal or distal tibia, proximal or distal humerus, and the sternum. The distal femur is also a common insertion site in pediatric patients. The dwell time for the IO device is 24 to 48 hours, after which an alternative route of access should be obtained.

Method

1. Monitor according to organizational policy, procedures, and practice guidelines.
2. Document response to therapy, i.e., vital signs improvement, urine output, site pain.
3. Maintain IO device placement, care, and maintenance.

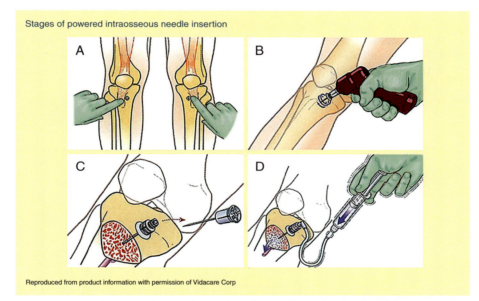

Stages of powered intraosseous needle insertion

A
B
C
D

Reproduced from product information with permission of Vidacare Corp

Figure 5-13 Intraosseous catheter insertion. **A,** Site is palpated. **B,** Catheter placed with drill device. **C,** Stylet is removed. **D,** Medication is infused. (Image courtesy Teleflex Incorporated. (c) 2015 Teleflex Incorporated. All rights reserved.)

INTRASPINAL ACCESS

Purpose

Intraspinal access devices are catheters and infusion pumps used for the delivery of narcotics, anesthetic agents, or antispasmodic medications to relieve pain or to control severe muscle spasms. The two access areas for intraspinal medication are the epidural space and the intrathecal space of the spine (Figure 5-14). The anesthesia provider inserts a needle in the subarachnoid space of the spine between the pia mater and the arachnoid mater for the intrathecal or spinal access and threads a catheter through the needle. For the epidural, the needle is placed between the dura mater and the flavum ligament, and a catheter is threaded into that area. Once the catheter is secured, medication is administered through the catheter via infusion pumps. Epidurals are given frequently for pain management in the labor and delivery setting, and both intrathecal and epidural procedures are used for surgical pain management.

Small implantable pumps can be surgically placed under the skin of the abdomen to deliver medication through an intrathecal catheter for chronic conditions (Figure 5-15). Medications such as baclofen, morphine, or ziconotide may be delivered in this manner to minimize the side effects often associated with the higher doses used in oral or intravenous delivery of these drugs. The goal of a drug pump is to better control symptoms and to reduce oral medications, thus reducing their associated side effects.

Method

1. Monitor according to the institution's policy, procedures, and practice guidelines.
2. Document responses to therapy (i.e., pain scale, sedation level, head or neck pain).
3. Maintain infusions according to physician orders and established policy and procedures.
4. Identify and label intraspinal access devices and administration sets to differentiate from other infusion administration systems.

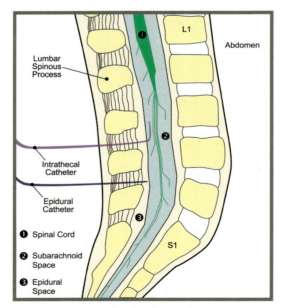

Figure 5-14 Intrathecal and epidural insertion sites.

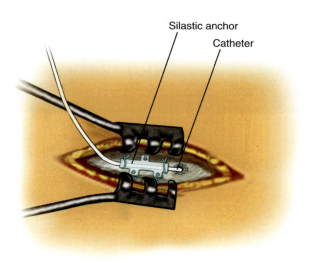

Silastic anchor

Catheter

A   Secure catheter with Silastic anchor and sutures

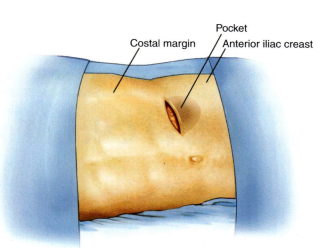

Costal margin

Pocket

Anterior iliac creast

B   Create pocket for pump

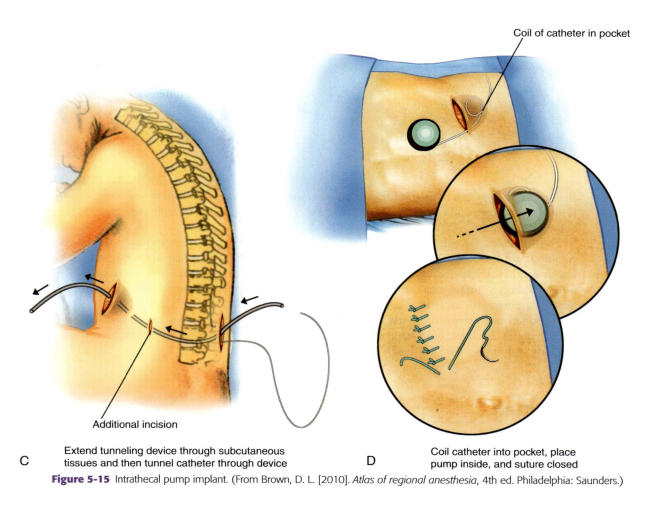

Coil of catheter in pocket

Additional incision

C   Extend tunneling device through subcutaneous tissues and then tunnel catheter through device

D   Coil catheter into pocket, place pump inside, and suture closed

Figure 5-15 Intrathecal pump implant. (From Brown, D. L. [2010]. *Atlas of regional anesthesia*, 4th ed. Philadelphia: Saunders.)

CHAPTER 6

Methods of Calculation

Objectives
- Determine the amount of drug needed for a specified time.
- Select a dosage formula, such as basic formula, ratio and proportion, fraction equation, or dimensional analysis, for solving drug dosage problems.
- Convert units of measurement to the same system and unit of measurement before calculating drug dosage.
- Calculate the dosage amount of tablets, capsules, and liquid volume (oral or parenteral) needed to administer the prescribed drug.

Outline **DRUG CALCULATION**
  Method 1: Basic Formula
  Method 2: Ratio and Proportion
  Method 3: Fractional Equation
  Method 4: Dimensional Analysis

Before drug dosage can be calculated, units of measurement must be converted to one system. If the drug is ordered in grams and comes in milligrams, then grams are converted to milligrams or milligrams are converted to grams.

Four methods for calculating drug dosages include basic formula, ratio and proportion, fractional equation, and dimensional analysis. The ratio and proportion and fractional equation methods are similar. For drugs that require individualized dosing, body weight and body surface area are used. When body weight and body surface area calculations are used, one of the first four methods for calculation is necessary to determine the amount of drug needed from the container.

At some institutions, the nurse orders enough medication doses for a designated period. If the order requires 2 tablets, qid (4 times a day) for 5 days, then the number of tablets needed would be 2 tablets × 4 times a day × 5 days = 40 tablets.

DRUG CALCULATION

The four methods as mentioned for drug calculations are (1) basic formula, (2) ratio and proportion, (3) fractional equation, and (4) dimensional analysis (factor labeling).

Method 1: Basic Formula

The following formula is often used to calculate drug dosages. The basic formula (BF) is the most commonly used method, and it is easy to remember.

$$\frac{D}{H} \times V = \text{Amount to give}$$

D or desired dose: drug dose ordered by physician or health care providers (HCPs)
H or on-hand dose: drug dose on label of container (bottle, vial, ampule)
V or vehicle: form and amount in which the drug comes (tablet, capsule, liquid)

EXAMPLES   **PROBLEM 1:**   Order: erythromycin (ERY-TAB) 0.5 g, po, q8h.
Drug available:

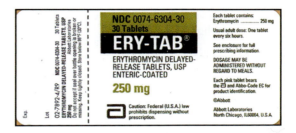

   a. Both the dosage of the drug ordered and the dosage on the bottle are in the metric system; however, the units of measurement are different. Conversion is needed. To convert grams to milligrams, move the decimal point three spaces to the right (see Chapter 1: Systems Used for Drug Administration and Temperature Conversion):

$$0.5 \text{ g} = 0.500 \text{ mg} = 500 \text{ mg}$$

   b. BF: $\dfrac{D}{H} \times V = \dfrac{\overset{2}{500} \text{ mg}}{\underset{1}{250} \text{ mg}} \times 1 \text{ tab} = 2 \text{ tablets}$

Answer: erythromycin 0.5 g = 2 tablets

PROBLEM 2:   Order: loracarbef (Lorabid) 0.5 g, po, q12h for 7 days.
Drug available:

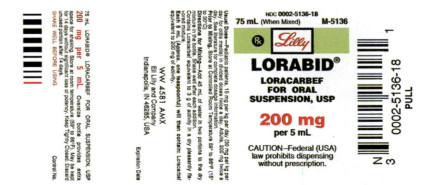

a. The unit of measurement ordered and the unit given on the bottle are in the same system but in different units; therefore conversion of units within the same system must be done first. To convert grams to milligrams, move the decimal point three spaces to the right (see Chapter 1).

$$0.5 \text{ g} = 0.500 \text{ mg} = 500 \text{ mg}$$

b. $\dfrac{D}{H} \times V = \dfrac{\overset{5}{\cancel{500}}}{\underset{2}{\cancel{200}}} \times 5 \text{ mL} = \dfrac{5}{2} \times 5 = \dfrac{25}{2} = 12.5 \text{ mL}$

Answer: Lorabid 0.5 g per dose = 12.5 mL

PROBLEM 3: Order: phenobarbital 120 mg, STAT.
Drug available: phenobarbital 30 mg per tablet.
a. Conversion of unit of measurement is NOT needed because both are of the same unit, milligrams.

b. BF: $\dfrac{D}{H} \times V = \dfrac{120}{30} \times 1 = \dfrac{120}{30} = 4 \text{ tablets}$

Answer: phenobarbital 120 mg = 4 tablets

PROBLEM 4: Order: meperidine (Demerol) 35 mg, IM, STAT
Drug available:

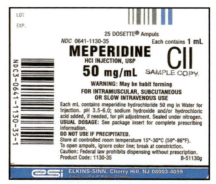

a. Conversion is not needed, because both are of the same unit of measurement.

b. BF: $\dfrac{D}{H} \times V = \dfrac{35}{50} \times 1 \text{ mL} = \dfrac{35}{50} = 0.7 \text{ mL}$

Answer: meperidine (Demerol) 35 mg = 0.7 mL

Method 2: Ratio and Proportion

Ratio and proportion (RP) is the oldest method used for calculating dosage problems:

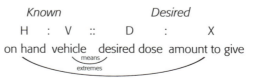

H and **V:** On the left side of the equation are the known quantities, which are dose on hand and vehicle.
D and **X:** On the right side of the equation are the desired dose and the unknown amount to give.
Multiply the means and the extremes. Solve for **X.**

EXAMPLES   PROBLEM 1:   Order: erythromycin (ERY-TAB) 0.5 g, po, q8h.
Drug available:

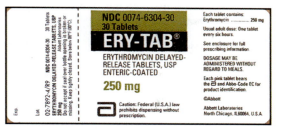

a. To convert grams to milligrams, move the decimal point three spaces to the right (see Chapter 1):

$$0.5 \text{ g} = 0.500 \text{ mg} = 500 \text{ mg}$$

b. RP: H : V ::   D   :   X
250 mg : 1 tab :: 500 mg : X tab

250 X = 500
X = 2 tablets

Answer: erythromycin 0.5 g = 2 tablets

Note: With RP, the ratio on the left (milligrams to tablets) has the same relation as the ratio on the right (milligrams to tablets); the only difference is values.

PROBLEM 2:   Order: aspirin (ASA) 650 mg, PRN.
Drug available: aspirin 325 mg per tablet.

RP: H : V ::   D   :   X
325 mg : 1 tablet :: 650 mg : X tablet
325 X = 650
X = 2 tablets

Answer: aspirin 650 mg = 2 tablets

PROBLEM 3:   Order: amoxicillin 75 mg, po, qid.
Drug available:

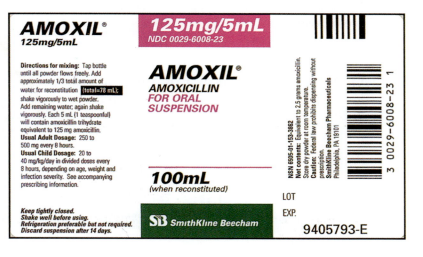

a. Conversion is not needed because both use the same unit of measurement.
b. RP: H : V :: D : X
125 mg : 5 mL :: 75 mg : X mL
125 X = 375
X = 3 mL

Answer: amoxicillin 75 mg = 3 mL

PROBLEM 4: Order: meperidine (Demerol) 60 mg, IM, STAT.
Drug available:

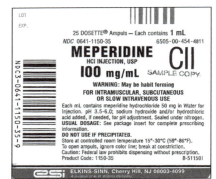

a. Conversion is not needed; the same unit of measurement is used.
b. RP: H : V :: D : X
100 mg : 1 mL :: 60 mg : X mL
100 X = 60
X = 0.6 mL

Answer: meperidine (Demerol) 60 mg = 0.6 mL

Method 3: Fractional Equation

The fractional equation (FE) method *is similar* to RP, except it is written as a fraction.

$$\frac{H}{V} = \frac{D}{X}$$

H: the dosage on hand or in the container
V: the vehicle or the form in which the drug comes (tablet, capsule, liquid)
D: the desired dosage
X: the unknown amount to give
Cross multiply and solve for X.

EXAMPLES PROBLEM 1: Order: erythromycin (ERY-TAB) 750 mg, po, q8h.
Drug available:

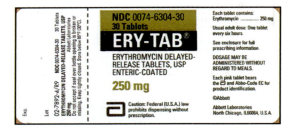

a. How many tablet(s) should the patient receive per dose? _____

$$FE: \frac{H}{V} = \frac{D}{X} \qquad \frac{250 \text{ mg}}{1 \text{ tab}} = \frac{750 \text{ mg}}{X} =$$

(Cross multiply) $\qquad 250 \text{ X} = 750$

$$X = 3 \text{ tablets per dose}$$

b. How many tablet(s) should the patient receive per day? _____

3 tablets per dose × 3 times per day = 9 tablets per day

Answer: erythromycin: 9 tablets per day

PROBLEM 2: Order: valproic acid (Depakene) 100 mg, po, tid.
Drug available: valproic acid (Depakene) 250 mg/5 mL suspension.
a. No unit conversion is needed.

b. $FE: \dfrac{H}{V} = \dfrac{D}{X} \qquad \dfrac{250}{5} = \dfrac{100}{X}$

(Cross multiply) $\qquad 250 \text{ X} = 500$

$$X = 2 \text{ mL}$$

Answer: valproic acid (Depakene) 100 mg = 2 mL

PROBLEM 3: Order: atropine 0.6 mg, IM, STAT.
Drug available:

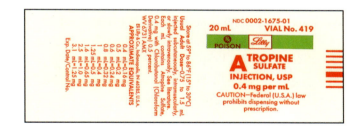

$$FE: \frac{H}{V} = \frac{D}{X} \qquad \frac{0.4 \text{ mg}}{1 \text{ mL}} = \frac{0.6 \text{ mg}}{X}$$

(Cross multiply) $\qquad 0.4 \text{ X} = 0.6$

$$X = 1.5 \text{ mL}$$

Answer: atropine 0.6 mg = 1.5 mL

Method 4: Dimensional Analysis

Dimensional analysis (DA) is a calculation method known as units and conversions. The advantage of DA is that it decreases the number of steps required to calculate a drug dosage. It is set up as one long equation to answer a desired unit (e.g., mL, tab, or cap).
1. Identify the unit/form (tablet, capsule, mL) of the drug to be calculated. If the drug comes in tablet (unit), then tablet = (equal sign).

2. The known dose and unit/form from the **drug label** follow the equal sign.
   Example order: Amoxicillin 500 mg. On the drug label: 250 mg per 1 capsule.

$$\text{capsule} = \frac{1 \text{ cap}}{250 \text{ mg}} \text{ (unit)}$$
$$\text{(drug label)}$$

3. The milligram value (250 mg) is the **denominator** and it must match the NEXT **numerator,** which is 500 mg (desired dose or order). The NEXT denominator would be 1 (one) or blank.

$$\text{capsule} = \frac{1 \text{ cap} \times \overset{2}{\cancel{500 \text{ mg}}}}{\underset{1}{\cancel{250 \text{ mg}}} \times 1} =$$

4. Cancel out the mg, and reduce the 250 and 500. What remains is the capsule and 2. Answer: 2 capsules.

When conversion is needed between milligrams (drug label) and grams (order), then a conversion factor is needed, which appears **between** the drug dose on hand (drug label) and the desired dose (order). You should REMEMBER the following:

Metric Equivalent

1 g = 1000 mg
1 mg = 1000 mcg

Also use Table 6-1 for metric and household conversions.

EXAMPLE   Order: Amoxicillin 0.5 g.
Available: 250 mg = 1 capsule (drug label). A conversion is needed between grams and milligrams. Remember, 250 mg is the denominator; therefore 1000 mg (conversion factor, which is 1000 mg = 1 g) is the NEXT numerator and 1 g becomes the NEXT denominator. The third numerator is 0.5 g (desired dose), and the denominator is 1 (one) or blank.

$$\text{capsule} = \frac{1 \text{ cap} \times \overset{4}{\cancel{1000 \text{ mg}}} \times 0.5 \cancel{g}}{\underset{1}{\cancel{250 \text{ mg}}} \times 1 \cancel{g} \times 1 \text{ (or blank)}} = 2 \text{ capsules}$$
$$\text{(drug label)} \quad \text{(conversion)} \quad \text{(drug order)}$$

If conversion from grams to milligrams is not needed, then the middle step can be omitted. The following are formulas for DA:

$$\text{V (form of drug)} = \frac{\text{V (drug form)} \times \text{D (desired dose)}}{\text{H (on hand)(drug label)} \times 1 \text{ or blank (drug order)}}$$

For conversion: V (form of drug) =

$$\frac{\text{V (drug form)} \times \text{C(H)} \times \text{D (desired dose)}}{\underset{\substack{\text{(drug label)} \quad \text{(conversion} \\ \text{factor)}}}{\text{H (on hand)}} \times \underset{}{\text{C(D)}} \times \underset{\text{(drug order)}}{1 \text{ (or blank)}}}$$

As with other methods for calculation, the three components are **D, H,** and **V.** With DA, the conversion factor is built into the equation and is included when the units of measurement of the drug order and the drug container differ. If the two are of the same units of measurement, the conversion factor is eliminated from the equation.

TABLE 6-1 Metric and Household Conversions*

METRIC	
Grams (g)	Milligrams (mg)
1	1000
0.5	500
0.3	300 (325)
0.1	100
0.06	60 (64 or 65)
0.03	30 (32)
0.015	15 (16)
0.010	10
0.0006	0.6
0.0004	0.4
0.0003	0.3

Liquid (Approximate)
30 mL = 1 oz = 2 tbsp (T) = 6 tsp (t)
15 mL = ½ oz = 1 T = 3 t
1000 mL = 1 quart (qt) = 1 liter (L)
500 mL = 1 pint (pt)
5 mL = 1 tsp (t)

EXAMPLES   **PROBLEM 1:**   Order: erythromycin (ERY-TAB) 1 g, po, q12h.
Drug available:

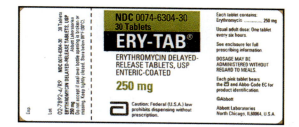

Drug label: 250 mg = 1 tablet
Drug order: 1 g
Conversion factor: 1 g = 1000 mg
a. How many tablets should the patient receive per dose? _____

$$\text{DA: tab} = \frac{1 \text{ tablet}}{250 \text{ mg}} \times \frac{\overset{4}{1000} \text{ mg}}{1 \text{ g}} \times \frac{1 \text{ g}}{1} = 4 \text{ tablets}$$

(drug label)   (conversion factor)   (drug order)

(cancel units and numbers from numerator and denominator)

Answer: erythromycin 1 g = 4 tablets
Give 4 tablets every 12 hours.

PROBLEM 2: Order: acetaminophen (Tylenol) 1 g, po, PRN.
Drug available:

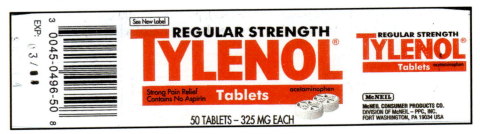

Drug label: 325 mg = 1 tablet
Conversion factor: 1000 mg = 1 g
How many tablet(s) would you give?

$$DA: tab = \frac{1\ tab \times 1000\ mg \times 1\ g}{325\ mg \times 1\ g \times 1} = \frac{1000}{325} = 3.07\ tab\ or\ 3\ tab\ (cannot\ round\ off\ in\ tenths\ for\ tablets)$$

Answer: acetaminophen 1 g = 3 tablets
Tylenol is also available in 500-mg (extra-strength) tablets.

PROBLEM 3: Order: ciprofloxacin (Cipro) 500 mg, po, q12h.
Drug available:

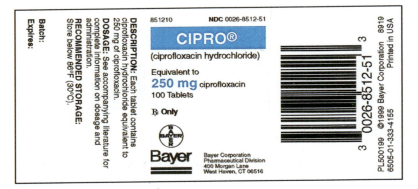

No conversion factor is needed because both are stated in milligrams (mg).

$$DA: tab = \frac{1\ tab \times \overset{2}{500}\ mg}{\underset{1}{250}\ mg \times 1} = 2\ tablets$$

Answer: Cipro 500 mg = 2 tablets

SUMMARY PRACTICE PROBLEMS

Answers can be found on pages 94 to 96.

Solve the following calculation problems using Method 1, 2, 3, or 4. To convert units within the metric system (grams to milligrams), refer to Chapter 1. To convert apothecary to metric units and vice versa, refer to Chapter 2, Table 2-1. For reading drug labels, refer to Chapter 3. Several of the calculation problems have drug labels. Drug dosage and drug form are printed on the drug label.

Extra practice problems are available in the chapters on oral drugs, injectable drugs, and pediatric drug administration.

1. **Order:** doxycycline hyclate (Vibra-Tabs), po, initially 200 mg; then 50 mg, po, bid.
   Drug available: Use one of the four methods to calculate dosage.

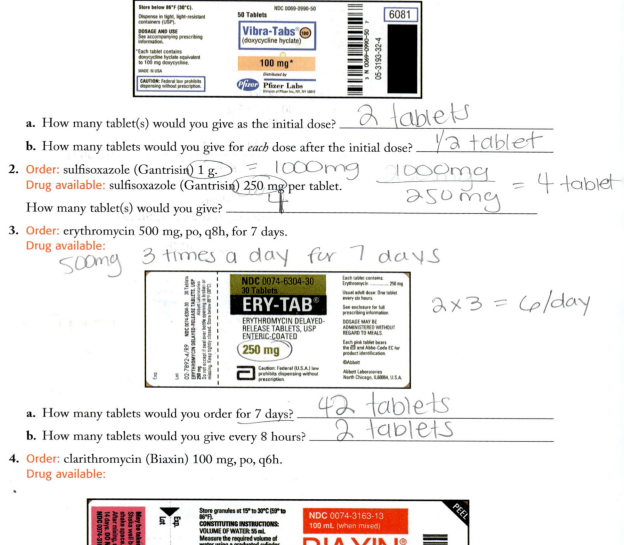

   a. How many tablet(s) would you give as the initial dose? _____ 2 tablets

   b. How many tablets would you give for *each* dose after the initial dose? _____ ½ tablet

2. **Order:** sulfisoxazole (Gantrisin) 1 g. = 1000mg $\frac{1000mg}{250mg}$ = 4 tablet
   Drug available: sulfisoxazole (Gantrisin) 250 mg per tablet.

   How many tablet(s) would you give? _____ 4

3. **Order:** erythromycin 500 mg, po, q8h, for 7 days.
   Drug available:
   500mg   3 times a day for 7 days

   2 × 3 = 6/day

   a. How many tablets would you order for 7 days? _____ 42 tablets

   b. How many tablets would you give every 8 hours? _____ 2 tablets

4. **Order:** clarithromycin (Biaxin) 100 mg, po, q6h.
   Drug available:

   How many milliliters should the patient receive per dose? _____ 4mL

   mL

5. Order: phenytoin (Dilantin) 50 mg, po, bid.
Drug available:

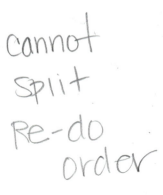

cannot split
Re-do order

Each capsule contains 100 mg phenytoin sodium, USP.

Usual dosage– Adults, 1 capsule three or four times daily or as directed.

See package insert for complete prescribing information.

Keep this and all drugs out of the reach of children.

NOTE TO PHARMACIST– Do not dispense capsules which are discolored.

Exp date and lot

0362G077

N 0071-0362-24
KAPSEALS®
Dilantin®
(Extended Phenytoin Sodium Capsules, USP)
100 mg
℞ only
100 CAPSULES
Ⓟ PARKE-DAVIS

Dispense in a tight, light-resistant container as defined in the USP.
Store below 30°C (86°F). Protect from light and moisture.
PARKE-DAVIS Div of Warner-Lambert Co., Morris Plains, NJ 07950 USA

0071-0362-24

Pediatric Dose–Initially, 5 mg/kg daily in two or three equally divided doses, with subsequent dosage individualized to a maximum of 300 mg daily.

See package insert for complete prescribing information.

Keep this and all drugs out of the reach of children.

NOTE TO PHARMACIST–Do not dispense capsules which are discolored.

Lot
Exp. date

0365G135

N 0071-0365-24
KAPSEALS®
Dilantin®
(Extended Phenytoin Sodium Capsules, USP)
30 mg
℞ only
100 CAPSULES
Ⓟ PARKE-DAVIS

Dispense in a tight, light-resistant container as defined in the USP.
Store below 30°C (86°F). Protect from light and moisture.
PARKE-DAVIS Div of Warner-Lambert Co Morris Plains, NJ 07950 USA

0071-0365-24

a. Which Dilantin container would you select? ___N/A___

b. How many Dilantin capsules would you give per dose? ___N/A___

6. Order: indomethacin (Indocin) 30 mg, po, tid.
Drug available:

3x a day

$$\frac{30}{25} \times \frac{5}{1} = \frac{150}{25}$$

6 mL

30 mg × 3 =

NDC 42211-101-11
INDOCIN®
(INDOMETHACIN)
ORAL SUSPENSION
25 mg per 5 mL
SHAKE WELL BEFORE USING
Alcohol 1%
Rx only
🌿 IROKO
PHARMACEUTICALS
PHILADELPHIA, PA 19112
237 mL

a. How many milliliters would you give per dose? ___6 mL___

b. How many milligrams would the patient receive per day? ___90 mg___

7. Order: dexamethasone (Decadron) 0.5 mg, po, qid.   *4 times a day*
Drug available:

USUAL ADULT DOSAGE: See accompanying circular. This is a bulk package and not intended for dispensing. Dispense in a well-closed container. CAUTION: Federal (USA) law prohibits dispensing without prescription.	NDC 0006-0020-68 **100 TABLETS** **Decadron® 0.25 mg** (Dexamethasone) Dist. by: **MERCK & CO., INC.** West Point, PA 19486, USA

100 No. 7592   7834109   Lot   Exp.

a. How many tablets would you give per dose? ___*2 tablets*___

b. How many milligrams would the patient receive per day? ___*2 mg*___

8. Order: diltiazem (Cardizem) SR 120 mg, po, bid for hypertension.   *twice/day*
Drugs available:

NDC 0088-1772-47   6505-01-146-4174
60 mg MARION MERRELL DOW INC.
CARDIZEM®
(diltiazem HCl)
60 mg
100 Tablets

NDC 0088-1777-47
60 mg **Hoechst Marion Roussel**
CARDIZEM® SR
(diltiazem HCl)   **SR**
60 mg SUSTAINED RELEASE
100 Capsules

NDC 0088-1796-30   6505-01-353-9846
180 mg **Hoechst Marion Roussel**
CARDIZEM® CD
(diltiazem HCl)   **CD**
180 mg ONCE-A-DAY DOSAGE
30 Capsules

a. Which drug bottle should be selected? ___*60 mg SR*___

b. How many tablet(s) should the patient receive per dose? ___*2*___

9. **Order:** cimetidine (Tagamet) 0.2 g, po, qid.
   Drug available:

[handwritten: 4/day]

[handwritten: 0.2g, 200mg]

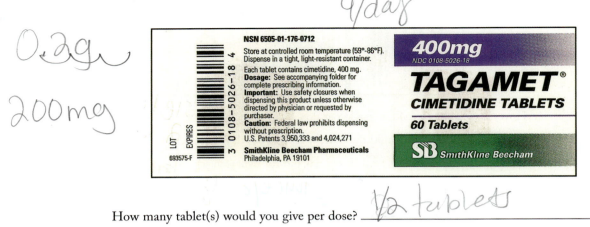

How many tablet(s) would you give per dose? _____ *[handwritten: 1/2 tablets]*

10. **Order:** bisoprolol (Zebeta) 5 mg, po, daily for the first week. Increase Zebeta to 15 mg, po, daily starting with the second week.
    Drug available:

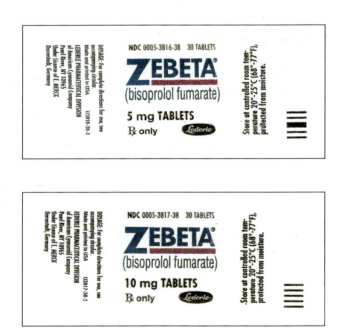

a. Which drug bottle(s) would you select the first week and how many tablet(s) would you give?
   [handwritten: 1st week = 5mg / 1 tablet for 7 days = 7 tablets]

b. The dose is increased to 15 mg the second week. Explain which drug bottle(s) you would select and how many tablets you would give? *[handwritten: 5mg so that I would not split the 10mg]*

11. **Order:** fluoxetine (Prozac) 25 mg, po, in the AM.
    Drug available:

Basic Formula

$$\frac{Desired}{Hand} \times V$$ ✓

$$\frac{25 mg}{20 mg} \times 5 ml$$

6.25

How many milliliters (mL) should the patient receive in the AM? ____6.25____

12. **Order:** methylprednisolone (Medrol) 75 mg, IM.
    Drug available: Medrol 125 mg per 2 mL per ampule.

$$\frac{75 mg}{125 mg} \times 2 ml = 1.2 mL$$

How many milliliters would you give? _____

13. **Order:** atropine sulfate 0.3 mg, IM, STAT.
    Drug available:

$$\frac{0.3 mg}{0.4 mg} \times 1$$

How many milliliters should the patient receive? ____0.75 mL____

14. **Order:** Cefobid (cefoperazone NA) 1 g, IM, q12h.
    Drug available:

According to the drug administration instructions, 3.4 mL of sterile water should be added to drug to yield 4 mL of drug solution. How many milliliters (mL) would you administer per dose? ____2 mL____

Additional Dimensional Analysis (Factor Labeling)

15. Order: aminocaproic acid 1.5 g, po, STAT.
Drug available: aminocaproic acid 500-mg tablet.
Drug label: 500 mg = tablet
Conversion factor: 1 g = 1000 mg

How many tablet(s) would you give? _____3 tablets_____

16. Order: ampicillin (Principen) 50 mg/kg/day, po, in 4 divided doses (q6h).
Patient weighs 88 pounds, or 40 kg (88 ÷ 2.2 = 40 kg).
Drug available:

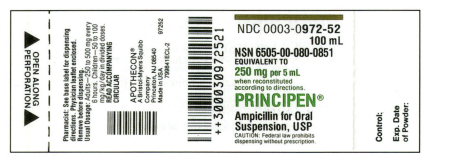

Drug label: 250 mg = 5 mL
Conversion factor: none (both are in milligrams)

a. How many milligrams per day should the patient receive? _____2000_____

b. How many milligrams per dose should the patient receive? _____500mg_____

c. How many milliliters should the patient receive per dose (q6h)? _____10ml_____

17. Order: cimetidine (Tagamet) 0.8 g, po, bedtime.
Drug available:

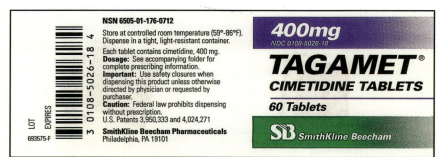

Drug label: 400 mg = 1 tablet
0.8 g (drug order)
Conversion factor: 1 g = 1000 mg (units of measurements are not the same; conversion factor is needed)

How many tablet(s) would you give? _____2 tablets_____

18. Order: Xanax (alprazolam) 0.25 mg, po, tid.
Drug available:

3 times a day

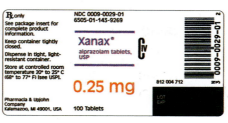

Xanax tablet is scored.

a. How many tablet(s) should the patient receive per dose? _____ 1/2

b. How many tablet(s) should the patient receive per day? _____ 1 1/2

19. Order: codeine gr i (1), po, STAT.
Drug available:

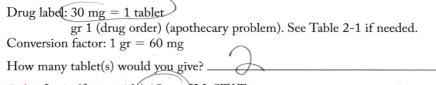

Drug label: 30 mg = 1 tablet
        gr 1 (drug order) (apothecary problem). See Table 2-1 if needed.
Conversion factor: 1 gr = 60 mg

How many tablet(s) would you give? _____ 2

20. Order: Lasix (furosemide) 15 mg, IM, STAT.
Drug available:

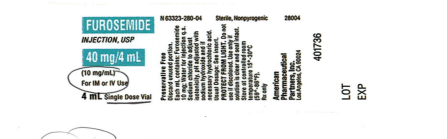

How many milliliters (mL) would you give? _____

ANSWERS   SUMMARY PRACTICE PROBLEMS

1. a. *Initially:*

$$BF: \frac{D}{H} \times V = \frac{200}{100} \times 1 =$$

2 tablets

or

$$FE = \frac{100}{1} = \frac{200}{X}$$

$$100\,X = 200$$
$$X = 2 \text{ tablets}$$

or

RP: H   :V:: D   :X
100 mg: 1 ::200 mg:X

$$100\,X = 200$$
$$X = 2 \text{ tablets}$$

or

DA: No conversion factor

$$\text{Tablet(s)} = \frac{1 \text{ tab} \times \overset{2}{\cancel{200}} \text{ mg}}{\underset{1}{\cancel{100}} \text{ mg} \times 1} = 2 \text{ tablets}$$

b. *Daily:*

$$BF: \frac{D}{H} \times V = \frac{50}{100} \times 1 =$$

½ tablet

or

$$FE = \frac{100}{1} = \frac{50}{X} =$$

(Cross multiply) $100\,X = 50$
$$X = \text{½ tablet}$$

or

RP: H   :V:: D   :X
100 mg: 1 ::50 mg:X

$$100\,X = 50$$
$$X = \text{½ tablet}$$

or

DA: No conversion factor

$$\text{Tablet(s)} = \frac{1 \text{ tab} \times \overset{1}{\cancel{50}} \text{ mg}}{\underset{2}{\cancel{100}} \text{ mg} \times 1} = \text{½ tablet}$$

2. 4 tablets

3. a. 2 tablets × 3 doses per day × 7 days = 42 tablets
   b. 2 tablets every 8 hours

4. $$BF: \frac{D}{H} \times V = \frac{100}{\underset{25}{\cancel{125}}} \times \overset{1}{\cancel{5}} = \frac{100}{25} = 4 \text{ mL}$$

or

RP: H :V:: D :X
125 : 5 ::100:X
$$125\,X = 500$$
$$X = \frac{500}{125} = 4 \text{ mL}$$

or

$$DA: mL = \frac{5 \text{ mL} \times \overset{4}{\cancel{100}} \text{ mg}}{\underset{5}{\cancel{125}} \text{ mg} \times 1} = \frac{20}{5} = 4 \text{ mL}$$

or

$$FE: \frac{125}{5} = \frac{100}{X} =$$

(Cross multiply) $125\,X = 500$
$$X = 4 \text{ mL}$$

5. a. The nurse could *not* use either of the Dilantins.
   b. A capsule *cannot* be cut in half. The physician should be notified. Dilantin dose should be changed.

6. a. $$BF: \frac{D}{H} \times V = \frac{30 \text{ mg}}{25 \text{ mg}} \times 5 \text{ mL} = 6 \text{ mL}$$

$$DA: mL = \frac{\overset{1}{\cancel{5}} \text{ mL} \times 30 \text{ mg}}{\underset{5}{\cancel{25}} \text{ mg} \times 1} = \frac{30}{5} = 6 \text{ mL}$$

RP: H   :   V   ::   D   : X
25 mg : 5 mL = 30 mg : X
$$25\,X = 150$$
$$X = 6 \text{ mL}$$

$$FE: \frac{H}{V} = \frac{D}{X} = \frac{25 \text{ mg}}{5 \text{ mL}} = \frac{30 \text{ mg}}{X}$$
$$25\,X = 150$$
$$X = 6 \text{ mL}$$

   b. 30 mg × 3 = 90 mg per day

7. a. BF: $\dfrac{D}{H} \times V = \dfrac{0.5}{0.25} \times 1$

$0.25\overline{)0.50}^{\,2.} = 2$ tablets

or

RP: H : V :: D : X
0.25 : 1 tablet :: 0.5 : X tablets
0.25 X = 0.5
X = 2 tablets

b. 2 mg

8. a. Cardizem SR 60 mg

b. 2 SR capsules per dose

9. Change grams to milligrams by moving the decimal three spaces to the right (see Chapter 1).

0.2 g = 0.200 mg = 200 mg

BF: $\dfrac{D}{H} \times V = \dfrac{200}{400} \times 1$ tablet

$= \dfrac{200}{400} = \tfrac{1}{2}$ tablet

or

RP: H : V :: D : X
400 mg : 1 tablet :: 200 mg : X tablet
400 X = 200
$X = \dfrac{200}{400} = 0.5$ or $\tfrac{1}{2}$ tablet

or

DA: With conversion factor

$\text{Tablets} = \dfrac{1 \text{ tab}}{400 \text{ mg}} \times \dfrac{\overset{10}{1000} \text{ mg}}{1 \text{ g}} \times \dfrac{0.2 \text{ g}}{1} = \dfrac{2.0}{4} = \tfrac{1}{2}$ tablet

10. a. Select Zebeta 5-mg bottle.

BF: $\dfrac{D}{H} \times V = \dfrac{5 \text{ mg}}{5 \text{ mg}} \times 1 = 1$ tablet of Zebeta 5-mg bottle

RP: H : V :: D : X
5 : 1 :: 5 : X
5 X = 5
X = 1 tablet of Zebeta

b. Select either Zebeta 5-mg bottle OR Zebeta 5-mg and Zebeta 10-mg bottles
FE: using Zebeta 5-mg bottle

$\dfrac{H}{V} = \dfrac{D}{X} = \dfrac{5 \text{ mg}}{1} = \dfrac{15 \text{ mg}}{X}$

(Cross multiply)   5 X = 15
X = 3 tablets of Zebeta

If only the Zebeta 10-mg bottle was available, then give 1½ tablets.

11. BF: $\dfrac{D}{H} \times V = \dfrac{\overset{5}{25} \text{ mg}}{\underset{4}{20} \text{ mg}} \times 5 \text{ mL} = \dfrac{25}{4} = $ 6.25 or 6.3 mL of Prozac

FE: $\dfrac{H}{V} = \dfrac{D}{X} = \dfrac{20 \text{ mg}}{5 \text{ mL}} = \dfrac{25 \text{ mg}}{X}$

(Cross multiply)   20 X = 125
X = 6.25 OR 6.3 mL of Prozac

12. BF: $\dfrac{D}{H} \times V = \dfrac{75}{125} \times 2$

$\dfrac{150}{125} = 1.2 \text{ mL}$

or

FE: $\dfrac{125}{2} = \dfrac{75}{X}$

$125\,X = 150$

$X = 1.2 \text{ mL}$

or

RP: $\quad$ H : $\quad$ V $\quad$ :: D : $\quad$ X

$\qquad$ 125 : $\quad$ 2 $\quad$ :: 75 : $\quad$ X

$\qquad\qquad$ 125 X = 150

$\qquad\qquad\qquad$ X = 1.2 mL

or

DA: No conversion factor needed

$\text{mL} = \dfrac{2 \text{ mL} \times \overset{3}{\cancel{75}} \text{ mg}}{\underset{5}{\cancel{125}} \text{ mg} \times 1} = \dfrac{6}{5} = 1.2 \text{ mL}$

13. BF: $\dfrac{D}{H} \times V = \dfrac{0.3 \text{ mg}}{0.4 \text{ mg}} \times 1 \text{ mL} =$

0.75 mL

or

FE: $\dfrac{0.4 \text{ mg}}{1} = \dfrac{0.3 \text{ mg}}{X} =$

$0.4 \text{ mg } X = 0.3 \text{ mg}$

$X = 0.75 \text{ mL}$

or

RP: $\quad$ H $\quad$: $\quad$ V $\quad$ :: $\quad$ D $\quad$: $\quad$ X

$\qquad$ 0.4 mg : 1 mL :: 0.3 mg : $\quad$ X

$\qquad\qquad$ 0.4 mg X = 0.3 mg

$\qquad\qquad\qquad$ X = 0.75 mL

or

DA: $\text{mL} = \dfrac{1 \text{ mL} \times 0.3 \text{ mg}}{0.4 \text{ mg} \times 1} = \dfrac{0.3}{0.4} = 0.75 \text{ mL}$

14. RP: $\quad$ H : $\quad$ V $\quad$ :: D : X

$\qquad$ 2 g : 4 mL :: 1 g : X

$\qquad\qquad$ 2 X = 4

$\qquad\qquad\quad$ X = 2 mL of Cefobid per dose

Additional Dimensional Analysis (Factor Labeling)

15. $\text{Tablets} = \dfrac{1 \text{ tablet} \times \overset{2}{\cancel{1000}} \text{ mg} \times 1.5 \text{ g}}{\underset{1}{\cancel{500}} \text{ mg} \times \quad 1 \text{ g} \quad \times \quad 1} = \dfrac{3.0}{1} = 3 \text{ tablets}$

16. **a.** 50 mg/kg/day

$50 \times 40 = 2000 \text{ mg}$

b. 2000 mg ÷ 4 = 500 mg per dose

c. $\text{mL} = \dfrac{5 \text{ mL} \times \overset{2}{\cancel{500}} \text{ mg}}{\underset{1}{\cancel{250}} \text{ mg} \times 1} = \dfrac{10}{1} = 10 \text{ mL}$

17. $\text{Tablets} = \dfrac{1 \text{ tablet} \times \overset{10}{\cancel{1000}} \text{ mg} \times 0.8 \text{ g}}{\underset{4}{\cancel{400}} \text{ mg} \times \quad 1 \text{ g} \quad \times \quad 1} = \dfrac{10 \times 0.8}{4} = \dfrac{8}{4} = 2 \text{ tablets}$

18. **a.** DA: $\text{tab} = \dfrac{1 \text{ tab} \times 0.25 \text{ mg}}{0.5 \text{ mg} \times \quad 1} = \dfrac{0.25}{0.5} = \text{½ tablet of Xanax}$

b. ½ tablet × 3 (tid) = 1½ tablets per day

19. $\text{Tablets} = \dfrac{1 \text{ tablet} \times \overset{2}{\cancel{60}} \text{ mg} \times 1 \text{ gr}}{\underset{1}{\cancel{30}} \text{ mg} \times \quad 1 \text{ gr} \quad \times \quad 1} = 2 \text{ tablets}$

20. DA: $\text{mL} = \dfrac{1 \text{ mL} \times \overset{3}{\cancel{15}} \text{ mg}}{\underset{2}{\cancel{10}} \text{ mg} \times 1} = \dfrac{3}{2} = 1.5 \text{ mL of furosemide (Lasix)}$

evolve $\quad$ Additional practice problems are available in the Methods of Calculating Dosages section of Drug Calculations Companion, version 5, on Evolve.

CHAPTER 7

Methods of Calculation for Individualized Drug Dosing

Objectives
- State the differences between the weight formulas used for drug calculations.
- Calculate drug dosages according to body surface area.
- Calculate drug dosages according to body weight.
- List indications for use of ideal body weight, adjusted body weight, and lean body weight formulas.

Outline **CALCULATION FOR INDIVIDUALIZED DRUG DOSING**

Body Weight (BW)
Body Surface Area (BSA or m²)
Ideal Body Weight (IBW)
Adjusted Body Weight (ABW)
Lean Body Weight (LBW)

CALCULATION FOR INDIVIDUALIZED DRUG DOSING

The two methods for individualizing drug dosing are body weight (BW) and body surface area (BSA). Other formulas that are associated with drug dosing, especially in bariatrics, are ideal body weight (IBW) and lean body weight (LBW).

Body Weight (BW)

Drug dosing by actual BW is the primary way medication is individualized for adults and children. Manufacturers supply dosing information in the package insert. The insert data provide the dosage based on the patient's weight in kilograms (kg). The first step is to convert pounds to kilograms (if necessary). The second step is to determine the drug dose per BW by multiplying drug dose × body weight (BW) × frequency (day or per day in divided doses). The third step is to choose one of the four methods of drug calculation for the amount of drug to be given.

EXAMPLES **PROBLEM 1:** Order: fluorouracil (5-FU), 12 mg/kg/day IV, not to exceed 800 mg/day. The adult weighs 140 pounds.

   a. Convert pounds to kilograms. Divide number of pounds by 2.2.
   Remember: 1 kg = 2.2 lb

   140 lb ÷ 2.2 lb/kg = 64 kg

    b. Dosage/BW: mg × kg × 1 day =

$$12 \times 64 \times 1 \quad = 768 \text{ mg IV per day}$$

Answer: fluorouracil (5-FU), 12 mg/kg/day = 768 mg or 770 mg

PROBLEM 2: Give cefaclor (Ceclor), 20 mg/kg/day in three divided doses. The child weighs 20 pounds.
Drug available:

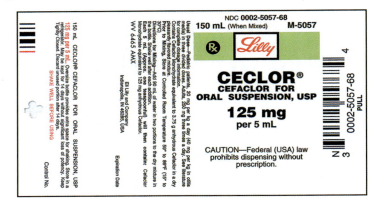

    a. Convert pounds to kilograms.

$$20 \text{ lbs} \div 2.2 \text{ lb/kg} = 9 \text{ kg}$$

    b. Dosage/BW: 20 mg × 9 kg × 1 day = 180 mg per day.

$$180 \text{ mg} \div 3 \text{ divided doses} = 60 \text{ mg}$$

BF: $\dfrac{D}{H} \times V = \dfrac{60 \text{ mg}}{125 \text{ mg}} \times 5 \text{ mL} =$

$$\dfrac{300}{125} = 2.4 \text{ mL}$$

or
RP: H : V :: D :X
125 mg: 5 mL :: 60 mg: X mL
125 X = 300
X = 2.4 mL

or
FE: $\dfrac{125 \text{ mg}}{5 \text{ mL}} = \dfrac{60 \text{ mg}}{X}$
125 X = 300
X = 2.4 mL

or
DA: mL $= \dfrac{\overset{1}{\cancel{5}} \text{ mL} \times \overset{12}{\cancel{60}} \text{ mg}}{\underset{\underset{5}{25}}{\cancel{125}} \text{ mg} \times 1} = \dfrac{12}{5} = 2.4 \text{ mL}$

Answer: cefaclor (Ceclor) 20 mg/kg/day = 2.4 mL per dose three times per day

Body Surface Area (BSA or m²)

Body surface area is an estimated mathematical function of height and weight. BSA is considered to be the most accurate way to calculate drug dosages in that the correct dosage is more proportional to the surface area. BSA is commonly used in chemotherapy and some drug dosages used for infants and children. There are two methods for calculating BSA. The first is the square root formula and the second is a nomogram derived from the square root formula.

YOU MUST REMEMBER

Rounding Off Rule: Since calculators are used for working problems, round off at the final answer and not the steps in between. For BSA problems, round off answers to the nearest hundredth.

BSA With the Square Root

BSA can be calculated by using the square root and a fractional formula of height and weight divided by a constant, one for the metric system and another for inches and pounds. Now that calculators are readily available, the square root formula is easier to calculate than the longhand version. But errors can be made with calculators too; therefore a BSA nomogram can prove useful to verify answers. Follow institutional policy regarding BSA methods of calculation. When solving BSA problems, it is necessary to convert weight and height to the same system of measure.

BSA: Inch and Pound (lb) Formula

$$BSA = \sqrt{\frac{ht(in) \times wt(lb)}{3131}}$$

BSA: Metric Formula by Centimeters (cm) and Kilograms (kg)

$$BSA = \sqrt{\frac{ht(cm) \times wt(kg)}{3600}}$$

EXAMPLES **PROBLEM 1:** Order: melphalon (Alkeran) 16 mg/m^2 q 2 weeks. Patient is 68 inches tall and weighs 172 pounds. Use the BSA inches and pounds formula.

a. $BSA = \sqrt{\dfrac{68 \text{ in} \times 172 \text{ lb}}{3131}}$

$BSA = \sqrt{\dfrac{11696}{3131}}$

$BSA = \sqrt{3.73}$

$BSA = 1.9 \text{ m}^2$

b. 16 mg $\times$ 1.9 m^2 = 30.4 mg/m^2 or 30 mg/m^2

PROBLEM 2: Order: cisplatin (Platinol) 50 mg/m^2/cycle IV. Patient weighs 84.5 kg and is 168 cm tall. Use the BSA metric formula.

a. $BSA = \sqrt{\dfrac{168 \text{ cm} \times 84.5 \text{ kg}}{3600}}$

$BSA = \sqrt{\dfrac{14196}{3600}}$

$BSA = \sqrt{3.94}$

$BSA = 1.99 \text{ m}^2$

b. 50 mg $\times$ 1.99 m^2 = 99.5 mg/m^2, or 100 mg/m^2

BSA With a Nomogram

The BSA in square meters (m^2) is determined by the person's height and weight and where these points intersect on the nomogram scale (Figures 7-1 and 7-2). The nomogram charts were developed from the square root formula and were correlated with heights and weights to provide a quick and simple method for drug dosing before calculators were readily available. There are separate nomograms for infants, children, and adults. When a nomogram is used, points on the scale must be carefully plotted. An error in plotting points or drawing intersecting lines can lead to reading of the incorrect BSA, resulting in dosing errors. Although there are slight discrepancies between the nomogram and square root method, the trend in medication safety is to use the nomogram to verify the calculator-generated square root.

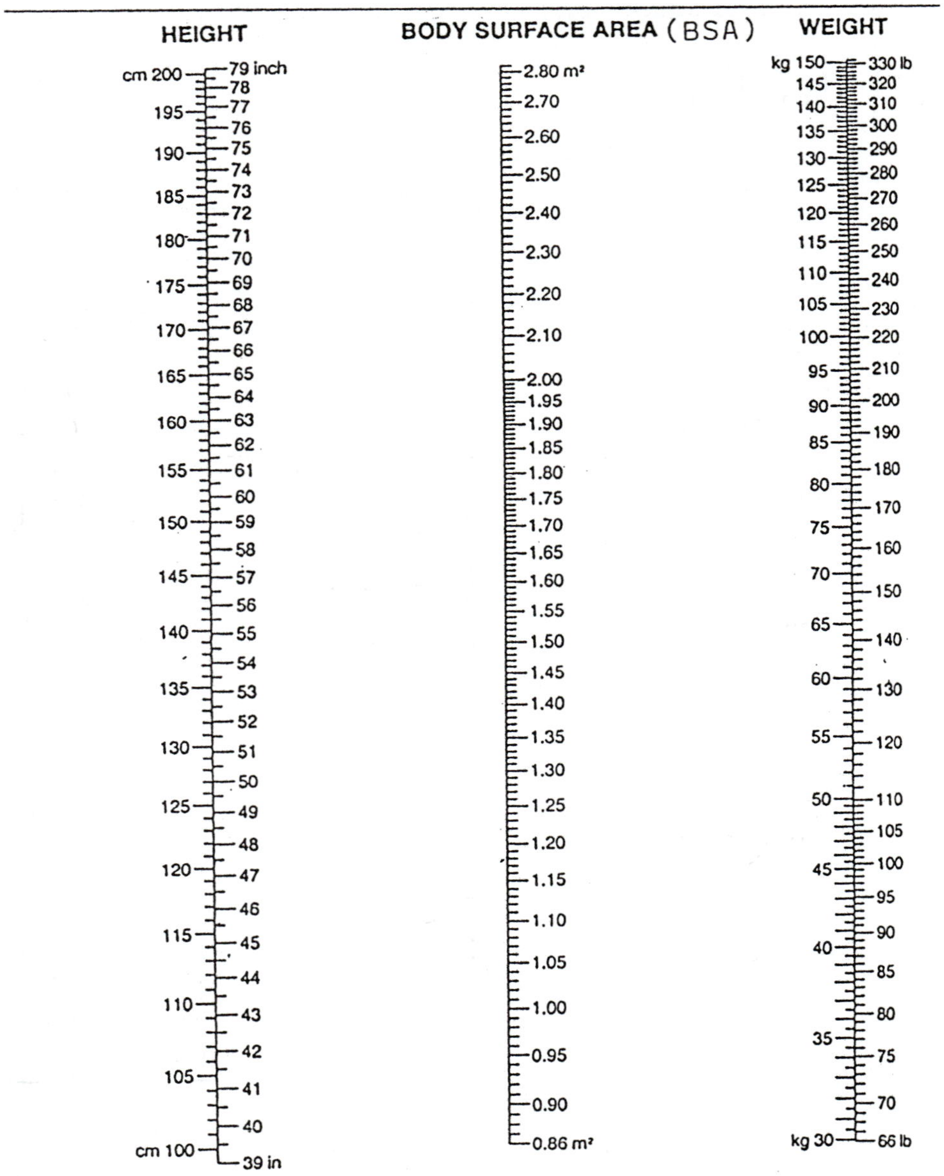

Figure 7-1 Body surface area (BSA) nomogram for adults. Directions: (1) find height, (2) find weight, (3) draw a straight line connecting the height and weight. Where the line intersects on the BSA column is the body surface area (m²). (From Deglin, H., Vallerand, A. H., & Russin, M. M. [1991]. *Davis' drug guide for nurses*, 2nd ed. Philadelphia: F. A. Davis, p. 1218. Used with permission from Lentner, C. [1991]. *Geigy scientific tables*, 8th ed., vol. 1, Basel, Switzerland: Ciba-Geigy, pp. 226-227.)

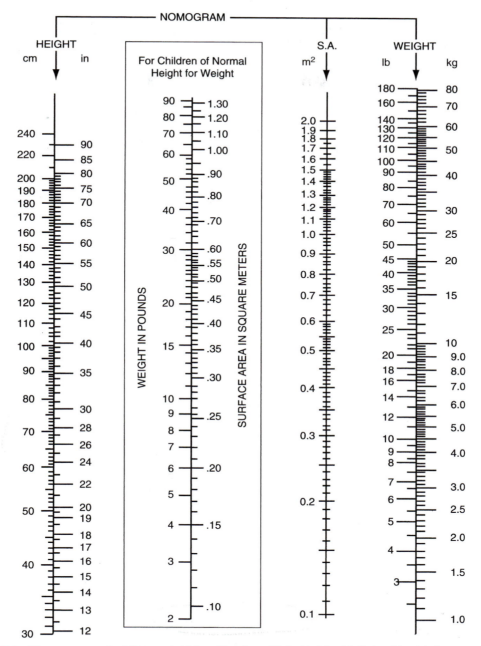

Figure 7-2   West nomogram for infants and children. Directions: (1) find height, (2) find weight, (3) draw a straight line connecting the height and weight. Where the line intersects on the SA column is the body surface area (m²). (From Behrman, R. E., Kliegman, R. M., & Jenson, H. B., editors. [2004]. *Nelson textbook of pediatrics,* 17th ed. Philadelphia: Saunders.)

To calculate the dosage by BSA obtained with nomogram, multiply the drug dose × m², e.g., 100 mg × 1.6 m² = 160 mg/m². The advantage of using the nomogram is that no conversions from pounds to kilograms or inches to centimeters are needed.

EXAMPLES   **PROBLEM 1:** Order: cyclophosphamide (Cytoxan) 100 mg/m²/day, po. Patient weighs 150 pounds and is 5′8″ (68 inches) tall.
   a. 68 inches and 150 pounds intersect the nomogram scale at 1.88 m² (BSA) (Figure 7-3).
   b. BSA: 100 mg × 1.9 m² = 190 mg/m²/day of Cytoxan

$$1.88 \text{ m}^2 = 188 \text{ mg/m}^2\text{/day or } 190 \text{ mg/m}^2\text{/day}$$

PROBLEM 2: Order: cytarabine (cytosine arabinoside) 200 mg/m²/day IV × 5 days for a patient with myelocytic leukemia. The patient is 64 inches tall and weighs 130 pounds.
   a. 64 inches and 130 pounds intersect the nomogram scale at 1.69 m² (BSA), or 1.7 m² (BSA) rounded off to the nearest tenth.
   b. BSA: 200 mg × 1.69 m² = 340 mg/m² IV daily for 5 days

$$1.69 \text{ m}^2 = 338 \text{ mg/m}^2 \text{ or } 340 \text{ mg/m}^2$$

Ideal Body Weight (IBW)

Drug dosing by ideal body weight (IBW) or lean body weight/mass (LBW)/(LBM) formulas is used for medications that are poorly absorbed and distributed throughout the body fat. The ideal body weight formula is based on height and can be adjusted for weight and is used for nutritional assessment. The lean body weight/mass formula is based upon height and weight but is less frequently used because it may predict insufficient doses in obese patients.

IBW Formula

Male: 50 kg + 2.3 kg for **EACH** inch over 5 feet
Female: 45.5 kg + 2.3 kg for **EACH** inch over 5 feet

EXAMPLE   Female is 5 feet 2 inches (2 inches × 2.3 kg)
IBW: 45.5 kg + 2 (2.3 kg) = 45.5 kg + 4.6 kg = 50.1 kg

Adjusted Body Weight (ABW)

Adjusted body weight (ABW) is used for dosing some medication for obese individuals or pregnant women. ABW is better for nutritional assessment of obese individuals because it prevents overfeeding. The ABW formula uses both the IBW and the actual body weight with adjustments for male and female.

ABW Formula

Male: IBW + 0.4 (Actual Body Weight [kg] − IBW [kg]) = ABW
Female: IBW + 0.4 (Actual Body Weight [kg] − IBW [kg]) = ABW

EXAMPLE   Female is 5 feet 2 inches and weighs 100.5 kg
   50.1 kg + 0.4 (100.5 − 50.1 kg) =
   50.1 kg + 0.4 (50.4 kg) =
   50.1 kg + 20.16 kg = 70.26 kg or 70.3 kg

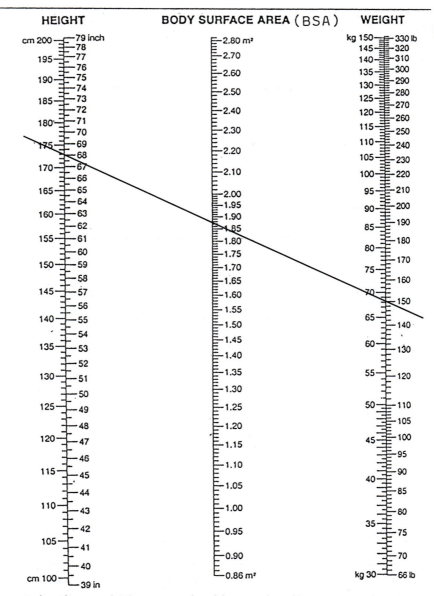

Figure 7-3 Body surface area (BSA) nomogram for adults. Example Problem 1: a. 68 inches and 150 pounds intersect the nomogram scale at 1.88 m² (BSA).

Lean Body Weight (LBW)

Lean body weight (LBW) is the weight of bone, muscle, and organs without any fat. LBW is used for the dosing of some medications and can be used as an indicator of overall health for patients with chronic diseases.

LBW Formula

Lean body weight in kilograms (males over 16 years of age) = (0.32810 × [body weight in kg] + 0.33929 × [height in centimeters]) − 29.5336

Lean body weight in kilograms (women over 30) = (0.29569 × [body weight in kg] + 0.41813 × [height in centimeters]) − 43.2933

EXAMPLE Female is 5 feet 2 inches, weighs 100.5 kg, and is 55 years old.

(0.29569 × [100.5 kg] + ([0.41813 × (62″ × 2.54 cm)]) − 43.2933 =

29.71 + (0.41813 × 157.48) − 43.2933 =

29.71 + 65.84 − 43.2933 =

95.55 − 43.2933 = 52.26 kg

SUMMARY PRACTICE PROBLEMS

Answers can be found on pages 108 to 111.

Body Weight

1. Order: trimethoprim-sulfamethoxazole 6 mg/kg/day, po, q12h.
   Patient weighs 44 pounds.

   How many milligrams should the patient receive per dose? _____

2. Order: azithromycin (Zithromax), po. First day: 10 mg/kg/day; next 4 days: 5 mg/kg/day. Patient weighs 44 pounds.
   Drug available:

   FOR ORAL USE ONLY.
   Store dry powder below 86°F (30°C).
   PROTECT FROM FREEZING.
   DOSAGE AND USE
   See accompanying prescribing information.
   MIXING DIRECTIONS:
   Tap bottle to loosen powder.
   Add 9 mL of water to the bottle.
   After mixing, store suspension at
   41° to 86°F (5° to 30°C).
   Oversized bottle provides extra space
   for shaking.
   After mixing, use within 10 days. Discard
   after full dosing is completed.
   SHAKE WELL BEFORE USING.
   Contains 600 mg azithromycin.

   NDC 0069-3120-19
   15 mL (when mixed)
   Zithromax®
   (azithromycin for
   oral suspension)
   CHERRY FLAVORED
   200 mg* per 5 mL
   Pfizer **Pfizer Labs**
   Division of Pfizer Inc, NY, NY 10017

   * When constituted as directed, each teaspoonful (5 mL) contains azithromycin dihydrate equivalent to 200 mg of azithromycin.

   Rx only
   05-5013-32-1

   6416
   MADE IN USA

   N 0069-3120-19   2

   a. How much does the child weigh in kilograms? _____

   b. How many milliliters should the child receive for the first day? _____

   c. How many milliliters should the child receive each day for the next 4 days (second to fifth days)? _____

3. **Order:** ticarcillin disodium (Ticar), 200 mg/kg/day in 4 divided doses, IV. Patient weighs 176 pounds.
   Max dose: 24 g every day
   Drug available:

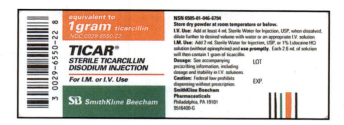

   a. How many kilograms does the patient weigh? _____

   b. How many milligrams per day should the patient receive? How many milligrams per dose?

   _____ mg, q6h. Or how many grams per dose? _____ g, q6h

4. **Order:** tobramycin 5.1 mg/kg/day in 3 divided doses (q8h), IV. The patient weighs 180 pounds.
   Drug available:

   a. How many kilograms does the patient weigh? _____

   b. How many milligrams should the patient receive per day? _____

   c. How many milliliters should the patient receive per dose? _____

5. **Order:** sulfisoxazole (Gantrisin) 2 g/m^2 daily in 4 divided doses (q6h). The patient weighs 110 pounds and is 60 inches tall. Use nomogram.
   How many milligrams should the patient receive per dose? _____

6. **Order:** doxorubicin (Adriamycin) 60 mg/m^2 IV per month. Patient weighs 120 pounds and is 5′2″ (62 inches) tall. Use nomogram.
   How many milligrams should the patient receive? _____

7. Order: etoposide (VePesid) 100 mg/m²/day × 5 days. Patient weighs 180 pounds and is 70 inches tall. Use nomogram.
Drug available:

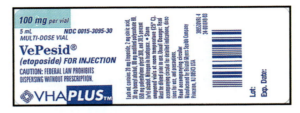

  a. What is the BSA? _____

  b. How many milligrams should the patient receive? _____

  c. How many milliliters are needed? _____

BSA by Square Root

8. Order: vinblastine sulfate (Velban) 7.4 mg/m² IV × 1. Patient's height is 115 cm and weight is 52 kg. Use the BSA metric formula to determine dosage.
Drug available:

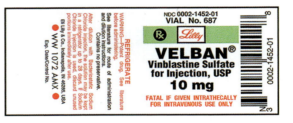

How many milligrams should the patient receive? _____

9. Order: etoposide (VePesid) 50 mg/m² day IV. Patient's height is 72 inches and weight is 180 pounds.

How many milligrams should the patient receive? _____

10. Patient with advanced colorectal cancer
Order: Fluorouracil 250 mg/m²/day × 7 days
Patient's height and weight: 6′2″, 218 lb

  a. What is patient's BSA in square meters? _____ (use square root)

  b. What is the daily dose? _____

  c. What is the total dosage for 7 days? _____

11. Order: docetaxel (Taxotene) 60 mg/m²/dose in 200 mL of normal saline solution over 60 minutes.
Patient's height and weight: 5′8″, 136 lb.

  a. What is patient's BSA in square meters? _____

  b. What is the total dosage of docetaxel? _____

  c. What is the concentration per milliliter? _____

12. Order: gemcitabine (Gemzar) 800 mg/m^2/dose in 100 mL of normal saline solution over 30 minutes. Patient's height and weight: 6'6", 150 lb.
    Drug available: 1 g/25 mL

    a. What is patient's BSA in square meters? _____

    b. What is the total dose of gemcitabine? _____

    c. How many milliliters should you prepare? _____

13. Order: Liposomal doxorubicin 20 mg/m^2 in 250 mL D$_5$W IV over 30 minutes. Patient's height and weight: 6', 129 lb.
    Drug available: Doxorubicin 20 mg/10 mL

    a. What is patient's BSA in square meters? _____

    b. What is the total dose of doxorubicin? _____

    c. How many milliliters should you prepare? _____

14. Order: irinotecan (Camptosar) 60 mg/m^2 in 500 mL D5 ½NS IV over 90 minutes. Patient's height and weight: 6', 202 lb.
    Drug available: Irinotecan 20 mg/mL

    a. What is patient's BSA in square meters? _____

    b. What is the total dose of irinotecan? _____

    c. How many milliliters should you prepare? _____

15. Order: Cisplatin 80 mg/m^2 in 500 mL normal saline solution over 90 minutes. Patient's height and weight: 6', 200 lb.
    Drug available: Cisplatin 1 mg/mL

    a. What is patient's BSA in square meters? _____

    b. What is the total dose of cisplatin? _____

16. Order: Adriamycin 50 mg/m^2 in 3 individual doses mixed with 1000 mL normal saline solution per dose continuous infusion over 24 hr. Patient's height and weight: 5'8", 139 lb.
    Drug available: Adriamycin 10 mg/5 mL

    a. What is patient's BSA in square meters? _____

    b. What is the total dosage? _____

    c. What is the divided dose? _____

Ideal Body Weight (IBW) and Adjusted Body Weight (ABW)

17. What is the IBW and ABW for a male weighing 385 lb and 5'8" tall? _____

18. What is the IBW and ABW for a female weighing 370 lb and 5'2" tall? _____

19. What is the IBW and ABW for a female weighing 290 lb and 5'3" tall? _____

20. What is the IBW and ABW for a male weighing 310 lb and 5'10" tall? _____

Lean Body Weight (LBW)

21. What is the LBW for a 50-year-old male weighing 385 lb and 5′8″ tall? _____

22. What is the LBW for a 60-year-old female weighing 385 lb and 5′2″ tall? _____

23. What is the LBW for a 30-year-old male weighing 134 lb and 6′ tall? _____

24. What is the LBW for a 65-year-old female weighing 99 lb and 5′2″ tall? _____

ANSWERS   SUMMARY PRACTICE PROBLEMS

Body Weight

1. 44 lb ÷ 2.2 lb/kg = 20 kg
   20 kg × 6 mg/kg/day = 120 mg ÷ 2 doses = 60 mg/dose trimethoprim-sulfamethoxazole
2. **a.** 20 kg
   b. First day: 10 mg × 20 kg = 200 mg

   $$BF: \frac{D}{H} \times V = \frac{\overset{1}{\cancel{200}} \text{ mg}}{\underset{1}{\cancel{200}} \text{ mg}} \times 5 \text{ mL} = 5 \text{ mL}$$

   or
   $$RP: \quad H \ : \ V \ :: \ D \ :X$$
   $$200 \text{ mg}:5 \text{ mL}::200 \text{ mg}:X$$
   $$200\,X = 1000$$
   $$X = 5 \text{ mL}$$

   $$DA: mL = \frac{5 \text{ mL} \times \overset{1}{\cancel{200}} \text{ mg}}{\underset{1}{\cancel{200}} \text{ mg} \times 1} = 5 \text{ mL}$$

   or
   $$FE = \frac{200 \text{ mg}}{5 \text{ mL}} = \frac{200 \text{ mg}}{X} = 200\,X = 1000$$
   $$X = 5 \text{ mL}$$

   First day give 5 mL
   c. Second to fifth days (next 4 days): 5 mg × 20 kg = 100 mg
   Give 2.5 mL/day.
3. **a.** Client weighs 80 kg
   b. 200 mg × 80 = 16,000 mg per day; 4000 mg per dose or 4 g per dose (q6h)
4. Tobramycin: 1.2 g = 1200 mg
   a. 180 lbs ÷ 2.2 kg = 81.8 kg
   5.1 mg × 81.8 kg = 417.2 mg/day
   b. 417.2 mg ÷ 3 doses/day = 139 mg/dose or 140 mg/dose

   c. $$BF: \frac{D}{H} \times V = \frac{140 \text{ mg}}{1200 \text{ mg}} \times 30 \text{ mL} = \frac{4200}{1200} = 3.5 \text{ mL}$$

   or
   $$RP: \quad H \ : \ V \ :: \ D \ :X$$
   $$1200 \text{ mg}:30 \text{ mL}::140 \text{ mg}:X$$
   $$1200\,X = 4200$$
   $$X = 3.5 \text{ mL of tobramycin}$$

   $$DA: mL = \frac{30 \text{ mL} \times 140 \text{ mg}}{1200 \text{ mg} \times 1} = \frac{4200}{1200} = 3.5 \text{ mL of tobramycin}$$

5. 60 inches and 110 pounds intersect the nomogram scale at 1.5 m².
   BSA: 2 g × 1.5 m² = 3 g or 3000 mg per day
   3000 mg ÷ 4 times per day = 750 mg

6. 62 inches and 120 pounds intersect the nomogram scale at 1.6 m².
   BSA: 60 mg × 1.6 m² = 96 mg of Adriamycin

7. **a.** With the use of the nomogram, the BSA is 2.06
   b. 100 mg $\times$ 2.06 = 206 mg or 200 mg.
   c. The amount of VePesid administered should be 10 mL.

$$\text{BF:} \frac{D}{H} \times V = \frac{200 \text{ mg}}{100 \text{ mg}} \times 5 \text{ mL} = 10 \text{ mL}$$

or

$$\text{RP: } 100 \text{ mg}:5 \text{ mL}::200 \text{ mg}:X$$
$$100\,X = 1000$$
$$X = 10 \text{ mL}$$

or

$$\text{DA: mL} = \frac{5 \text{ mL} \times \overset{2}{\cancel{200}} \text{ mg}}{\underset{1}{\cancel{100}} \text{ mg} \times 1} = 10 \text{ mL}$$

BSA by Square Root

8. $\text{BSA} = \sqrt{\dfrac{115 \text{ cm} \times 52 \text{ kg}}{3600}}$

   $\text{BSA} = \sqrt{\dfrac{5980}{3600}}$

   $\text{BSA} = \sqrt{1.66}$
   $\text{BSA} = 1.29 \text{ m}^2$
   $7.4 \text{ mg} \times 1.29 \text{ m}^2 = 9.5 \text{ mg/m}^2$

9. $\text{BSA} = \sqrt{\dfrac{72 \text{ in} \times 180 \text{ lb}}{3131}}$

   $\text{BSA} = \sqrt{\dfrac{12960}{3131}}$

   $\text{BSA} = \sqrt{4.13}$
   $\text{BSA} = 2.0 \text{ m}^2$
   $50 \text{ mg/m}^2 \times 2 \text{ m}^2 = 100 \text{ mg}$

10. **a.** $\sqrt{\dfrac{74 \times 218}{3131}} = 2.27 \text{ m}^2$

    b. 250 mg $\times$ 2.27 m^2 = 567.5 or 568 mg
    c. 568 mg $\times$ 7 = 3976 mg

11. **a.** $\sqrt{\dfrac{68 \times 136}{3131}} = 1.7 \text{ m}^2$

    b. 60 mg/m^2 $\times$ 1.7 m^2 = 102 mg

    c. $\dfrac{102 \text{ mg}}{200 \text{ mL}} = 0.51 \text{ mg/mL}$

12. a. $\sqrt{\dfrac{78 \times 150}{3131}} = 1.9 \text{ m}^2$

    b. 800 mg/m² × 1.9 m² = 1520 mg

    c.   1 g = 1000 mg

         BF: $\dfrac{D}{H} \times V = \dfrac{1520 \text{ mg}}{1000 \text{ mg}} \times \dfrac{25 \text{ mL}}{1} =$

         $\dfrac{38000}{1000} = 38 \text{ mL}$

         or

         DA: mL $= \dfrac{25 \text{ mL} \times 1520 \text{ mg}}{1000 \text{ mg} \times 1} = 38 \text{ mL}$

     or

     RP: 1000 mg : 25 mL :: 1520 mg : X

           1000 X = 38000

               X = 38 mL

     or

     FE: $\dfrac{1000 \text{ mg}}{25 \text{ mL}} = \dfrac{1520 \text{ mg}}{X}$

         1000 X = 3800

             X = 38 mL

13. a. $\sqrt{\dfrac{72 \times 129}{3131}} = 1.72 \text{ m}^2$

    b. 20 mg/m² × 1.72 m² = 34 mg

    c. BF: $\dfrac{D}{H} \times V = \dfrac{34 \text{ mg}}{20 \text{ mg}} \times 10 \text{ mL}$

         $\dfrac{340}{20} = 17 \text{ mL}$

         or

         DA: mL $= \dfrac{10 \text{ mL} \times 34 \text{ mg}}{20 \text{ mg} \times 1} = 17 \text{ mL}$

     or

     RP: 20 mg : 10 mL :: 34 mg : X

           20 X = 340

             X = 17 mL

     or

     FE: $\dfrac{20 \text{ mg}}{10 \text{ mL}} = \dfrac{34 \text{ mg}}{X} = 20x = 340$

                  X = 17 mL

14. a. $\sqrt{\dfrac{72 \times 202}{3131}} = 2.15 \text{ m}^2$

    b. 60 mg × 2.15 m² = 129 mg or 130 mg/m²

    c. BF: $\dfrac{D}{H} \times V = \dfrac{130 \text{ mg}}{20 \text{ mg}} \times 1 \text{ mL} =$

         $\dfrac{130}{20} = 6.5 \text{ mL}$

         or

         DA: mL $= \dfrac{1 \text{ mL} \times 130 \text{ mg}}{20 \text{ mg} \times 1} = 6.5 \text{ mL}$

     or

     RP: 20 mg : 1 mL :: 130 mg : X

           20 X = 130

             X = 6.5 mL

     or

     FE: $\dfrac{20 \text{ mg}}{1 \text{ mL}} = \dfrac{130 \text{ mg}}{X}$

         20 X = 130

             X = 6.5 mL

15. a. $\sqrt{\dfrac{72 \times 200}{3131}} = 2.14 \text{ m}^2$ **b.** 80 mg/m² × 2.14 m² = 171 mg or 170 mg

16. a. $\sqrt{\dfrac{68 \times 139}{3131}} = 1.73 \text{ m}^2$ **b.** 50 mg/m² × 1.73 m² = 86.5 mg

    c. 86.5 mg/3 doses = 28.8 mg

Ideal Body Weight (IBW) and Adjusted Body Weight (ABW)

17. 385 lb ÷ 2.2 = 175 kg
    IBW = 50 kg + 2.3 kg (8 inches) =
         50 kg + 18.4 kg = 68.4 kg
    Adjusted Body Weight 68.4 kg + 0.4 (175 kg − 68.4) =
                 68.4 kg + 0.4 (106.6 kg) =
                 68.4 kg + 42.64 kg = 111.04 kg

18. 370 lb ÷ 2.2 = 168.2 kg
    IBW = 45.5 kg + 2.3 (2 inches) =
         45.5 kg + 4.6 kg = 50.1 kg
    Adjusted Body Weight 50.1 kg + 0.4 (168.2 kg − 50.1) =
                 50.1 kg + 0.4 (118.1 kg) =
                 50.1 kg + 47.24 kg = 97.34 kg

19. 290 lb ÷ 2.2 = 131.8 kg
    IBW = 45.5 kg + 2.3 (3 inches) =
         45.5 kg + 6.9 kg = 52.4 kg
    Adjusted Body Weight 52.4 kg + 0.4 (131.8 kg − 52.4) =
                 52.4 kg + 0.4 (79.4 kg) =
                 52.4 kg + 31.76 = 84.16 or 84.2 kg

20. 310 lb ÷ 2.2 = 141 kg
    IBW = 50 kg + 2.3 kg (10 inches) =
         50 kg + 23 kg = 73 kg
    Adjusted Body Weight 73 kg + 0.4 (141 kg − 73) =
                 73 kg + 0.4 (68) =
                 73 kg + 27.2 = 100.2 kg

Lean Body Weight (LBW)

21. 0.32810 × (385 lb ÷ 2.2) + 0.33929 × (68″ × 2.54) − 29.5336 =
    0.32810 × (175 kg) + 0.33929 × (172.72 cm) − 29.5336 =
            57.4 + 58.6 − 29.5336 =
                116 − 29.5336 = 86.46 kg

22. 0.29569 × (385 lb ÷ 2.2) + 0.41813 × (62″ × 2.54) − 43.2933 =
    0.29569 × (175 kg) + 0.41813 × (157.48 cm) − 43.2933 =
            51.7 + 65.84 − 43.2933 =
                117.54 − 43.2933 = 74.246, or 74.25 kg

23. (0.32810 × [135 lb ÷ 2.2] + 0.33929 × [72″ × 2.54]) − 29.5336 =
    0.32810 × (61.3 kg) + 0.33929 × (182.9 cm) − 29.5336 =
            20.11253 + 62.05614 − 29.5336 =
                82.16867 − 29.5336 = 52.63507 kg or 52.64 kg

24. (0.29569 × [99 lb ÷ 2.2] + 0.41813 × [60″ × 2.54]) − 43.2933 =
    0.29569 × (45 kg) + 0.41813 × (152.4 cm) − 43.2933 =
            13.306 + 63.7230 − 43.2933 =
                77.0290 − 43.2933 = 33.7357 kg or 33.74 kg

PART III

CALCULATIONS FOR ORAL, INJECTABLE, AND INTRAVENOUS DRUGS

CHAPTER 8

Oral and Enteral Preparations With Clinical Applications

Objectives
- State the advantages and disadvantages of administering oral medications.
- Calculate oral dosages from tablets, capsules, and liquids using given formulas.
- Give the rationale for diluting and not diluting oral liquid medications.
- Explain the method for administering sublingual medication.
- Calculate the amount of oral drug to be given per day in divided doses.

Oral administration of drugs is considered a convenient, less invasive, and economical method of giving medications. Oral drugs are available as tablets, capsules, powders, and liquids. Oral medications are referred to as po (per os, or by mouth) drugs and are absorbed by the gastrointestinal tract, mainly from the small intestine.

There are some disadvantages in administering oral medications, such as (1) variation in absorption rate caused by gastric and intestinal pH and food consumption within the gastrointestinal tract; (2) irritation of the gastric mucosa causing nausea, vomiting, or ulceration (e.g., with oral potassium chloride); (3) retention or inactivation of the drug in the body because of reduced liver function; (4) destruction of drugs by digestive enzymes; (5) aspiration of drugs into the lungs by seriously ill or confused patients; and (6) discoloration of tooth enamel (e.g., with a saturated solution of potassium iodide [SSKI]). Oral administration is an effective way to give medications in many instances, and at times it is the route of choice.

Body weight and body surface area are discussed in Chapter 7. When solving drug problems that require body weight or body surface area, refer to Chapter 7.

Enteral nutrition and enteral medication are discussed toward the end of the chapter.

TABLETS, CAPSULES, FLUID, AND FILM STRIPS

Most tablets are scored and can be broken in halves and sometimes in quarters (Figure 8-1). Half of a tablet may be indicated when the drug does not come in a lesser strength. If a half-tablet is not broken equally, the patient may receive less than or more than the required dose. Also, crushing a drug tablet does not ensure that the patient will receive the entire drug dose. Some of the crushed tablet could be lost. Instead of halving or crushing a drug tablet, use the liquid form of the drug, if available, to ensure proper drug dosage. If a tablet or pill is not scored, then it should NOT be broken or altered.

Capsules are gelatin shells containing powder or time pellets. Caplets (solid-looking capsules) are hard-shell capsules. Sprinkle capsules have small granules inside that may be opened and sprinkled on food. They may also be swallowed whole. Time-release capsules should remain intact and not be divided in any way. Many drugs that come in capsules also come in liquid form. When a smaller dose is indicated and is not available in tablet or capsule form, the liquid form of the drug is used (Figure 8-2).

Drug films are strips of medication that dissolve in seconds when in contact with wet mucosa. They were originally designed for children and the elderly or for anyone who has difficulty swallowing. Films are convenient, have a high dosage accuracy, and improve compliance. Strips are not to be cut or torn. Examples of drugs that come in film form are Benadryl and Klonopin.

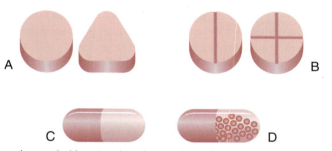

Figure 8-1 **A** and **B,** Some shapes of tablets. **C** and **D,** Shapes of capsules. (From Kee, J. L., Hayes, E. R., & McCuistion, L. E. [2015]. *Pharmacology: a patient-centered nursing process approach,* 8th ed. Philadelphia: Elsevier.)

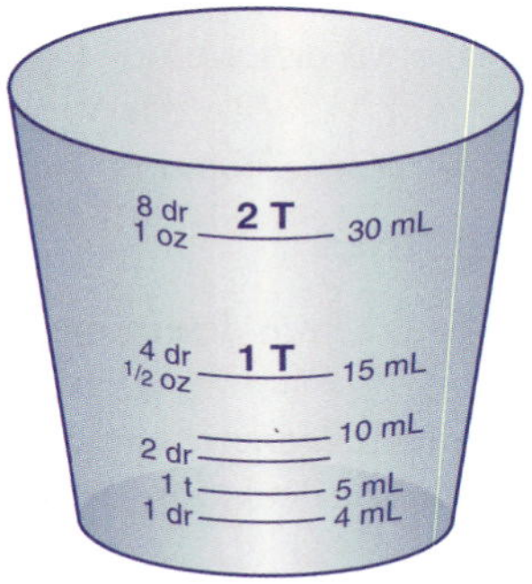

Figure 8-2 Medicine cup for liquid measurement. (From Kee, J. L., Hayes, E. R., & McCuistion, L. E. [2015]. *Pharmacology: a patient-centered nursing process approach,* 8th ed. Philadelphia: Elsevier.)

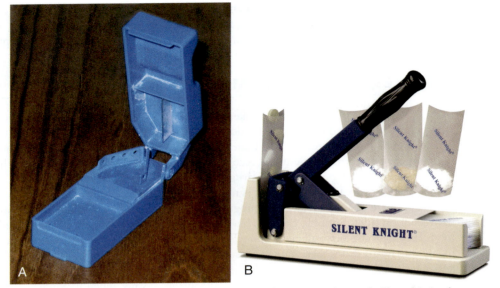

Figure 8-3 A, Pill/tablet cutter. **B,** Silent Knight tablet crushing system. (**B,** Used with permission from Links Medical Products, Inc., Irvine, California.)

Pill/Tablet Cutter and Crusher

A pill or tablet cutter can be used to evenly split or divide a scored or unscored tablet. The pill cutter *cannot* be used to cut/divide enteric-coated tablets or capsules, time-released, sustained-released, or controlled-released capsules. Pill/tablet cutters can be purchased at a drug-store (Figure 8-3). If the patient cannot swallow pills or tablets, best practice is to consult with the prescriber or pharmacist to find if a liquid form of the drug is available. If the medication is not manufactured in liquid form, then a pill crusher (Figure 8-3, *B*) can be used to reduce tablets to a powdered form that can be mixed with water, juice, fruit sauce, or ice cream. Not all pills can be crushed; see Caution below.

> **! CAUTION**
>
> - Enteric-coated tablets have a special coating that allows them to move through the stomach and be dissolved in the small intestine so that the medication doesn't irritate the gastric mucosa.
> - Time-released, sustained-release, or controlled-release tablets slowly release drug over a period of time.
> - Layered tablets have medications that may be released at different times. The outer coating dissolves quickly, and the tablet core will dissolve slowly.

Calculation of Tablets and Capsules

The following steps should be taken to determine the drug dose:
1. Check the drug order.
2. Determine the drug available (generic name, brand name, and dosage per drug form).
3. Set up the method for drug calculation (basic formula, ratio and proportion, fraction equation, or dimensional analysis).
4. Convert to like units of measurement within the same system before solving the problem. Use the unit of measure on the drug container to calculate the drug dose.
5. Solve for the unknown (X).

Decide which of the methods of calculation you wish to use, and then use that same method for calculating all dosages. In the following examples, the basic formula, the ratio and proportion, fraction equation, and dimensional analysis methods are used (see Chapter 6).

Basic Formula (BF)

$$\frac{D \text{ (desired dose)}}{H \text{ (on-hand dose)}} \times V \text{ (vehicle)} = X$$

Fraction Equation (FE)

$$\frac{H \text{ (on hand)}}{V \text{ (Vehicle)}} = \frac{D \text{ (desired dose)}}{X \text{ (unknown)}}$$

(Cross multiply)

Ratio and Proportion (RP)

$$\begin{array}{ccccc} H & : & V & :: & D & : X \\ \text{on hand} & & \text{vehicle} & & \text{desired dose} & X \end{array}$$

Dimensional Analysis (DA)

$$V = \frac{V \times C(H) \times D}{H \times C(D) \times 1}$$

Note: C = conversion factor if needed.

EXAMPLES   **PROBLEM 1:**   Order: pravastatin sodium (Pravachol) 20 mg, daily.
Drug available:

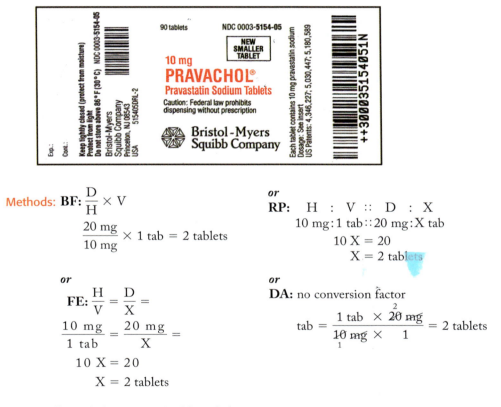

Methods: **BF:** $\dfrac{D}{H} \times V$

$$\frac{20 \text{ mg}}{10 \text{ mg}} \times 1 \text{ tab} = 2 \text{ tablets}$$

or

FE: $\dfrac{H}{V} = \dfrac{D}{X} =$

$$\frac{10 \text{ mg}}{1 \text{ tab}} = \frac{20 \text{ mg}}{X} =$$

$$10 \text{ X} = 20$$

$$X = 2 \text{ tablets}$$

or

RP: H : V :: D : X

10 mg : 1 tab :: 20 mg : X tab

$$10 \text{ X} = 20$$

$$X = 2 \text{ tablets}$$

or

DA: no conversion factor

$$\text{tab} = \frac{1 \text{ tab} \times \overset{2}{20} \text{ mg}}{\underset{1}{10} \text{ mg} \times 1} = 2 \text{ tablets}$$

Answer: Pravachol 20 mg = 2 tablets, daily.

PROBLEM 2:   Order: erythromycin (ERY-TAB) 0.5 g, qid (four times a day).
Drug available:

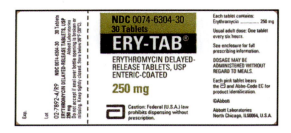

Note: Grams (g) and milligrams (mg) are units in the metric system. *Remember:* When changing grams (larger unit) to milligrams (smaller unit), move the decimal point three spaces to the right. Refer to Chapter 1, Table 1-2. Because the drug dose on the drug label is in milligrams, conversion should be from grams to milligrams.

Methods: 0.5 g = 0.500 mg or 500 mg

BF: $\dfrac{D}{H} \times V = \dfrac{500 \text{ mg}}{250 \text{ mg}} \times 1 \text{ tab}$

$= \dfrac{500}{250} = 2$ tablets

or
RP: H : V :: D : X
250 mg : 1 tab :: 500 mg : X tab
250 X = 500
X = 2 tablets

or
FE: $\dfrac{250 \text{ mg}}{1 \text{ tab}} = \dfrac{500 \text{ mg}}{X}$

250 X = 500
X = 2 tablets

or
DA: tablet $= \dfrac{1 \text{ tab} \times \overset{4}{\cancel{1000}} \text{ mg} \times 0.5 \text{ g}}{\underset{1}{\cancel{250}} \text{ mg} \times 1 \text{ g} \times 1}$

$4 \times 0.5 = 2$ tablets

Answer: ERY-TAB 0.5 g = 2 tablets

PROBLEM 3:   Order: aspirin 650 mg, po, STAT.
Drug available: aspirin 325 mg per tablet.
Methods:

BF: $\dfrac{D}{H} \times V = \dfrac{\overset{2}{\cancel{650}} \text{ mg}}{\underset{1}{\cancel{325}} \text{ mg}} \times 1 = \dfrac{2}{1} = 2$ tablets

or
RP: H : V :: D : X
325 mg : 1 tab :: 650 mg : X tab
325 X = 650
X = 2 tablets

or
FE: $\dfrac{H}{V} = \dfrac{D}{X} =$

$\dfrac{325 \text{ mg}}{1} = \dfrac{650 \text{ mg}}{X} =$

325X = 650
X = 2 tablets

or
DA: tablet $= \dfrac{1 \text{ tab} \times \overset{2}{\cancel{650}} \text{ mg}}{\underset{1}{\cancel{325}} \text{ mg} \times 1} = 2$ tablets

Answer: Aspirin 650 mg = 2 tablets.

LIQUIDS

Liquid medications come as tinctures, extracts, elixirs, suspensions, and syrups. Some liquid medications are irritating to the gastric mucosa and must be well diluted before being given (e.g., potassium chloride [KCl]). Medications in tincture form are always diluted or should be diluted. Liquid medication can be poured into a calibrated measuring cup or drawn up into a syringe when greater accuracy is required (i.e., liquid narcotics).

Liquids are designed to be taken orally or through an enteral tube and are made palatable by the addition of sweeteners such as suctrose, aspartame, saccharin, fructose, and sorbitol. Unpalatable liquid drugs can be mixed with 30 to 60 mL of fruit juice. Grapefruit juice interacts with many medications. Check with the pharmacist before choosing which juice to mix with the drug.

! CAUTION

- Concentrated liquid medication that can irritate the gastric mucosa should be diluted in *at least* 6 ounces of fluid, preferably 8 ounces of fluid.
- Liquid medication that can discolor the teeth *should be well diluted* and taken through a drinking straw.

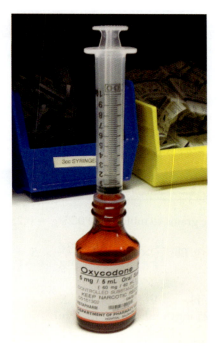

Figure 8-4 Liquid medication drawn up into a syringe.

Calculation of Liquid Medications

EXAMPLES **PROBLEM 1:** Order: potassium chloride (KCl) 20 mEq, po, bid.

Drug available: liquid potassium chloride 10 mEq per 5 mL.

Methods: **BF:** $\dfrac{D}{H} \times V = \dfrac{20 \text{ mEq}}{10 \text{ mEq}} \times 5 \text{ mL} = \dfrac{100}{10} = 10 \text{ mL}$

or

RP: H : V :: D : X

10 mEq : 5 mL :: 20 mEq : X mL

10 X = 100

X = 10 mL

or

FE: $\dfrac{H}{V} = \dfrac{D}{X} =$

$\dfrac{10 \text{ mEq}}{5 \text{ mL}} = \dfrac{20 \text{ mEq}}{X}$

10 X = 100

X = 10 mL

or

DA: no conversion factor

$mL = \dfrac{5 \text{ mL} \times \overset{2}{\cancel{20}} \text{ mEq}}{\underset{1}{\cancel{10}} \text{ mEq} \times \quad 1} = 10 \text{ mL}$

Answer: Potassium chloride 20 mEq = 10 mL

PROBLEM 2: Order: amoxicillin (Amoxil) 0.25 g, po, tid.

Drug available:

Change grams to milligrams: 0.25 g = 0.250 mg or 250 mg

Methods: **BF:** $\dfrac{D}{H} \times V = \dfrac{250 \text{ mg}}{125 \text{ mg}} \times 5 = \dfrac{1250}{125} = 10 \text{ mL}$

or

RP: H : V :: D : X

125 mg : 5 mL :: 250 mg : X mL

125 X = 1250

X = 10 mL

or

FE: $\dfrac{H}{V} = \dfrac{D}{X} =$

$\dfrac{125 \text{ mg}}{5} = \dfrac{250 \text{ mg}}{X} =$

125X = 1250

X = 10 mL

or

DA: $mL = \dfrac{5 \text{ mL} \times \overset{8}{\cancel{1000}} \text{ mg} \times \overset{1}{\cancel{0.25}} \text{ g}}{\underset{1}{\cancel{125}} \text{ mg} \times \underset{4}{\cancel{1}} \text{ g} \times 1} = \dfrac{40}{4} = 10 \text{ mL}$

Answer: Amoxil 0.25 g = 10 mL

PROBLEM 3: Give SSKI 300 mg, q6h, diluted in water.
Drug available: saturated solution of potassium iodide, 50 mg per drop (gt).

Methods: **BF:** $\dfrac{D}{H} \times V = \dfrac{300 \text{ mg}}{50 \text{ mg}} \times 1 \text{ drop} = \dfrac{300}{50} = 6 \text{ drops}$

or

RP: $\quad$ H $\quad$: V $\quad$ :: $\quad$ D $\quad$:X
$\qquad$ 50 mg : 1 drop :: 300 mg : X drop
$\qquad\qquad$ 50 X = 300
$\qquad\qquad\qquad$ X = 6 drops

or

FE: $\dfrac{H}{V} = \dfrac{D}{X} =$

$\dfrac{50 \text{ mg}}{1 \text{ drop}} = \dfrac{300 \text{ mg}}{X} =$

$\qquad$ 50 X = 300
$\qquad\qquad$ X = 6 drops

or

DA: $\text{gtt} = \dfrac{1 \text{ gt} \times \overset{6}{\cancel{300}} \text{ mg}}{\underset{1}{\cancel{50}} \cancel{\text{ mg}} \times 1} = 6 \text{ drops}$

Answer: SSKI 300 mg = 6 drops (gtt)

BUCCAL TABLETS

Buccal tablets are dissolved when held between the cheek and gum, permitting direct absorption of the active ingredient through the oral mucosa. The buccal tablet should be placed in the buccal cavity, above the rear molar between the upper cheek and gum.

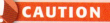

CAUTION

The patient should not split, crush, or chew the tablet.

EXAMPLE **PROBLEM 1:** **Order:** fentanyl buccal tablet, 100 mcg, STAT.
Drug available: 4 fentanyl, 100-mcg tablet each in a blister package. Dissolve 1 tablet in the buccal cavity over 30 minutes; then swallow any remaining pieces.

SUBLINGUAL TABLETS

Few drugs are administered sublingually (tablet placed under the tongue). Sublingual tablets are small and soluble and are quickly absorbed by the numerous capillaries on the underside of the tongue. Sublingual tablet may be called "orally disintegrating" tablet. Today some sublingual medications may include steroids, enzymes, antipsychotics, and cardiovascular drugs.

CAUTION

- A sublingual tablet (e.g., nitroglycerin [NTG]) should not be swallowed. If the drug is swallowed, the desired immediate action of the drug is decreased or lost.
- Fluids *should not* be taken until the drug has dissolved.

Calculation of Sublingual Medications

EXAMPLES **PROBLEM 1:** Order: nitroglycerin (Nitrostat) 0.6 mg, sublingually (SL).
Drug available:

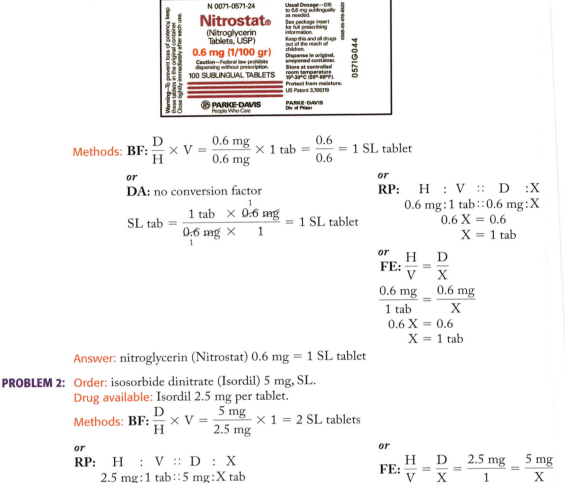

Methods: **BF:** $\dfrac{D}{H} \times V = \dfrac{0.6 \text{ mg}}{0.6 \text{ mg}} \times 1 \text{ tab} = \dfrac{0.6}{0.6} = 1 \text{ SL tablet}$

or
DA: no conversion factor

$$\text{SL tab} = \dfrac{1 \text{ tab} \times \overset{1}{\cancel{0.6 \text{ mg}}}}{\underset{1}{\cancel{0.6 \text{ mg}}} \times 1} = 1 \text{ SL tablet}$$

or
RP: H : V :: D :X
0.6 mg : 1 tab :: 0.6 mg : X
0.6 X = 0.6
X = 1 tab

or
FE: $\dfrac{H}{V} = \dfrac{D}{X}$

$$\dfrac{0.6 \text{ mg}}{1 \text{ tab}} = \dfrac{0.6 \text{ mg}}{X}$$

0.6 X = 0.6
X = 1 tab

Answer: nitroglycerin (Nitrostat) 0.6 mg = 1 SL tablet

PROBLEM 2: Order: isosorbide dinitrate (Isordil) 5 mg, SL.
Drug available: Isordil 2.5 mg per tablet.
Methods: **BF:** $\dfrac{D}{H} \times V = \dfrac{5 \text{ mg}}{2.5 \text{ mg}} \times 1 = 2 \text{ SL tablets}$

or
RP: H : V :: D : X
2.5 mg : 1 tab :: 5 mg : X tab
2.5 X = 5
X = 2 SL tablets

or
FE: $\dfrac{H}{V} = \dfrac{D}{X} = \dfrac{2.5 \text{ mg}}{1} = \dfrac{5 \text{ mg}}{X}$

2.5 X = 5
X = 2 tablets

or
DA: no conversion factor

$$\text{SL tablets} = \dfrac{1 \text{ SL tab} \times \overset{2}{\cancel{5 \text{ mg}}}}{\underset{1}{\cancel{2.5 \text{ mg}}} \times 1} = 2 \text{ SL tablets}$$

Answer: Isordil 5 mg = 2 SL tablets

PROBLEM 3: Order: olanzapine (Zyprexa, Zydis) 5 mg, SL daily.
Drug available: olanzapine 2.5-, 5-, 7.5-, 10-, 20-mg orally disintegrating blister packet.
a. Which tablet in the blister pack of olanzapine would you select?
b. Explain how the orally disintegrating (SL) olanzapine tablet is administered.

Answer
a. Select 5-mg tablet from the olanzapine blister pack.
b. Have the patient place the sublingual tablet under the tongue, where it will be dissolved
and absorbed by the oral mucosa.

Answers can be found on pages 142 to 147.

Note: Tablets: Round off tenths to whole numbers; Liquid: Round off to hundredths and then to tenths.

For each question, calculate the correct dosage that should be administered.

1. Order: doxycycline hyclate (Vibra-Tabs) 50 mg, po, q12h.
   Drug available:

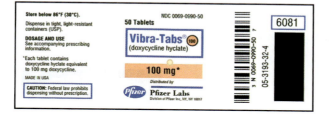

How many tablets(s) would you give for each dose? _____

2. Order: trimethoprim/sulfamethexazole (Septra) 40 mg/200 mg, po, bid.
   Drug available:

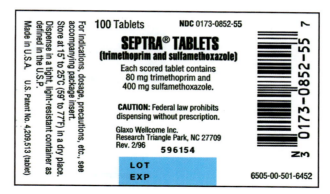

a. The drug label states that each tablet is _____.

b. How many tablet(s) would you give? _____

3. Order: digoxin (Lanoxin) 0.5 mg.
   Drug available:

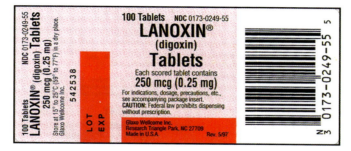

How many tablets should the patient receive? _____

4. **Order:** furosemide (Lasix) 20 mg, po, daily.

   Drug available: Drug is scored.

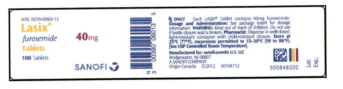

How many tablet(s) would you give? _____

5. **Order:** Diovan HCT (valsartan and hydrochlorothiazide) 160 mg/25 mg, po, daily.
   Drug available:

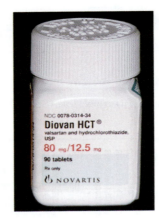

How many tablets would you give? _____

6. **Order:** potassium chloride 20 mEq, po.
   Drug available:

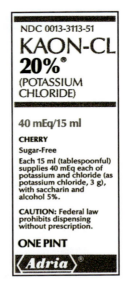

How many milliliters should the patient receive? _____

7. Order: cefaclor (Ceclor) 250 mg, q8h.

Drug available:

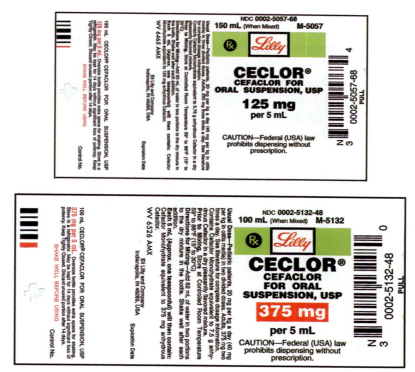

a. Which Ceclor bottle would you select? Why? _____

b. How many milliliters per dose should the patient receive? _____

8. Order: ProSom (estazolam) 2 mg, po, at bedtime.

Drug available: 1-mg tablet.

How many tablet(s) should be given? _____

9. Order: cefuroxime axetil (Ceftin) 400 mg, po, q12h.
   Drug available:

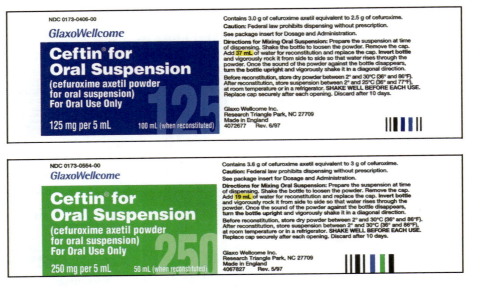

a. How many milliliters should the patient receive? _____

b. Which drug bottle would you use? _____

   Why? _____

10. Order: zidovudine (Retrovir) 300 mg, po, q12h.
   Drug available:

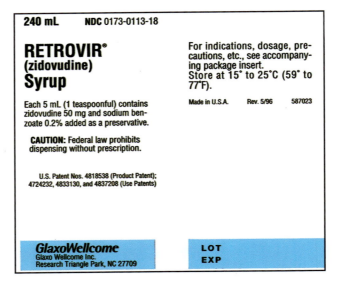

a. How many milligrams would you give per day? _____

b. How many milliliters would you give per dose? _____

11. Order: Depakene 750 mg, po, daily.
    Drug available:

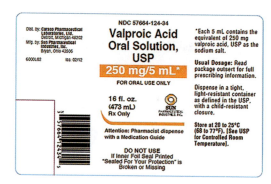

How many milliliters would the patient receive? _____

12. Order: HydroDiuril 50 mg, po, daily.
    Drug available:

a. Which drug bottle would you use? _____

b. How many tablet(s) would you give, if the tablet(s) are not scored?

   _____

   Explain. _____

13. Order: simvastatin (Zocor) 30 mg, po, daily.
Drug available:

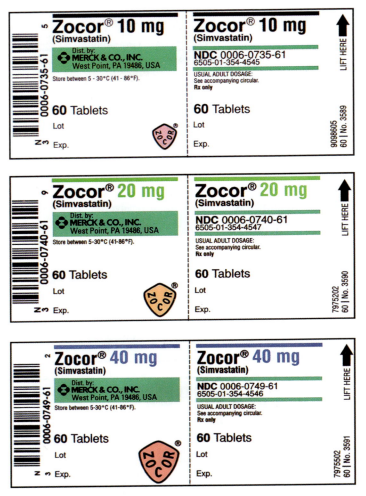

a. Which bottle(s) of Zocor would you select? Why? _____

b. How many tablet(s) should the patient receive? _____

14. **Order:** oxycodone hydrochloride, 15 mg, po, q6h, PRN for pain.
   Drug available:

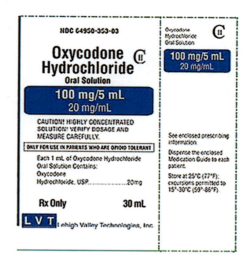

How many milliliters (mL) should the patient receive? _____

15. **Order:** phenobarbital gr ½ (apothecary system). See Table 2-1.
   Drug available: phenobarbital 15 mg per tablet.

How many tablet(s) should the patient receive? _____

16. **Order:** cefprozil (Cefzil) 100 mg, po, q12h.
   Drug available:

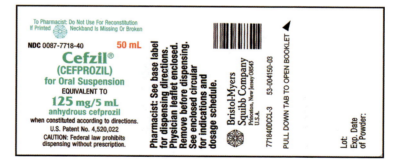

How many milliliters should the patient receive per dose? _____

17. Order: Crestor 20 mg, po, daily.
Drug available:

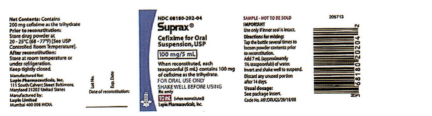

a. Which Crestor bottle(s) would you select? _____

b. How many tablet(s) would you give? _____

18. Order: nitroglycerin 0.4 mg SL, STAT.
Drug available:

Usual Dosage–0.3 to 0.6 mg sublingually as needed. See package insert for full prescribing information. Keep this and all drugs out of the reach of children. Dispense in original unopened container. Store up to 25°C (77°F). Protect from moisture. See lot number and expiration date on bottom.	N 0071-0569-24 **Nitrostat®** (Nitroglycerin Tablets, USP) 0.3 mg (1/200 gr) ℞ only 100 TABLETS	Usual Dosage–0.3 to 0.6 mg sublingually as needed. See package insert for full prescribing information. Keep this and all drugs out of the reach of children. Dispense in original unopened container. Store up to 25°C (77°F). Protect from moisture. See lot number and expiration date on bottom.	N 0071-0570-24 **Nitrostat®** (Nitroglycerin Tablets,USP) 0.4 mg (1/150 gr) ℞ only 100 TABLETS	Usual Dosage–0.3 to 0.6 mg sublingually as needed. See package insert for full prescribing information. Keep this and all drugs out of the reach of children. Dispense in original unopened container. Store up to 25°C (77°F). Protect from moisture. See lot number and expiration date on bottom.	N 0071-0571-24 **Nitrostat®** (Nitroglycerin Tablets,USP) 0.6 mg (1/100 gr) ℞ only 100 TABLETS
© 1997-'98, Warner-Lambert Co. **PARKE-DAVIS** Div of Warner-Lambert Co Morris Plains, NJ 07950 USA	Ⓟ PARKE-DAVIS	© 1997-'98, Warner-Lambert Co. **PARKE-DAVIS** Div of Warner-Lambert Co Morris Plains, NJ 07950 USA	Ⓟ PARKE-DAVIS	© 1997-'98, Warner-Lambert Co. **PARKE-DAVIS** Div of Warner-Lambert Co Morris Plains, NJ 07950 USA	Ⓟ PARKE-DAVIS

Which Nitrostat SL tablet would you give? _____

19. Order: cefixime 0.4 g, po, daily.
Drug available:

Net Contents: Contains 200 mg cefixime as the trihydrate
Prior to reconstitution:
Store drug powder at 20 - 25°C (68 -77°F) [See USP Controlled Room Temperature].
After reconstitution:
Store at room temperature or under refrigeration.
Keep tightly closed.
Manufactured for:
Lupin Pharmaceuticals, Inc.
111 South Calvert Street Baltimore, Maryland 21202 United States
Manufactured by:
Lupin Limited
Mumbai 400 098 INDIA

NDC 68180-202-04
Suprax®
Cefixime for Oral Suspension, USP
100 mg/5 mL
When reconstituted, each teaspoonful (5 mL) contains 100 mg of cefixime as the trihydrate.
FOR ORAL USE ONLY
SHAKE WELL BEFORE USING
Rx only
Usual dosage:
See package insert.
Code No. MP/DRUGS/20/18/08

SAMPLE - NOT TO BE SOLD   205713
IMPORTANT
Use only if inner seal is intact.
Directions for mixing:
Tap the bottle several times to loosen powder contents prior to reconstitution.
Add 7 mL (approximately 1½ teaspoonful) of water.
Invert and shake well to suspend.
Discard any unused portion after 14 days.

How many milliliters would the patient receive? _____

20. Order: digoxin (Lanoxin) 0.25 mg, po, daily.
    Drug available:

   a. Which Lanoxin bottle would you select? _____

   b. How many tablet(s) would you give? _____

21. Order: diazepam (Valium) 2½ mg.
    Drug available: Valium 5-mg scored tablet.

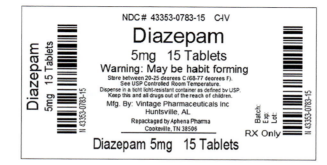

   How many tablet(s) would you give? _____

22. Order: ondansetron HCl (Zofran) 6 mg, po, 30 min before chemotherapy, then q8h × 2 more
    doses.
    Drug available:

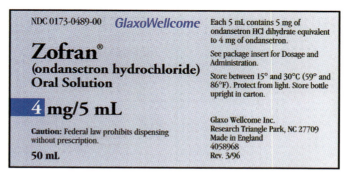

   How many milliliters would you give per dose?_____

23. Order: allopurinol 450 mg, po, daily.

   Drug available: allopurinol 300 mg scored tablet.

   How many tablet(s) would you give? _____

24. Order: captopril (Capoten) 25 mg, po, bid, for an elderly patient with heart failure.
Drug available:

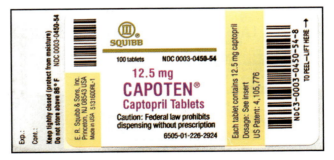

a. How many milligrams should the patient receive per day? _____

b. How many tablet(s) would you give? _____

25. Order: Cogentin 1.5 mg, initially (first day); then 1 mg, po, daily starting second day.
Drug available:

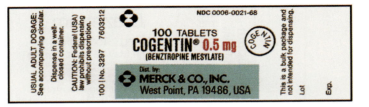

a. How many tablet(s) should the patient receive initially (first day)? _____

b. How many tablet(s) should the patient receive the second day? _____

26. Order: fluconazole (Diflucan) 120 mg, po, daily for 4 weeks.
Drug available:

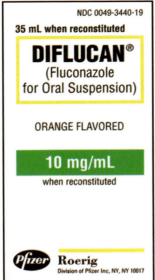

How many milliliters should the patient receive per dose? _____

27. Order: lithium carbonate 600 mg, po, tid.
    Drug available:

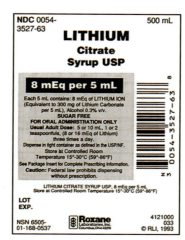

   a. Drug label states that 8 mEq per 5 mL of lithium citrate is equivalent to _____ of lithium carbonate.

   b. How many milliliters per dose should the patient receive? _____

   c. How many milligrams should the patient receive per day? _____

28. Order: furosemide 100 mg, po, as a loading dose, then furosemide 20 mg, po, q12h.
    Drug available:

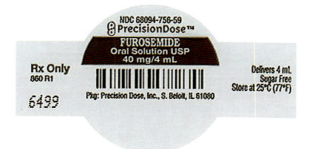

   a. How many milliliters would be given as the loading dose? _____

   b. How many milliliters would be given for the next scheduled dose? _____

29. **Order:** amoxicillin/clavulanate potassium (Augmentin) 0.5 g, po, q8h.
    Drug available:

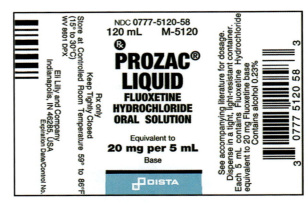

How many milliliters should the patient receive per dose? _____

30. **Order:** Prozac 30 mg, po, daily.
    Drug available:

How many milliliters should the client receive? _____

Solve **questions 31 to 39** with Additional Dimensional Analysis (factor labeling). Refer to Chapter 6 as necessary.

31. Order: Ativan 1.5 mg, po, bid.
Drug available:

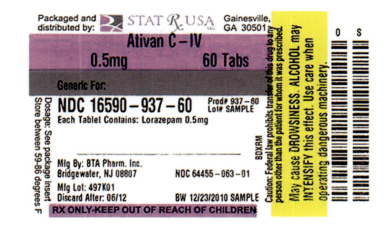

How many milligrams should the patient receive per dose? _____

32. Order: Vasotec 5 mg, po, bid.
Drug available:

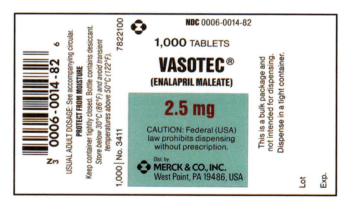

Factors: 2.5 mg = 1 tablet (drug label); 5 mg/1 (drug order)

Conversion factor: none.

How many tablet(s) should the patient receive? _____

33. Order: fluoxetine (Prozac) 60 mg, po, daily in the AM for bulimia nervosa.
Drug available:

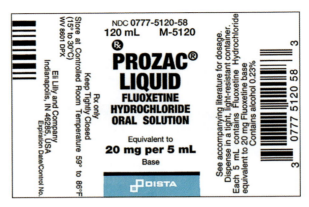

Conversion factor: None

How many milliliters of fluoxetine should the patient receive per day? _____

34. Order: cephalexin (Keflex) 1 g, po, 1 hour before dental cleaning.
Drug available:

a. Conversion factor: 1 g = 1000 mg

b. How many capsules would you give 1 hour before dental cleaning? _____

35. **Order:** metoprolol (Lopressor) 0.1 g, po, daily.
    Drug available:

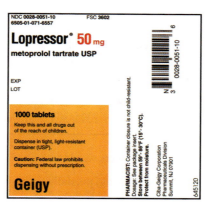

Conversion factor: 1 g = 1000 mg

How many tablet(s) would you give? _____

36. **Order:** amoxicillin (Amoxil) 0.4 g, po, q6h.
    Drug available:

Factors: 250 mg/5 mL (drug label); 0.4 g/1 (drug order)

Conversion factor: 1 g = 1000 mg

How many milliliters would you give? _____

37. Order: acetaminophen (Tylenol) 650 mg, po.
Drug available:

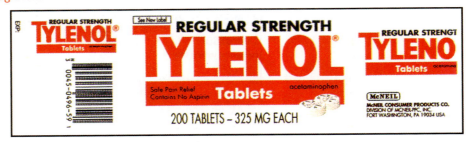

How many acetaminophen tablets would you give? _____

38. Order: atenolol (Tenormin) 50 mg, po, daily for the first 2 weeks and then increase to 100 mg, po, daily starting the third week.
Drug available:

Conversion factor: None

a. How many tablet(s) should the patient receive for the first 2 weeks? _____

b. How many tablet(s) should the patient receive after the second week? _____

39. Order: lactulose 25 g, po × 1 dose.
Drug available:

How many milliliters would the patient receive? _____

Questions 40 to 44 relate to body weight and body surface area. Refer to Chapter 7 as necessary.

40. **Order:** valproic acid (Depakene) 10 mg/kg/day in three divided doses (tid), po. Patient weighs 165 pounds. How much Depakene should be administered tid? _____

41. **Order:** cyclophosphamide (Cytoxan) 4 mg/kg/day, po. Patient weighs 154 pounds. How much Cytoxan would you give per day? _____

42. **Order:** mercaptopurine 2.5 mg/kg/day po or 100 mg/m² body surface area po. The patient weighs 132 pounds and is 64 inches tall. The estimated body surface area according to the nomogram is 1.7 m². The amount of drug the patient should receive according to body weight is _____ and according to body surface area is _____.

43. **Order:** ethosuximide (Zarontin) 20 mg/kg/day in 2 divided doses (q12h). Patient weighs 110 pounds (110 ÷ 2.2 = 50 kg).
    Drug available:

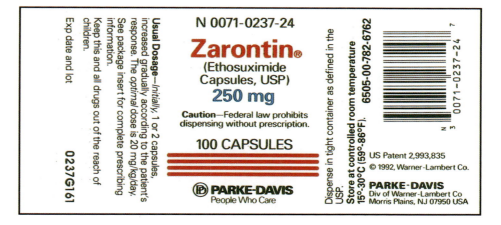

    a. How many milligrams should the patient receive per day? _____

    b. How many tablet(s) should the patient receive per dose? _____

44. **Order:** minocycline HCl (Minocin) 4 mg/kg/day in 2 divided doses (q12h). Patient weighs 132 pounds (132 ÷ 2.2 = 60 kg).

    Drug available: Minocin 50 mg/5 mL.

    a. How many milligrams should the patient receive per day? _____

    b. How many milliliters should the patient receive per dose? _____

45. **Order:** Pradaxa 150 mg, po, q12h.

    Drug available: Pradaxa 75-mg tablet.

    How many tablets should the patient receive? _____

46. **Order:** Xarelto 10 mg, po, daily.

    Drug available: Xarelto 20-mg tablet.

    How many tablets should the patient receive? _____

ENTERAL NUTRITION AND DRUG ADMINISTRATION

When the patient is unable to take nourishment by mouth, enteral feeding (tube feeding) is usually preferred over parenteral (intravenous) nutrition. Candidates for enteral feedings include patients who suffer from neurological deficits and have swallowing problems; patients who are debilitated; have burns; suffer from malnutrition disorders; and those who have undergone radical head and neck surgery. The cost of enteral nutrition is much less than the use of intravenous therapy. Enteral nutrition also carries considerably less risk of infection.

Drugs that can be administered orally (with the exception of sustained-release and extended-release drugs) can also be given through the enteral feeding tube. The drug must be in liquid form or dissolved into a liquid.

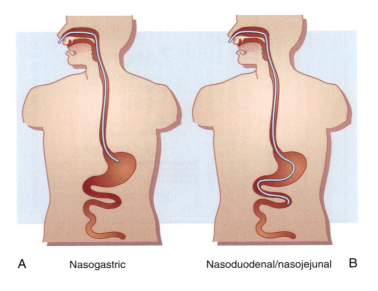

A   Nasogastric   Nasoduodenal/nasojejunal   B

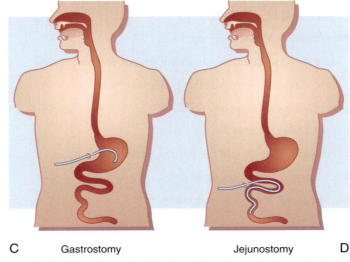

C   Gastrostomy   Jejunostomy   D

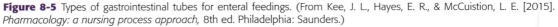

Figure 8-5 Types of gastrointestinal tubes for enteral feedings. (From Kee, J. L., Hayes, E. R., & McCuistion, L. E. [2015]. *Pharmacology: a nursing process approach,* 8th ed. Philadelphia: Saunders.)

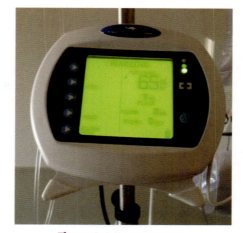

Figure 8-6 Kangaroo pump.

Enteral Feedings

Enteral nutrition may be provided by a gastric, jejunal, or nasogastric tube. Enteral feeding tubes can be identified by their anatomical insertion site and the location of the tip. Gastrostomy and jejunostomy routes are used for long-term feeding and require a surgical procedure for insertion. There are two types of nasogastric tubes: the flexible small-bore tube that has a small diameter (4-8 Fr), and the rigid large bore tube with a larger diameter (10-18 Fr). All tubes inserted orally or nasally are primarily for short-term use and may cause nasal or pharyngeal irritation if the use is prolonged. Large-bore tubes are less likely to clog than small-bore tubes. It is essential to flush any feeding tube before and after feedings and between medications.

Enteral feedings may be given as a bolus (intermittent) or as a continuous drip feeding over a specific time period. Continuous feedings can be given by gravity flow from a bag or by infusion pump. With bolus feedings, the amount of solution administered is approximately 200 mL or less and feeding times per day are more frequent.

Although enteral feeding solutions are formulated to be given at full strength, this may not be tolerated. Solutions that are highly concentrated (hyperosmolar or hypertonic) when given in full strength can cause vomiting, cramping, or excessive diarrhea. In many situations, clients have better gastrointestinal tolerance when the strength of the solution is gradually increased. Continuous feedings are usually started slowly and advanced as tolerated by approximately 10 mL/hr to the goal feeding rate.

If diarrhea continues, changing to a fiber-containing formula may decrease or eliminate it. With some patients, hypoalbuminemia could be a cause of diarrhea, which can lead to malabsorption in the intestines. The prealbumin level is a better indicator of hypoalbuminemia than is the serum albumin test. Other causes of diarrhea may include fecal impaction, *Clostridium difficile,* pseudomembranous colitis, and gut atrophy.

Blood sugar levels should be monitored during enteral therapy. This is important for patients who are acutely ill, have septic conditions, are recovering from acute trauma, or who are receiving steroids. If hyperglycemia occurs, decreasing the tube feeding rate or concentration may help.

TABLE 8-1 Common Enteral Formulations

Ensure	Isocal	Nephro
Ensure Plus	Sustacal	Ultracal
Ensure HN	Sustacal HC	Jevity
Osmolite	Vital	Criticare
Osmolite HN	Pulmocare	Promote

Enteral Medications

Oral medications in liquid, tablet, or capsule form may be administered through a feeding tube when diluted with 30 to 60 mL of water. Tablets or capsules than can be crushed should be pulverized into a fine powder and then mixed in enough water to form a slurry. The slurry can be given through a large-bore feeding tube with a catheter-tip syringe; 30 to 60 mL of water is flushed through the feeding tube between medications. Some new feeding pumps are designed to include a flush bag that periodically clears the feeding tube and prevents clogging.

> **! CAUTION**
>
> - Use caution with crushing devices, such as a mortar and pestle, to avoid cross-contamination and possible allergic reactions, which may occur if the device is not cleaned or if the medication being crushed is not shielded.

> **! CAUTION**
>
> - Medications in time-released, enteric-coated, or sublingual form and bulk-forming laxatives cannot be crushed or administered enterally.

ANSWERS

Oral Medications

1. BF: $\dfrac{D}{H} \times V = \dfrac{50 \text{ mg}}{100 \text{ mg}} \times 1 \text{ tab} = 0.5 = \tfrac{1}{2} \text{ tablet}$

FE: $\dfrac{H}{V} = \dfrac{D}{X} = \dfrac{100 \text{ mg}}{1} = \dfrac{50 \text{ mg}}{X}$

$$100 \, X = 50$$
$$X = 0.5 \text{ or } \tfrac{1}{2} \text{ tablet}$$

or
RP: H : V :: D : X
   100 mg : 1 tab :: 50 mg : X tab
         $100 \, X = 50$
         $X = 0.5$ or $\tfrac{1}{2}$ tablet

or
DA: no conversion factor

$\text{tab} = \dfrac{1 \text{ tab} \times \overset{1}{\cancel{50 \text{ mg}}}}{\underset{2}{\cancel{100 \text{ mg}}} \times 1} = \tfrac{1}{2}$ tablet

2. a. scored
   b. $\tfrac{1}{2}$ tablet
3. 2 tablets

4. BF: $\dfrac{D}{H} \times V = \dfrac{\overset{1}{\cancel{20 \text{ mg}}}}{\underset{2}{\cancel{40 \text{ mg}}}} \times 1 = \tfrac{1}{2}$ tablet of Lasix

RP: H : V :: D : X
   40 mg : 1 tab :: 20 mg : X
         $40 \, X = 20$
         $X = \tfrac{1}{2}$ tablet of Lasix

FE: $\dfrac{H}{V} = \dfrac{D}{X} = \dfrac{40 \text{ mg}}{1} = \dfrac{20 \text{ mg}}{X}$

   $40 \, X = 20$
   $X = \tfrac{1}{2}$ tablet of Lasix
5. 2 tablets daily

6. 7.5 mL

7. a. Select the 125-mg/5-mL bottle. It is a fractional dosage with the 375-mg/5-mL bottle (3.3 mL).

b. BF: $\dfrac{D}{H} \times V = \dfrac{250 \text{ mg}}{125 \text{ mg}} \times 5 \text{ mL} = \dfrac{1250}{125} = 10 \text{ mL of Ceclor}$

or

RP: H : V :: D   :X
        125 mg : 5 mL :: 250 mg : X
               125 X = 1250
                   X = 10 mL of Ceclor

or

DA: mL $= \dfrac{5 \text{ mL} \times \overset{2}{\cancel{250 \text{ mg}}}}{\underset{1}{\cancel{125 \text{ mg}}} \times 1} = 10 \text{ mL of Ceclor}$

8. 2 tablets of ProSom

9. a. BF: $\dfrac{D}{H} \times V = \dfrac{400 \text{ mg}}{125 \text{ mg}} \times 5 \text{ mL} = \dfrac{2000}{125} = 16 \text{ mL of Ceftin}$

or

BF: $\dfrac{D}{H} \times V = \dfrac{400 \text{ mg}}{250 \text{ mg}} \times 5 \text{ mL} = \dfrac{2000}{250} = 8 \text{ mL of Ceftin}$

b. Either Ceftin bottle could be used. For fewer milliliters, select the 250-mg/5-mL bottle.

10. a. 600 mg per day

b. BF: $\dfrac{D}{H} \times V = \dfrac{300 \text{ mg}}{50 \text{ mg}} \times 5 \text{ mL}$
$= 30 \text{ mL per dose}$

or

RP: H : V :: D   :X
        50 mg : 5 mL :: 300 mg : X mL
              50 X = 1500
                 X = 30 mL

or

FE: $\dfrac{H}{V} = \dfrac{D}{X} = \dfrac{50 \text{ mg}}{5 \text{ mL}} = \dfrac{300 \text{ mg}}{X} =$

50 X = 1500
   X = 30 mL per dose

or

DA: mL $= \dfrac{5 \text{ mL} \times \overset{6}{\cancel{300 \text{ mg}}}}{\underset{1}{\cancel{50 \text{ mg}}} \times 1} = 30 \text{ mL per dose}$

11. BF: $\dfrac{D}{H} \times V = \dfrac{750 \text{ mg}}{250 \text{ mg}} \times 5 \text{ mL} = 15 \text{ mL}$

or

RP: H : V :: D : X
     250 : 5 :: 750 : X
     250 X = 3750
         X = 15 mL

or

FE: $\dfrac{H}{V} = \dfrac{D}{H} = \dfrac{250 \text{ mg}}{5 \text{ mL}} = \dfrac{750 \text{ mg}}{X}$

250 X = 3750
    X = 15 mL

or

DA: mL $= \dfrac{5 \text{ mL} \times 750 \text{ mg}}{250 \text{ mg} \times 1} = 15 \text{ mg}$

12. a. The HydroDiuril 25-mg tablet bottle is preferred. A half-tablet from the HydroDiuril 100-mg tablet bottle can be used; however, breaking or cutting the 100-mg tablet can result in an inaccurate dose.

b. From the HydroDiuril 25-mg bottle, give 2 tablets. From the HydroDiuril 100-mg bottle, give ½ tablet (if the tablet is scored).

13. a. Select a 10-mg and 20-mg Zocor bottle. The 40-mg tablet would not be selected because breaking or cutting the tablet can result in an inaccurate dose.

b. Give 1 tablet from each bottle.

14. BF: $\dfrac{D}{H} \times V = \dfrac{15 \text{ mg}}{20 \text{ mg}} \times 1 \text{ mL} = 0.75 \text{ mL}$

   or
   RP: H :V:: D :X
   20 mg : 1 :: 15 mg : X
   20 X = 15
   X = 0.75 mL

   or
   FE: $\dfrac{H}{V} = \dfrac{D}{X} = \dfrac{20 \text{ mg}}{1} = \dfrac{15 \text{ mg}}{X}$
   20 X = 15
   X = 0.75 mL

   or
   DA: mL $= \dfrac{1 \text{ mL} \times 15 \text{ mg}}{20 \text{ mg} \times \quad 1} = 0.75 \text{ mL}$

15. Use the metric system. Give 2 tablets (gr ½ = 30 mg).

16. BF: $\dfrac{D}{H} \times V = \dfrac{100}{125} \times 5 \text{ mL} = \dfrac{500}{125} = 4 \text{ mL}$

   or
   RP: H : V :: D :X
   125 mg : 5 mL :: 100 mg : X
   125 X = 500
   X = 4 mL

   or
   FE: $\dfrac{125 \text{ mg}}{5 \text{ mL}} = \dfrac{100 \text{ mg}}{X} = 125X = 500$
   X = 4 mL

   or
   DA: no conversion factor
   mL $= \dfrac{5 \text{ mL} \times \overset{4}{\cancel{100 \text{ mg}}}}{\underset{5}{\cancel{125 \text{ mg}}} \times \quad 1} = \dfrac{20}{5} = 4 \text{ mL}$

17. **a.** Preferred the selection of Crestor 10-mg bottle. Could select Crestor 5-mg bottle; however, the number of tablets given would have to be increased.
   b. 2 tablets from Crestor 10-mg bottle. If Crestor 5-mg bottle was selected, then 4 tablets.

18. Nitrostat 0.4 mg

19. Change grams to milligrams: 0.400 g = 400 mg

   BF: $\dfrac{D}{H} \times V = \dfrac{400 \text{ mg}}{100 \text{ mg}} \times 5 \text{ mL} = 20 \text{ mL}$

   or
   RP: H :V :: D : X
   100 : 5 :: 400 : X
   100 X = 2000
   X = 20 mL

   or
   FE: $\dfrac{H}{V} = \dfrac{D}{X} = \dfrac{100 \text{ mg}}{5 \text{ mL}} = \dfrac{400 \text{ mg}}{X}$
   100 X = 2000
   X = 20 mL

   or
   DA: mL $= \dfrac{5 \text{ mL} \times 400 \text{ mg}}{100 \text{ mg} \times \quad 1} = 20 \text{ mL}$

20. **a.** Preferred: the selection of Lanoxin 0.125-mg (125-mcg) bottle. Could select Lanoxin 0.5-mg (500-mcg) bottle because the tablets are scored.
   b. 2 tablets from the Lanoxin 0.125-mg bottle or ½ tablet from the Lanoxin 0.5-mg bottle.

21. ½ tablet

22. BF: $\dfrac{D}{H} \times V = \dfrac{6 \text{ mg}}{4 \text{ mg}} \times 5 \text{ mL} = \dfrac{30}{4} = 7.5 \text{ mL of Zofran}$

23. 1½ tablets

24. **a.** 50 mg per day

b. BF: $\dfrac{D}{H} \times V = \dfrac{25 \text{ mg}}{12.5 \text{ mg}} \times 1 \text{ tab} = 2 \text{ tablets}$

or
RP: H : V :: D : X
12.5 mg : 1 tab :: 25 mg : X tab
12.5 mg X = 25 mg
X = 2 tablets

or
FE: $\dfrac{H}{V} = \dfrac{D}{X} = \dfrac{12.5 \text{ mg}}{1 \text{ tablet}} = \dfrac{25 \text{ mg}}{X} =$
12.5 X = 25
     X = 2 tablets

or
DA: tablets $= \dfrac{1 \text{ tab} \times \overset{2}{\cancel{25}} \text{ mg}}{\underset{1}{\cancel{12.5}} \text{ mg} \times 1} = 2 \text{ tablets}$

25. **a.** Initially, first day

BF: $\dfrac{D}{H} \times V = \dfrac{\overset{3}{\cancel{1.5}} \text{ mg}}{\underset{1}{\cancel{0.5}} \text{ mg}} \times 1 = 3 \text{ tablets}$

or
RP: H : V :: D : X
0.5 mg : 1 tab :: 1.5 mg : X
0.5 X = 1.5
     X = 3 tablets of Cogentin

b. Second day and ON

FE: $\dfrac{H}{V} = \dfrac{D}{X} = \dfrac{0.5 \text{ mg}}{1} = \dfrac{1 \text{ mg}}{X}$
0.5 X = 1
     X = 2 tablets

or
DA: tablet $= \dfrac{1 \text{ tab} \times \overset{2}{\cancel{1}} \text{ mg}}{\underset{1}{\cancel{0.5}} \text{ mg} \times 1} = 2 \text{ tablets of Cogentin}$

26. 12 mL of Diflucan

27. **a.** 300 mg per 5 mL

b. BF: $\dfrac{D}{H} \times V = \dfrac{\overset{2}{\cancel{600}} \text{ mg}}{\underset{1}{\cancel{300}} \text{ mg}} \times 5 \text{ mL} = 10 \text{ mL of lithium}$

or
RP: H : V :: D : X
300 mg : 5 mL :: 600 mg : X
300 X = 3000
     X = 10 mL

or
FE: $\dfrac{H}{V} = \dfrac{D}{X} = \dfrac{300 \text{ mg}}{5 \text{ mL}} = \dfrac{600 \text{ mg}}{X}$
300 X = 3000
     X = 10 mL of lithium

or
DA: mL $= \dfrac{5 \text{ mL} \times \overset{2}{\cancel{600}} \text{ mg}}{\underset{1}{\cancel{300}} \text{ mg} \times 1} = 10 \text{ mL}$

c. 600 mg × 3 (tid) = 1800 mg per day

28. **a.** Loading dose

BF: $\dfrac{D}{H} \times V = \dfrac{100 \text{ mg}}{40 \text{ mg}} \times 4 \text{ mL} =$

$\dfrac{400}{40} = 10 \text{ mL of furosemide}$

or
RP: H : V :: D : X
40 mg : 4 mL :: 100 mg : X
40 X = 400
     X = 10 mL

b. Per dose

FE: $\dfrac{H}{V} = \dfrac{D}{X} = \dfrac{40 \text{ mg}}{4 \text{ mL}} = \dfrac{20 \text{ mg}}{X}$
40 X = 80
     X = 2 mL

or
DA: mL $= \dfrac{4 \text{ mL} \times \overset{1}{\cancel{20}} \text{ mg}}{\underset{2}{\cancel{40}} \text{ mg} \times 1} = \dfrac{4}{2} = 2 \text{ mL of furosemide}$

29. 10 mL

30. BF: $\dfrac{D}{H} \times V = \dfrac{30 \text{ mg}}{20 \text{ mg}} \times 5 \text{ mL} =$

$\dfrac{150}{20} = 7.5 \text{ mL of Prozac}$

or

DA: mL $= \dfrac{5 \text{ mL} \times \overset{3}{\cancel{30}} \text{ mg}}{\underset{2}{\cancel{20}} \text{ mg} \times 1} = \dfrac{15}{2} = 7.5 \text{ mL of Prozac}$

Additional Dimensional Analysis

31. DA: tab $= \dfrac{1 \text{ tab} \times 1.5 \text{ mg}}{0.5 \text{ mg} \times 1} = \dfrac{1.5}{0.5} = 3 \text{ tablets of Ativan}$

32. tablets $= \dfrac{1 \times \overset{2}{\cancel{5.0}} \text{ mg}}{\underset{1}{\cancel{2.5}} \text{ mg} \times 1} = 2 \text{ tablets of Vasotec}$

33. DA: mL $= \dfrac{5 \text{ mL} \times \overset{3}{\cancel{60}} \text{ mg}}{\underset{1}{\cancel{20}} \text{ mg} \times 1} = 15 \text{ mL of Prozac}$

34. DA: cap $= \dfrac{1 \text{ cap} \times \overset{4}{\cancel{1000}} \text{ mg} \times 1 \text{ g}}{\underset{1}{\cancel{250}} \text{ mg} \times 1 \text{ g} \times 1} = 4 \text{ capsules of Keflex}$

35. DA: tab $= \dfrac{1 \text{ tab} \times \overset{20}{\cancel{1000}} \text{ mg} \times 0.1 \text{ g}}{\underset{1}{\cancel{50}} \text{ mg} \times 1 \text{ g} \times 1} = \dfrac{20 \times 0.1}{1} = 2 \text{ tablets of Lopressor}$

36. mL $= \dfrac{5 \text{ mL} \times \overset{4}{\cancel{1000}} \text{ mg} \times 0.4 \text{ g}}{\underset{1}{\cancel{250}} \text{ mg} \times 1 \text{ g} \times 1} = 8 \text{ mL}$

Give 8 mL per dose of amoxicillin.

37. Drug label: 325 mg = 1 tablet

DA: tablet $= \dfrac{1 \text{ tab} \times \overset{2}{\cancel{650}} \text{ mg}}{\underset{1}{\cancel{325}} \text{ mg} \times 1} = 2 \text{ tablets}$

38. a. 1 tablet of Tenormin

b. DA: tablet $= \dfrac{1 \text{ tablet} \times \overset{2}{\cancel{100}} \text{ mg}}{\underset{1}{\cancel{50}} \text{ mg} \times 1} = 2 \text{ tablets of Tenormin}$

39. BF: $\dfrac{D}{H} \times V = \dfrac{25 \text{ g}}{10 \text{ g}} \times 15 \text{ mL} = 37.5 \text{ mL}$

or

RP: H : V :: D :X

10 g : 15 mL :: 25 g : X

10 X = 375

X = 37.5 mL

or

FE: $\dfrac{H}{V} = \dfrac{D}{X} = \dfrac{10 \text{ g}}{15 \text{ mL}} = \dfrac{25 \text{ g}}{X}$

(Cross multiply) 10 X = 375

X = 37.5 mL

or

DA: mL $= \dfrac{15 \text{ mL} \times 25 \text{ mg}}{10 \text{ mg} \times 1} = 37.5 \text{ mL}$

40. 165 lb = 75 kg (change pounds to kilograms by dividing by 2.2 into 165 pounds, or 165 ÷ 2.2)

10 mg/kg/day × 75 = 750 mg/day

750 ÷ 3 = 250 mg, tid

41. 154 lb = 70 kg

4 mg/kg/day × 70 kg = 280 mg/day

42. 132 lb = 60 kg

2.5 mg/kg/day $\times$ 60 kg = 150 mg **or** 100 mg/m² $\times$ 1.7 m² = 170 mg

43. a. 20 mg/50 kg/day = 20 $\times$ 50 = 1000 mg per day

b. 2 tablets of Zarontin per dose (500 mg per dose)

44. a. 4 mg/60 kg/day = 4 $\times$ 60 = 240 mg per day **or** 120 mg, q12h

b. BF: $\dfrac{D}{H} \times V = \dfrac{120 \text{ mg}}{\underset{10}{\cancel{50} \text{ mg}}} \times \overset{1}{\cancel{5}} \text{ mL} = \dfrac{120}{10} = 12 \text{ mL}$

or

RP: H : V ::   D   :X

50 mg : 5 mL :: 120 mg : X

50 X = 600

$X = \dfrac{600}{50} = 12 \text{ mL}$

or

DA: mL $= \dfrac{5 \text{ mL} \times \overset{12}{\cancel{120} \text{ mg}}}{\underset{5}{\cancel{50} \text{ mg}} \times 1} = \dfrac{60}{5} = 12 \text{ mL}$

Give 12 mL per dose of minocycline.

45. BF: $\dfrac{D}{H} \times V = \dfrac{150 \text{ mg}}{75 \text{ mg}} \times 1 \text{ tab} = 2 \text{ tablets}$

or

H : V ::   D   :X

75 mg : 1 tab :: 150 mg : X

75 X = 150

X = 2 tablets

46. BF: $\dfrac{D}{H} \times V = \dfrac{10 \text{ mg}}{20 \text{ mg}} \times 1 \text{ tab} = 0.5 \text{ or } \frac{1}{2} \text{ tablet}$

or

H : V ::   D   :X

20 mg : 1 tab :: 10 mg : X

20 X = 10

X = 0.5 or ½ tablet

---

evolve   Additional practice problems are available in the Basic Calculations section of Drug Calculations Companion, version 5 on Evolve.

CHAPTER 9

Injectable Preparations With Clinical Applications

Medications administered by injection are given through four routes. In the first method, intradermal, the needle is inserted just under the epidermis in the dermal layer of the skin. In the second route, subcutaneous, the needle is placed farther into the fatty tissue. In the third route, intramuscular, the injection goes directly into the muscle. In the fourth route, intravenous, the medication is directly injected into a vein. (Intravenous injectables are discussed in Chapter 11.) Because these routes are commonly used in drug orders they are frequently abbreviated: intradermal as ID; subcutaneous as subcut, subQ, SC, and SQ; intramuscular as IM; and intravenous as IV. It is essential that injectable drugs be given by the correct route. Any use of abbreviations should follow institutional policies and protocols.

Injectable drugs are ordered in grams, milligrams, micrograms, or international units. The drug manufacturer prepares the medication as either a liquid or a powder according to the stability of the compound. The nurse's responsibility is to have working knowledge of all types of injectable preparations, the equipment for injections, and the routes of administration.

INJECTABLE PREPARATIONS

Vials and Ampules

Drugs are packaged in vials (sealed rubber-top containers) for single and multiple doses and in ampules (sealed glass containers) for a single dose. Multiple-dose vials can be used more than once because of their self-sealing rubber top; however, ampules are used only once after the glass-necked container is opened. A 15-gauge filtered needle should be used with a glass ampule to prevent aspiration of small glass particles. The drug is available in either liquid or powder form in vials and ampules. When drugs in solution deteriorate rapidly, they are packaged in dry form, and solvent (diluent) is added before administration. If the drug is in powdered form, mixing instructions and dose equivalents such as milligrams (mg) per milliliter (mL) are usually given; if not, check the drug information insert. After the dry form of the drug is reconstituted with sterile water, bacteriostatic water (sterile water with a small amount of benzyl alcohol to prevent bacterial growth), or saline solution, the drug must be used immediately or refrigerated. Usually, the reconstituted drug in the vial is used within 48 hours to 1 week; check the drug information insert. A Mix-O-Vial has two containers, one holding a diluent and the other holding a powdered drug. When pressure is applied to the top of the vial, the liquid is released, which dissolves the powdered drug. A vial, a Mix-O-Vial and an ampule are shown in Figure 9-1.

The route by which the injectable drug can be given, such as subcut or SQ, IM, or IV, is printed on the drug label.

Syringes

Types of syringes used for injection include 3-mL and 5-mL calibrated syringes, metal and plastic syringes for pre-filled cartridges, and tuberculin syringes. Insulin syringes are discussed in detail in Chapter 10. There are 10-mL, 20-mL, and 50-mL syringes that are used mostly for drug preparations. A syringe is composed of a barrel (outer shell), a plunger (inner part), and the tip, where the needle joins the syringe (Figure 9-2).

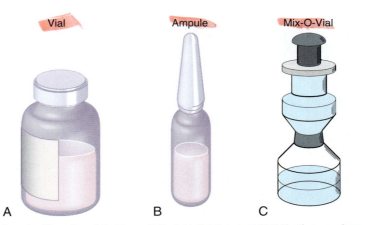

Vial   Ampule   Mix-O-Vial

A   B   C

Figure 9-1 A, Vial. **B,** Ampule. (From Kee, J. L., Hayes, E. R., & McCuistion, L. E. [2015]. *Pharmacology: a patient-centered nursing process approach,* 8th ed., Philadelphia: Elsevier.) **C,** Mix-o-vial. (From Clayton B. D., & Willihnganz M. J. [2013]: *Basic pharmacology for nurses,* 16th ed., St Louis: Elsevier.)

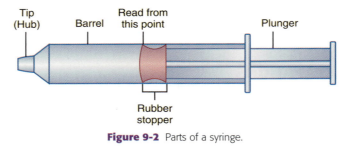

Figure 9-2 Parts of a syringe.

Three-Milliliter Syringe

The 3-mL syringe is calibrated in tenths (0.1 mL). The amount of fluid in the syringe is determined by the rubber end of the plunger that is closer to the tip of the syringe (Figure 9-3). An advance in safety needle technology is the SafetyGlide shielding hypodermic needle (Figure 9-4). The purpose of this type of needle is to reduce needlestick injuries. Needles should never be recapped by hand and should always be disposed of in a sharps container (Figure 9-5).

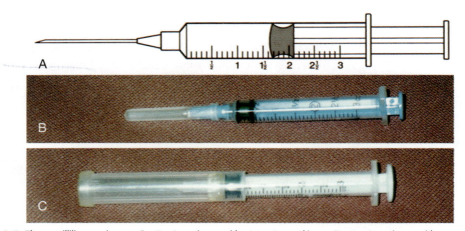

Figure 9-3 Three-milliliter syringes: **A,** 3-mL syringe with 0.1-mL markings. **B,** 3-mL syringe with a needle cover. **C,** 3-mL syringe with a protective cover over the needle after injection. (**B** and **C** from Kee, J. L., Hayes, E. R., & McCuistion, L. E. [2015]. *Pharmacology: a patient-centered nursing process approach.* 8th ed., Philadelphia: Elsevier.)

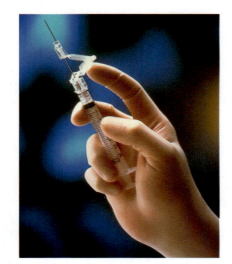

Figure 9-4 BD SafetyGlide™ needle. (From Becton, Dickinson and Company, Franklin Lakes, N.J.)

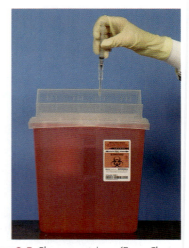

Figure 9-5 Sharps container. (From Clayton, B. D., & Willihnganz, M. J. [2013]. *Basic pharmacology for nurses,* 16th ed., St. Louis: Elsevier.)

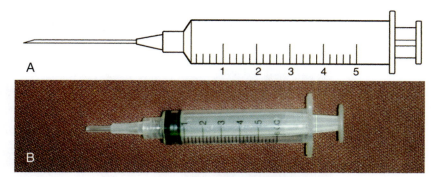

Figure 9-6 Five-milliliter syringes. **A,** 5-mL syringe with 0.2-mL markings. **B,** Needleless 5-mL syringe that can penetrate a rubber-top vial. (**B** from Kee, J. L., Hayes, E. R., & McCuistion, L. E. [2015]. *Pharmacology: a patient-centered nursing process approach.* 8th ed., Philadelphia: Elsevier.)

Five-Milliliter Syringe

The 5-mL syringe is calibrated in 0.2 mL increments. A 5-mL syringe usually is used when the fluid needed is more than 2½ mL. This syringe is frequently used to draw up appropriate solution to dilute the dry form of a drug in a vial because the volume needed for reconstitution is generally more than $2^1/_2$ mL. Figure 9-6 shows the 5-mL syringe and its markings and the 5-mL needleless syringe.

Tuberculin Syringe

The tuberculin syringe is a 1-mL slender syringe that is calibrated in tenths (0.1 mL), hundredths (0.01 mL), and minims (Figure 9-7). This syringe is used when the amount of drug solution to be administered is less than 1 mL and for pediatric and heparin dosages. The tuberculin syringe is also available in a $^1/_2$-milliliter (mL) syringe. Figure 9-8 shows the ½-mL and the 1-mL tuberculin syringes.

Pre-filled Drug Cartridge and Syringe

Many injectable drugs are packaged in pre-filled disposable cartridges. The disposable cartridge is placed into a reusable metal or plastic holder. A pre-filled cartridge usually contains 0.1 to 0.2 mL of excess drug solution. On the basis of the amount of drug to be administered, the excess solution must be expelled before administration. Injectables are also supplied by pharmaceutical companies in ready-to-use

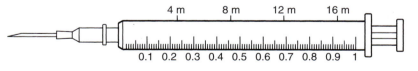

Figure 9-7 Tuberculin syringe.

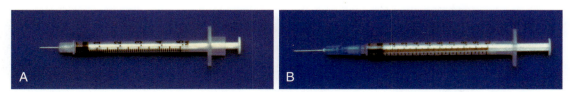

Figure 9-8 Two types of tuberculin syringes: **A,** ½-mL tuberculin syringe with a permanently attached needle. **B,** 1-mL tuberculin syringe with a detachable needle. (From Becton, Dickinson and Company, Franklin Lakes, N.J.)

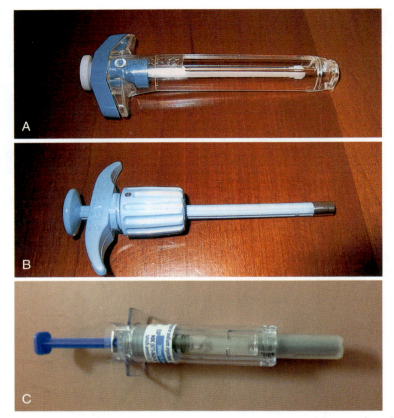

Figure 9-9 **A,** Carpuject syringe. **B,** Tubex syringe. (From Kee, J. L., Hayes, E. R., & McCuistion, L. E. [2015]. *Pharmacology: a patient-centered nursing process approach.* 8th ed., Elsevier: Saunders.) **C,** Lovenox syringe.

pre-filled syringes that do not require a holder. Figure 9-9, *A*, shows a Carpuject syringe. Figure 9-9, *B*, shows a Tubex syringe. Figure 9-9, *C*, shows a pre-filled Lovenox syringe.

Needles

A needle consists of (1) a hub (large metal or plastic part attached to the tip of the syringe), (2) a shaft (thin needle length), and (3) a bevel (end of the needle). Figure 9-10 shows the parts of a needle.

Needle size is determined by gauge (diameter of the shaft) and by length. The larger the gauge number, the smaller the diameter of the lumen. The smaller the gauge number, the larger the diameter of the lumen. The usual range of needle gauges is from 18 to 26. Needle length varies from $\frac{3}{8}$ inch to 2 inches. Table 9-1 lists the sizes and lengths of needles used in intradermal, subcutaneous, and intramuscular injections.

When choosing the needle length for an intramuscular injection, the nurse must consider the size of the patient and the amount of fatty tissue. A patient with minimal fatty tissue may need a needle length of 1 inch. For an obese patient, the length of the needle for an intramuscular injection may be $1\frac{1}{2}$ to 2 inches.

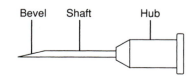

Figure 9-10 Parts of a needle. (From Kee, J. L., Hayes, E. R., & McCuistion, L. E. [2015]. *Pharmacology: a patient-centered nursing process approach.* 8th ed., Philadelphia: Elsevier.)

TABLE 9-1 Needle Size and Length		
Type of Injection	**Needle Gauge**	**Needle Lengths (inch)**
Intradermal	25, 26	$^3/_8$, $^1/_2$, $^5/_8$
Subcutaneous	23, 25, 26	$^3/_8$, $^1/_2$, $^5/_8$
Intramuscular	19, 20, 21, 22	1, 1$^1/_2$, 2

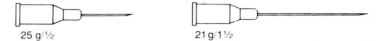

25 g/$^1/_2$ 21 g/1$^1/_2$

Figure 9-11 Two combinations of needle gauge and length.

Pre-filled cartridges have permanently attached needles. With other syringes, needle sizes can be changed. Needle gauge and length are indicated on the syringe package or on the top cover of the syringe. These values appear as gauge/length, such as 21 g/1½ inch. Figure 9-11 shows two types of needle gauge and length.

Research has shown that after an injection, medication remains in the hub of the syringe, where the needle joins the syringe. This volume can be as much as 0.2 mL. There is controversy as to whether air should be added to the syringe before administration to ensure that the total volume is given. The best practice is to follow the institution's policy.

Angles for Injection

For injections, the needle enters the skin at different angles. Intradermal injections are given at a 10- to 15-degree angle; subcutaneous injections, at a 45- to 90-degree angle; and intramuscular injections, at a 90-degree angle. Figure 9-12 shows the angles for intradermal, subcutaneous, and intramuscular injections.

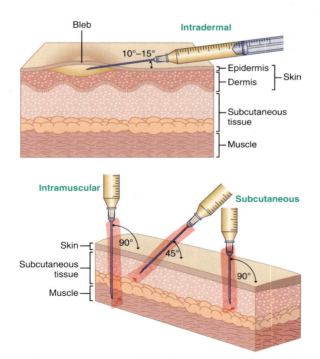

Figure 9-12 Angles of injection. (From Kee, J. L., Hayes, E. R., & McCuistion, L. E. [2015]. *Pharmacology: a patient-centered nursing process approach.*. 8th ed., Philadelphia: Elsevier.)

Answers can be found on page 179.

1. Which would have the larger needle lumen: a 21-gauge needle or a 25-gauge needle?

   _____

2. Which would have the smaller needle lumen: an 18-gauge needle or a 26-gauge needle?

   _____

3. Which needle would have a length of 1½ inches: a 20-gauge needle or a 25-gauge needle?

   _____

4. Which needle would have a length of ⅝ inch: a 21-gauge needle or a 25-gauge needle?

   _____

5. Which needle would be used for an intramuscular injection: a 21-gauge needle with a 1½-inch length or a 25-gauge needle with a ⅝-inch length?

   _____

INTRADERMAL INJECTIONS

Intradermal injections are shallow and designed to deliver medication between the dermis and epidermis. Usually, an intradermal injection is used for skin testing. Primary uses are for tuberculin and allergy testing. The tuberculin syringe (25 g/½ inch) holds 1 mL (16 minims) and is calibrated in 0.1 to 0.01 mL.

The inner aspect of the forearm is often used for diagnostic testing because there is less hair in the area and the test results are easily seen. The upper back can also be used as a testing site. The needle is inserted with the bevel upward at a 10- to 15-degree angle. Do not aspirate. The injected fluid creates a wheal or bleb that is slowly absorbed. For allergy testing, results are usually read in minutes to 24 hours after the injection. For tuberculin testing, results are read 48 to 72 hours after the injection. A reddened or raised hardened area, called the area of induration, indicates a positive reaction.

SUBCUTANEOUS INJECTIONS

Drugs injected into the subcutaneous (fatty) tissue are absorbed slowly because there are fewer blood vessels in the fatty tissue. The amount of drug solution administered subcutaneously is generally 0.5 to 1 mL at a 45-, 60-, or 90-degree angle. Irritating drug solutions are given intramuscularly because they could cause sloughing of the subcutaneous tissue.

The two types of syringes used for subcutaneous injection are the tuberculin syringe (1 mL), which is calibrated in 0.1 and 0.01 mL, and the 3-mL syringe, which is calibrated in 0.1 mL (Figure 9-13). The needle gauge commonly used is 25 or 26 gauge, and the length is usually ⅜ to ⅝ inch. Insulin is also administered subcutaneously and is discussed in Chapter 10.

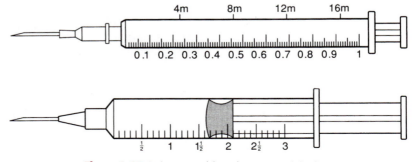

Figure 9-13 Syringes used for subcutaneous injections.

Calculations for Subcutaneous Injections

Types of formulas for calculating small dosages include the following: (1) basic formula, (2) ratio and proportion, (3) fractional equation, and (4) dimensional analysis (see Chapter 6).

EXAMPLES   **PROBLEM 1:**   Order: heparin 5000 units, subcut.
Drug available:

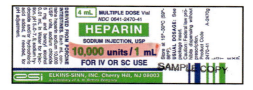

Methods:

Basic formula (BF)

$$\frac{D}{H} \times V = \frac{5000 \text{ units}}{10{,}000 \text{ units}} \times 1 \text{ mL} = \frac{5}{10} = 0.5 \text{ mL}$$

or

Ratio and proportion (RP)

$$H \quad : \quad V \quad :: \quad D \quad : \quad X$$
$$10{,}000 \text{ units} : 1 \text{ mL} :: 5000 \text{ units} : X \text{ mL}$$

$$10{,}000 \, X = 5000$$

$$X = \frac{5000}{10{,}000} = \frac{5}{10} = 0.5 \text{ mL}$$

or

Fractional equation (FE)

$$\text{FE:} \frac{H}{V} = \frac{D}{X} = \frac{10{,}000 \text{ units}}{1 \text{ mL}} = \frac{5000 \text{ units}}{X} =$$

$$(\text{Cross multiply}) \; 10{,}000 \, X = 5000$$

$$X = 0.5 \text{ mL}$$

or

Dimensional analysis (DA)

$$V = \frac{V \times C(H) \times D}{H \times C(D) \times 1}$$

$$\text{mL} = \frac{1 \text{ mL} \times \overset{1}{5000} \text{ units}}{\underset{2}{10{,}000} \text{ units} \times \quad 1} = \frac{1}{2} \text{ or } 0.5 \text{ mL}$$

Answer: heparin 5000 units = 0.5 mL

PROBLEM 2:   Order: morphine 10 mg, subcut.
Drug available:

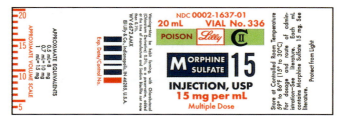

See label with approximate equivalents.

Methods: BF: $\dfrac{D}{H} \times V = \dfrac{10 \text{ mg}}{15 \text{ mg}} \times 1 \text{ mL} = \dfrac{2}{3} = 0.67 \text{ mL or } 0.7 \text{ mL (round off in tenths)}$

or

RP: H : V :: D : X
  15 mg : 1 mL :: 10 mg : X mL

$$15 X = 10$$

$$X = \dfrac{\overset{2}{\cancel{10}}}{\underset{3}{\cancel{15}}} = \dfrac{2}{3} = 0.67 \text{ mL or } 0.7 \text{ mL}$$

or

FE: $\dfrac{H}{V} = \dfrac{D}{X} = \dfrac{15 \text{ mg}}{1 \text{ mL}} = \dfrac{10 \text{ mg}}{X} =$

(Cross multiply) $15 X = 10$

$$X = \dfrac{10}{15} = \dfrac{2}{3} =$$

0.67 or 0.7 mL

or

DA: no conversion factor

$$mL = \dfrac{1 \text{ mL} \times \overset{2}{\cancel{10} \text{ mg}}}{\underset{3}{\cancel{15} \text{ mg}} \times 1} = \dfrac{2}{3} \text{ or } 0.7 \text{ mL}$$

Answer: morphine 10 mg = 0.67 or 0.7 mL (use a tuberculin syringe or a 3-mL syringe). (Round off in tenths.)

PRACTICE PROBLEMS ▶ II SUBCUTANEOUS INJECTIONS

Answers can be found on pages 179 to 181.

Use the formula you chose for calculating oral drug dosages in Chapter 8.

Note: Answers should be rounded off in tenths or whole numbers.

1. Which needle gauge and length should be used for a subcutaneous injection:

 a. 25 g/⅝ inch or 26 g/⅜ inch? _____

2. Order: heparin 4000 units, subcut.
 Drug available:

 a. How many milliliters of heparin would you give? _____

 b. At what angle would you administer the drug? _____

3. Order: heparin 7500 units, subcut.
 Drug available:

How many milliliters of heparin would you give? _____

4. Order: Lovenox (enoxaparin sodium) 30 mg, subcut, q12h. Lovenox is a low-molecular-weight heparin (LMWH).
   Drug available:

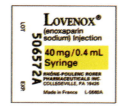

   How many milliliters would you give? _____

5. Order: atropine sulfate 0.6 mg, subcut.
   Drug available:

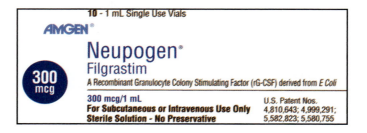

   How many milliliters of atropine would you give? _____

6. Order: epoetin alfa (Epogen) 50 units/kg, subcut.
   Drug available: Epogen 10,000 units/mL.
   Patient weighs 65 kg.

   a. What is the correct dosage? _____

   b. How many milliliters would you give? _____

7. Order: filgrastim (Neupogen) 6 mcg/kg, subcut, bid.
   Drug available:

   Patient weighs 198 pounds.

   a. How many kilograms does the patient weigh? _____

   b. How many micrograms (mcg) would you give? _____

   c. How many milliliters would you give? _____

   d. Explain how the drug should be drawn up. _____

8. Order: enoxaparin (Lovenox) 1 mg/kg, subcut, q12h, for 3 days (treatment of deep vein thrombosis [DVT]).
Drug available: Lovenox in pre-filled syringes: 40 mg per 0.4 mL; 60 mg per 0.6 mL; 80 mg per 0.8 mL.
Patient weighs: 70 kg

a. Which Lovenox dosage would you select? _____

b. How many milliliters should the patient receive? _____

9. Order: morphine 8 mg, subcut, × 1 dose.
Drug available:

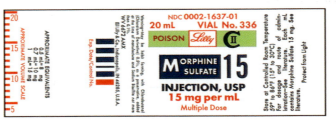

How many milliliters would the patient receive? _____

10. Order: Fragmin 120 units/kg, subcut, q12h.
Drug available:

Patient weighs 165 kg.

a. How many international units (IU) would the patient receive per dose? _____

b. How many milliliters would the patient receive per dose? _____

INTRAMUSCULAR INJECTIONS

The IM injection is a common method of administering injectable drugs. The muscle has many blood vessels (more than fatty tissue), so medications given by IM injection are absorbed more rapidly than those given by subcutaneous injection. The volume of solution for an IM injection is 0.5 to 3.0 mL, with the average being 1 to 2 mL. A volume of drug solution greater than 3 mL causes increased muscle tissue displacement and possible tissue damage. Occasionally, 5 mL of certain drugs, such as magnesium sulfate, may be injected into a large muscle, such as the ventrogluteal. Dosages greater than 3 mL are usually divided and are given at two different sites.

Needle gauges for IM injections containing thick solutions are 19 gauge and 20 gauge, and for thin solutions, 20 gauge to 21 gauge. IM injections are administered at a 90-degree angle. The needle length depends on the amount of adipose (fat) and muscle tissue; the average needle length is 1½ inches.

The *Z*-track injection technique delivers medication intramuscularly in a method that prevents the drug from leaking back into the subcutaneous tissue (Figure 9-14). This method is ordered for medications that could cause irritation to the subcutaneous tissue or discoloration to the skin. When preparing the medication, a needle change is made after the drug has been drawn up into the syringe and before it is injected into the patient. The large gluteal muscle is frequently used for *Z*-track injections.

Common sites for IM injections are the deltoid, dorsogluteal, ventrogluteal, and vastus lateralis muscles. Figure 9-15 displays the sites for each muscle used with IM injection. Table 9-2 gives the volume for drug administration, common needle size, patient's position, and angle of injection for the four IM injection sites.

> **Note:** Some institutions may prohibit using the dorsogluteal for intramuscular injections due to the close proximity of the sciatic nerve to the injection site. Always check institutional policy and procedures.

Drug Solutions for Injection

Commercially premixed drug solutions are stored in vials and ampules for immediate use. At times, enough drug solution may be left in a vial for another dose, and the vial may be saved. The balance of a drug solution in an ampule is *always* discarded after the ampule has been opened and used.

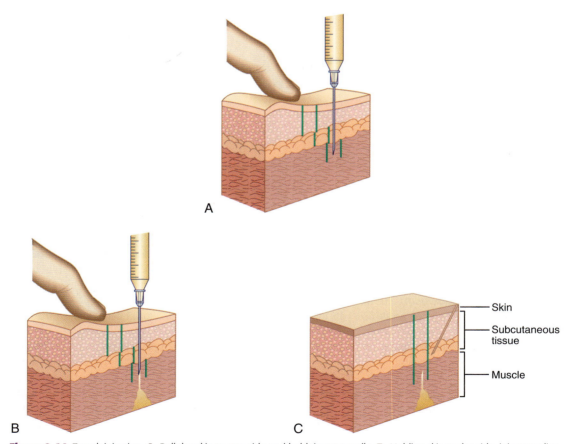

Skin

Subcutaneous tissue

Muscle

Figure 9-14 Z-track injection. **A,** Pull the skin to one side and hold; insert needle. **B,** Holding skin to the side, inject medication. **C,** Withdraw needle and release skin. This technique prevents medication from entering subcutaneous tissue. (From Kee, J. L., Hayes, E. R., & McCuistion, L. E. [2015]. *Pharmacology: a patient-centered nursing process approach.,* 8th ed., Philadelphia:Elsevier).

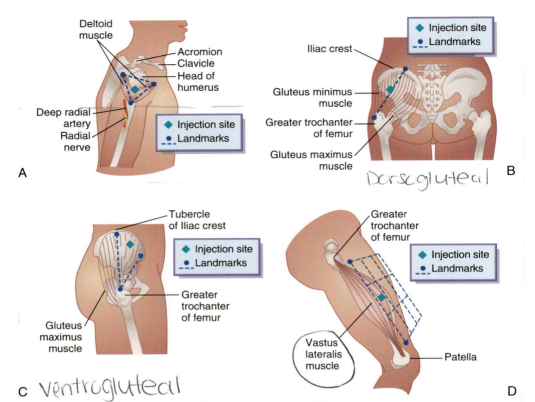

Figure 9-15 Intramuscular injection sites. **A,** Deltoid. **B,** Dorsogluteal. **C,** Ventrogluteal. **D,** Vastus lateralis. (From Kee, J. L., Hayes, E. R., & McCuistion, L. E. [2015]. *Pharmacology: a patient-centered nursing process approach.,* 8th ed., Philadelphia: Elsevier).

TABLE 9-2 Intramuscular Injection Sites in the Adult

	Deltoid	Dorsogluteal	Ventrogluteal	Vastus Lateralis
Volume for drug administration	*Usual:* 0.5 to 1 mL *Maximum:* 2.0 mL	*Usual:* 1.0 to 3 mL *Maximum:* 3 mL; 5 mL gamma globulin	*Usual:* 1 to 3 mL *Maximum:* 3 to 4 mL	*Usual:* 1 to 3 mL *Maximum:* 3 to 4 mL
Common needle size	23 to 25 gauge; $5/8$ to $1\frac{1}{2}$ inches	18 to 23 gauge; $1\frac{1}{4}$ to 3 inches	20 to 23 gauge; $1\frac{1}{4}$ to $2\frac{1}{2}$ inches	20 to 23 gauge; $1\frac{1}{4}$ to $1\frac{1}{2}$ inches
Patient's position	Sitting; supine; prone	Prone	Supine; lateral	Sitting (dorsiflex foot); supine
Angle of injection	90-degree angle, angled slightly toward the acromion	90-degree angle to flat surface; upper outer quadrant of the buttock *or* outer aspect of line from the posterior iliac crest to the greater trochanter of the femur	80- to 90-degree angle; angle the needle slightly toward the iliac crest	80- to 90-degree angle For thin person: 60- to 75-degree angle

EXAMPLES Here are two problems for calculating IM dosage, using all four methods and rounded to the nearest tenths.

PROBLEM 1: Order: gentamycin (Garamycin) 60 mg, IM, q12h.
Drug available:

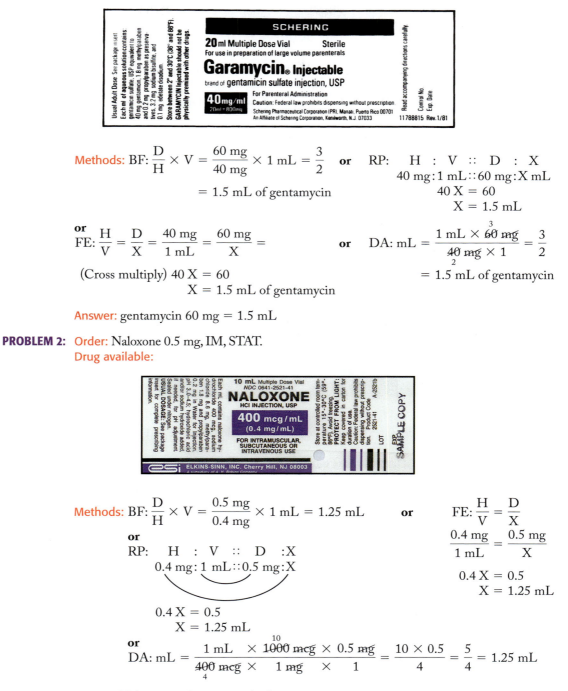

Methods: BF: $\dfrac{D}{H} \times V = \dfrac{60 \text{ mg}}{40 \text{ mg}} \times 1 \text{ mL} = \dfrac{3}{2}$ or   RP: $\begin{array}{ccccc} H & : & V & :: & D & : & X \\ 40 \text{ mg} & : & 1 \text{ mL} & :: & 60 \text{ mg} & : & X \text{ mL} \end{array}$

$= 1.5 \text{ mL of gentamycin}$ $40\,X = 60$
$X = 1.5 \text{ mL}$

or
FE: $\dfrac{H}{V} = \dfrac{D}{X} = \dfrac{40 \text{ mg}}{1 \text{ mL}} = \dfrac{60 \text{ mg}}{X} =$ or   DA: mL $= \dfrac{1 \text{ mL} \times \overset{3}{\cancel{60 \text{ mg}}}}{\underset{2}{\cancel{40 \text{ mg}}} \times 1} = \dfrac{3}{2}$

(Cross multiply) $40\,X = 60$ $= 1.5 \text{ mL of gentamycin}$
$X = 1.5 \text{ mL of gentamycin}$

Answer: gentamycin 60 mg $= 1.5$ mL

PROBLEM 2: Order: Naloxone 0.5 mg, IM, STAT.
Drug available:

Methods: BF: $\dfrac{D}{H} \times V = \dfrac{0.5 \text{ mg}}{0.4 \text{ mg}} \times 1 \text{ mL} = 1.25 \text{ mL}$ or   FE: $\dfrac{H}{V} = \dfrac{D}{X}$

or
RP: $\begin{array}{ccccc} H & : & V & :: & D & : & X \\ 0.4 \text{ mg} & : & 1 \text{ mL} & :: & 0.5 \text{ mg} & : & X \end{array}$ $\dfrac{0.4 \text{ mg}}{1 \text{ mL}} = \dfrac{0.5 \text{ mg}}{X}$

$0.4\,X = 0.5$
$X = 1.25 \text{ mL}$

$0.4\,X = 0.5$
$X = 1.25 \text{ mL}$

or
DA: mL $= \dfrac{1 \text{ mL} \times \overset{10}{\cancel{1000 \text{ mcg}}} \times 0.5 \text{ mg}}{\underset{4}{\cancel{400 \text{ mcg}}} \times 1 \text{ mg} \times 1} = \dfrac{10 \times 0.5}{4} = \dfrac{5}{4} = 1.25 \text{ mL}$

Answer: Naloxone 0.5 mg $= 1.25$ mL

Reconstitution of Powdered Drugs

Certain drugs lose their potency in liquid form. Therefore manufacturers package these drugs in powdered form, and they are reconstituted before administration. To reconstitute a drug, look on the drug label or in the drug information insert (circular or pamphlet) for the type and amount of diluent to use. Sterile water, bacteriostatic water, and normal saline solution are the primary diluents. If the type and amount of diluent are not specified on the drug label or in the drug information insert, call the pharmacy.

The powdered drug occupies space and therefore increases the volume of drug solution. Usually, manufacturers determine the amount of diluent to mix with the drug powder to yield 1 to 2 mL per desired dose. After the powdered drug has been reconstituted, the unused drug solution should be dated, initialed, and refrigerated. Most drugs retain their potency for 48 hours to 1 week when refrigerated. Check the drug information insert or drug label to see how long the reconstituted drug may be used.

EXAMPLES PROBLEM 1: Order: Tazicef 500 mg, IM, q8h.
Drug available:

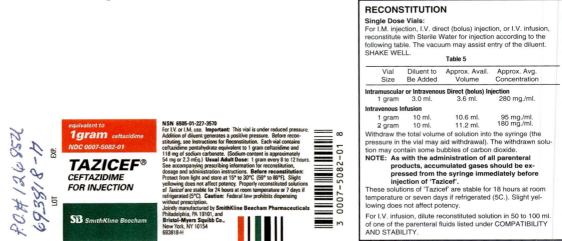

According to the label, the amount of powdered drug is 1 g. The drug label states for IM injection add 3 mL of sterile water (diluent) to the vial to yield a volume of 1 g/3.6 mL or 280 mg/mL.

Note: the diluent amount is different for IM versus IV formulation.

Milligrams

BF: $\dfrac{D}{H} \times V = \dfrac{500 \text{ mg}}{280 \text{ mg}} \times 1 \text{ mL} = 1.78 \text{ mL}$ **or**   RP: H : V :: D :X

or 1.8 mL

$$280 \text{ mg} : 1 \text{ mL} :: 500 \text{ mg} : X$$
$$280 X = 500$$
$$X = 1.78 \text{ mL or } 1.8 \text{ mL}$$

Grams

DA: $mL = \dfrac{3.6 \text{ mL} \times \quad \overset{1}{\cancel{1 \text{ g}}} \quad \times \overset{1}{\cancel{500 \text{ mg}}}}{\cancel{1 \text{ g}} \quad \times \underset{2}{\cancel{1000 \text{ mg}}} \times \quad 1} = \dfrac{3.6}{2}$ **or**   FE: $\dfrac{H}{V} = \dfrac{D}{X} = \dfrac{280 \text{ mg}}{1 \text{ mL}} = \dfrac{500 \text{ mg}}{X}$

$= 1.8 \text{ mL}$

(Cross multiply)
$$280 X = 500$$
$$X = 1.78 \text{ mL}$$
$$\text{or } 1.8 \text{ mL}$$

Answer: Tazicef 500 mg = 1.8 mL

PROBLEM 2: Order: methylprednisolone 250 mg IM × 1 dose.
Drug available:

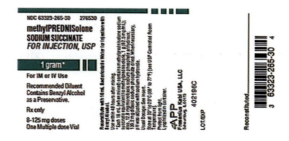

The drug label says to add 16 mL bacteriostatic water to reconstitute 1 g of methylprednisolone.

Change grams to milligrams (1 g = 1000 mg).

BF: $\dfrac{D}{H} \times V = \dfrac{250 \text{ mg}}{1000 \text{ mg}} \times 16 \text{ mL} = 4 \text{ mL}$ **or**   RP: $\text{H}\ :\ \text{V}\ ::\ \text{D}\ :\text{X}$
$$1000 \text{ mg}:16 \text{ mg}::250 \text{ mg}:\text{X}$$
$$1000 \text{ X} = 4000$$
$$\text{X} = 4 \text{ mL}$$

FE: $\dfrac{H}{V} = \dfrac{D}{X}$ **or**   DA: mL $= \dfrac{16 \text{ mL} \times \quad \overset{1}{\cancel{1\text{g}}} \quad \times \overset{1}{\cancel{250 \text{ mg}}}}{\underset{4}{\cancel{1\text{g}}} \times \cancel{1000 \text{ mg}} \times \quad 1} = \dfrac{16}{4} = 4 \text{ mL}$

$$\dfrac{1000 \text{ mg}}{16 \text{ mL}} = \dfrac{250 \text{ mg}}{X}$$

$$1000 \text{ X} = 4000$$
$$\text{X} = 4 \text{ mL}$$

Answer: methylprednisolone 250 mg = 4 mL. Since the volume of the ordered drug is greater than 3 mL, the dose should be divided into 2 mL per injection site.

MIXING OF INJECTABLE DRUGS

Drugs mixed together in the same syringe must be compatible to prevent precipitation. To determine drug compatibility, check drug references or check with a pharmacist. When in doubt about compatibility, do *not* mix drugs.

The three methods of drug mixing are (1) mixing two drugs in the same syringe from two vials, (2) mixing two drugs in the same syringe from one vial and one ampule, and (3) mixing two drugs in a pre-filled cartridge from a vial.

▶ Method 1
Mixing Two Drugs in the Same Syringe From Two Vials
1. Draw air into the syringe to equal the amount of solution to be withdrawn from the first vial, and inject the air into the first vial. Do *not* allow the needle to come into contact with the solution. Remove the needle.
2. Draw air into the syringe to equal the amount of solution to be withdrawn from the second vial. Invert the second vial and inject the air.
3. Withdraw the desired amount of solution from the second vial.
4. Change the needle unless you will use the entire volume in the first vial.
5. Invert the first vial and withdraw the desired amount of solution.

or

1. Draw air into the syringe to equal the amount of solution to be withdrawn, and inject the air into the first vial. Withdraw the desired drug dose.
2. Insert a 25-gauge needle into the rubber top (not in the center) of the second vial. This acts as an air vent. Injecting air into the second vial is *not* necessary.
3. Insert the needle in the center of the rubber-top vial (beside the 25-g needle–air vent), invert the second vial, and withdraw the desired drug dose.

▶ Method 2
Mixing Two Drugs in the Same Syringe From One Vial and One Ampule (same "prep" as Method 1).
1. Remove the amount of desired solution from the vial.
2. Aspirate the amount of desired solution from the ampule.

▶ Method 3
Mixing Two Drugs in a Pre-filled Cartridge From a Vial
1. Check the drug dose and the amount of solution in the pre-filled cartridge. If a smaller dose is needed, expel the excess solution.
2. Draw air into the cartridge to equal the amount of solution to be withdrawn from the vial. Invert the vial and inject the air.
3. Withdraw the desired amount of solution from the vial. Make sure the needle remains in the fluid and do *not* take more solution than needed.

EXAMPLES Mixing drugs in the same syringe.

PROBLEM 1: Order: meperidine (Demerol) 60 mg and atropine sulfate 0.4 mg IM.
The two drugs are compatible.
Drugs available:

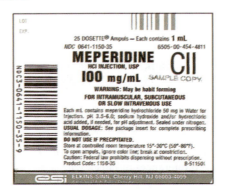

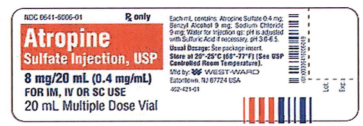

Note: Meperidine is in an ampule and atropine sulfate is in a vial.

How many milliliters of each drug would you give? Explain how to mix the two drugs.

Methods: meperidine

$$BF: \frac{D}{H} \times V = \frac{60 \text{ mg}}{100 \text{ mg}} \times 1 \text{ mL} = 0.6 \text{ mL}$$

or

RP: H : V :: D : X
      100 mg : 1 mL :: 60 mg : X mL
      100 X = 60
          X = 0.6 mL

or

$$FE: \frac{H}{V} = \frac{D}{X} = \frac{100 \text{ mg}}{1 \text{ mL}} = \frac{60 \text{ mg}}{X}$$

(Cross multiply) 100 X = 60
                     X = 0.6 mL

or

DA: no conversion factor

$$mL = \frac{1 \text{ mL} \times 60 \text{ mg}}{100 \text{ mg} \times 1} = \frac{60}{100} = 0.6 \text{ mL}$$

atropine SO_4 = 0.4 mg

Answer: meperidine (Demerol) 60 mg = 0.6 mL
        atropine 0.4 mg = 1 mL

Procedure: Mix two drugs in a syringe for IM injection:
1. Remove 1 mL of atropine solution from the vial.
2. Withdraw 0.6 mL of meperidine (Demerol) from the ampule into the syringe containing atropine solution.
3. Syringe contains atropine 1 mL and meperidine 0.6 mL = total 1.6 mL.

PROBLEM 2: Order: meperidine 25 mg, Vistaril 25 mg, and Robinul 0.1 mg, IM. All three drugs are compatible.
Drugs available: meperidine (Demerol) is in a 2-mL Tubex cartridge labeled 50 mg/mL. Hydroxyzine (Vistaril) is in a 50-mg/mL ampule. Glycopyrrolate (Robinul) is available in a 0.2-mg/mL vial.

How many milliliters of each drug would you give?
Explain how the drugs could be mixed together.
Methods:
a. meperidine 25 mg. Label: 50 mg/mL.

$$BF: \frac{D}{H} \times V = \frac{25 \text{ mg}}{50 \text{ mg}} \times 1 \text{ mL} = 0.5 \text{ mL}$$

or

RP: H : V :: D : X
      50 mg : 1 mL :: 25 mg : X mL
          50 X = 25
              X = ½ mL or 0.5 mL

or

$$FE: \frac{H}{V} = \frac{D}{X} = \frac{50 \text{ mg}}{1 \text{ mL}} = \frac{25 \text{ mg}}{X}$$

(Cross multiply) 50 X = 25
                     X = 0.5 mL

or

$$DA: mL = \frac{1 \text{ mL} \times \overset{1}{25} \text{ mg}}{\underset{2}{50} \text{ mg} \times 1} = \frac{1}{2} \text{ mL or 0.5 mL meperidine}$$

b. Vistaril 25 mg. Label: 50 mg/mL ampule.

$$BF: \frac{D}{H} \times V = \frac{25 \text{ mg}}{50 \text{ mg}} \times 1 \text{ mL} = 0.5 \text{ mL}$$

or

RP: H : V :: D : X
50 mg : 1 mL :: 25 mg : X mL
$$50\,X = 25$$
$$X = \tfrac{1}{2}\text{ mL or } 0.5\text{ mL}$$

or

FE: $\dfrac{H}{V} = \dfrac{D}{X} = \dfrac{50\text{ mg}}{1\text{ mL}} = \dfrac{25\text{ mg}}{X}$
$$50\,X = 25$$
$$X = 0.5\text{ mL}$$

c. Robinul 0.1 mg. Label: 0.2 mg/mL.

BF: $\dfrac{D}{H} \times V = \dfrac{0.1\text{ mg}}{0.2\text{ mg}} \times 1\text{ mL} = 0.5\text{ mL Robinul}$

or

FE: $\dfrac{H}{V} = \dfrac{D}{X} = \dfrac{0.2\text{ mg}}{1\text{ mL}} = \dfrac{0.1\text{ mg}}{X}$
$$0.2\,X = 0.1$$
$$X = 0.5\text{ mL}$$

or

RP: H : V :: D : X
0.2 mg : 1 mL :: 0.1 mg : X mL
$$0.2\,X = 0.1$$
$$X = 0.5\text{ mL}$$

or

DA: mL $= \dfrac{1\text{ mL} \times 0.1\text{ mg}}{0.2\text{ mg} \times 1} = \dfrac{0.1}{0.2} = \dfrac{1}{2}\text{ or } 0.5\text{ mL}$

Answer: meperidine (Demerol) 25 mg = 0.5 mL; Vistaril 25 mg = 0.5 mL; Robinul 0.1 mg = 0.5 mL

Procedure: Mix three drugs in the cartridge:
1. Check drug dose and volume on pre-filled cartridge. Expel 0.5 mL of meperidine and any excess of drug solution from cartridge.
2. Draw 0.5 mL of air into the cartridge and inject into the vial containing the Robinul.
3. Withdraw 0.5 mL of Robinul from the vial into the pre-filled cartridge containing meperidine.
4. Withdraw 0.5 mL of Vistaril from the ampule into the cartridge.

PRACTICE PROBLEMS ▶ **III INTRAMUSCULAR INJECTIONS**

Answers can be found on pages 181 to 187.

Round off to the nearest tenths.

1. **Order:** tobramycin (Nebcin) 50 mg, IM, q8h.
   Drug available:

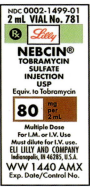

How many milliliters of tobramycin would you give? _____

2. Order: methylprednisolone (Solu-Medrol) 75 mg, IM, daily.
Drug available: 125 mg/2 mL in vial.

How many milliliters would you give? _____

3. Order: vitamin B$_{12}$ (cyanocobalamin) 300 mcg, IM, daily.
Drug available:

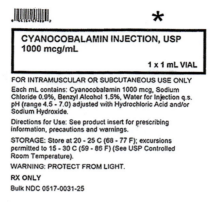

How many milliliters of cyanocobalamin would you give? _____

4. Order: naloxone 0.2 mg, IM, STAT.
Drug available:

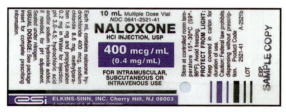

How many milliliters would you give? _____

5. Order: diazepam 4 mg, IM, q6h.
Drug available:

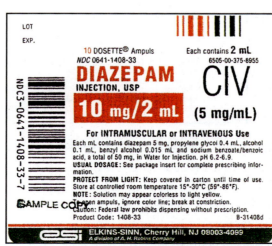

How many milliliters would you give? _____

6. **Order:** cefepime HCl (Maxipime) 500 mg, IM, q12h.
   Drug available:

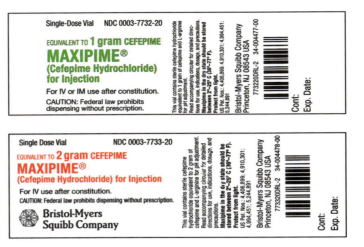

   a. Which single-dose vial of Maxipime would you select? _____

   Explain. _____

   b. How many milliliters (mL) of diluent should you use for reconstitution of the drug?

   _____

   > **Note:** The drug label does not indicate the amount of diluent to use. This may be found in the drug information insert. Usually, if you inject 2.6 mL of diluent, the amount of drug solution may be 3.0 mL. If you inject 3.4 or 3.5 mL of diluent, the amount of drug solution should be 4.0 mL.

   c. How many milliliters of drug solution should the patient receive? _____

7. **Order:** prochlorperazine (Compazine) 4 mg, IM, q8h, as needed.
   Drug available:

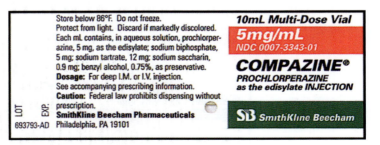

   How many milliliters should the patient receive? _____

8. **Order:** secobarbital (Seconal) 125 mg, IM, 1 hour before surgery.
   Drug available: Seconal 50 mg/mL.

   How many milliliters would you give? _____

9. Order: thiamine HCl 75 mg, IM, daily.
Drug available: 100 and 200 mg/mL vials.

    a. Which vial would you use? _____

    b. How many milliliters would you give? _____

10. Order: hydroxyzine (Vistaril) 25 mg, deep IM, STAT.
Drug available: Vistaril 100 mg/2 mL in a vial.

How many milliliters would you give? _____

11. Order: loxapine HCl (Loxitane) 25 mg, IM, q6h until desired response and then 50 mg.
Drug available:

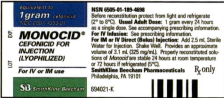

How many milliliters would you administer intramuscularly for the initial dose? _____

12. Order: penicillin G potassium (Pfizerpen) 250,000 units, IM, q6h.
Drug available:

    a. Select the appropriate dilution for the ordered dose. How many milliliters of diluent would you add? _____

    b. How many milliliters should the patient receive per dose? _____

13. Order: cefonicid (Monocid) 750 mg, IM, daily.
Drug available:

Change grams to milligrams (3 spaces to the right) or milligrams to gram (3 spaces to the left).

$$1.000 \text{ g} = 1000 \text{ mg or } 1000 \text{ mg} = 1 \text{ g}$$

    a. How many gram(s) is 750 mg, IM, daily? _____

    b. How many milliliters of diluent should be injected into the vial (see drug label)? _____

    c. How many milliliters of cefonicid (Monocid) should the patient receive per day? _____

14. Order: meperidine (Demerol) 35 mg and promethazine (Phenergan) 10 mg, IM.
Drugs available: meperidine 50 mg/mL in an ampule; promethazine 25 mg/mL in an ampule.

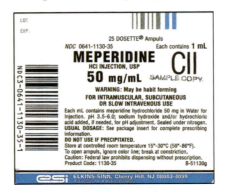

a. How many milliliters of meperidine would you give? _____

b. How many milliliters of promethazine would you give? _____

c. Explain how the two drugs should be mixed. _____

_____

15. Order: meperidine (Demerol) 50 mg and atropine sulfate 0.3 mg, IM.
Drugs available:

a. How many milliliters of meperidine would you give? _____

b. How many milliliters of atropine would you give? _____

c. Explain how the two drugs should be mixed.

_____

16. Order: codeine phosphate 20 mg IM × 1 dose.
Drug available:

How many milliliters would the patient receive? _____

17. Order: heparin 2500 units, subcut, q6h.
Drug available:

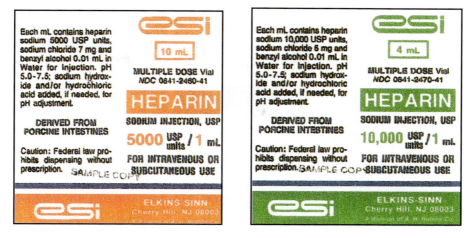

a. Which drug vial would you use? _____

b. How many milliliters of heparin would you give? _____

18. Order: chlordiazepoxide HCl (Librium) 50 mg, IM, STAT.
Drug available: Librium (100 mg) powder in ampule.
Add 2 mL of special intramuscular diluent to the ampule. When diluted, the powder content may increase the volume.

How many milliliters would be equivalent to 50 mg? _____

Explain. _____

19. Order: cefamandole (Mandol) 500 mg, IM, q6h.
Drug available:

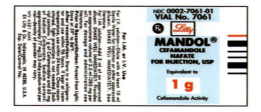

a. Change milligrams to grams (see Chapter 1).

_____

b. How many milliliters of diluent would you add (see drug label)? _____

c. What size syringe would you use? _____

d. How many milliliters should the patient receive? _____

20. Order: ticarcillin (Ticar), 400 mg, IM, q6h.
Drug available:

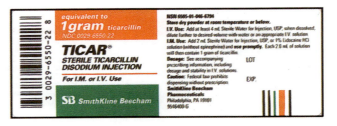

a. Drug label reads to add 2 mL of diluent. Total volume of solution is _____

b. How many milliliters of ticarcillin should be withdrawn? _____

21. Order: morphine 10 mg IM, STAT.
Drug available:

How many milliliters of morphine would you give? _____

22. Order: hydroxyzine (Vistaril) 25 mg, deep IM, q4–6h, PRN for nausea.
Drug available:

How many milliliters should the patient receive per dose? _____

23. Order: Decadron (dexamethasone) 2 mg, IM, q6h.
Adult parameters: 0.75–9 mg/day in 2 to 4 divided doses.
Drug available:

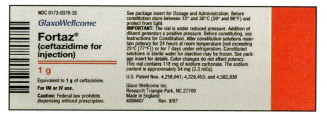

a. Is the dose according to adult parameters? _____

b. How many milliliters would you give? _____

c. What type of syringe could be used? _____

d. Can the Decadron vial be used again? Explain. _____

24. Order: ceftazidime (Fortaz) 500 mg, IM, q8h.
Add 2 mL of diluent = 2.6 mL drug solution. Check the drug information insert.
Drug available:

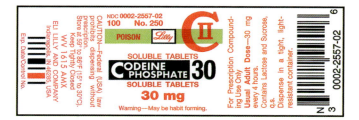

a. How many gram(s) of ceftazidime (Fortaz) should the patient receive per day?

_____

b. How many milliliters of ceftazidime would you give per dose?

_____

25. Order: streptomycin sulfate 1500 mg IM × 1 dose.
Drug available:

Change milligrams to grams or change grams to milligrams
1500 mg = 1.5 g or 5 g = 5000 mg

a. How many milliliters of diluent would you add to the vial? _____

b. How many milliliters would the patient receive? _____

26. Order: diazepam 8 mg, IM, STAT and repeat in 4 hours if necessary.
   Drug available:

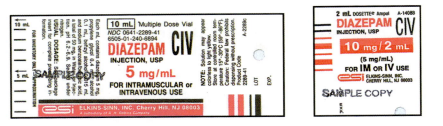

   a. Which ampule or vial of diazepam would you select? _____

   b. How many milliliters (mL) of diazepam should the patient receive? _____

27. Order: benztropine mesylate (Cogentin) 1.5 mg, IM, daily.
   Drug available:

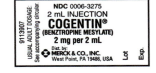

   How many milliliters (mL) of Cogentin should the patient receive?_____

28. Order: cefotaxime Na (Claforan) 750 mg, IM, bid.
   Drug available: Pamphlet states to add 3 mL of diluent equal 3.4 mL.

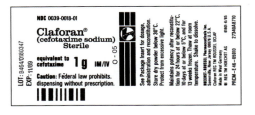

   a. 1 g = _____ mg

   b. How many milligrams should the patient receive per day? _____

   c. How many milliliters would you give per dose? _____

29. Order: diphenhydramine HCl 30 mg, IM, STAT.
   Drug available:

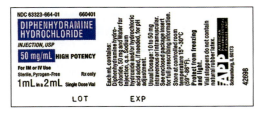

   How many milliliters should the patient receive? _____

30. Order: interferon alfa-2b (Intron A) 10 million international units IM 3 × week.
    Drug available: interferon alfa-2b (Intron A) 25 million international units/5 mL vials.

    How many milliliters would you give per dose? _____

31. Order: vitamin K (AquaMEPHYTON) 2.5 mg IM × 1.
    Drug available:

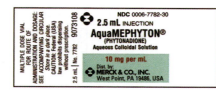

    How many milliliters would you give? _____

32. Order: ampicillin/sulbactam (Unasyn) 1 g, IM, q8h.
    Drug available:
    (add 3.6 mL of diluent to the vial; drug and diluent equals 4 mL)

    a. Unasyn 3 g vial equals _____.

    b. How many milliliters of Unasyn would you give every 8 hours? _____.

Questions 33 through 38 relate to additional dimensional analysis. Refer to Chapter 6.

33. Order: droperidol 2 mg, IM, STAT.
    Drug available: droperidol 5 mg/2 mL.
    Factors: 5 mg/2 mL; 2 mg/1
    Conversion factor: *none;* order and drug are both available in milligrams.

    How many milliliters of droperidol should be given? _____

34. Order: dexamethasone 5 mg, IM, daily.
    Drug available:

    How many milliliters should be administered daily? _____

35. **Order:** levothyroxine (Synthroid) 100 mcg, IM, STAT then 0.025 mg, po, daily.
    Drug available: levothyroxine 200 mcg/mL for IM; levothyroxine 12.5 mcg/tablet, po

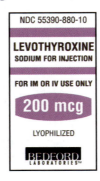

NDC 55390-880-10

LEVOTHYROXINE
SODIUM FOR INJECTION

FOR IM OR IV USE ONLY

200 mcg

LYOPHILIZED

BEDFORD
LABORATORIES™

a. How many milliliters would you give IM? _____

b. How many tablets would you give per dose? _____

36. **Order:** cefobid 500 mg, IM, q6h.
    Add 2 mL of diluent to equal 2.4 mL solution.
    Drug available:

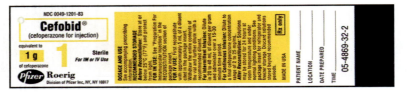

NDC 0049-1201-83

Cefobid®
(cefoperazone for injection)

equivalent to
1 g

1

Sterile
For IM or IV Use

of cefoperazone

Pfizer **Roerig**
Division of Pfizer Inc, NY, NY 10017

05-4869-32-2

a. Cefobid 1 g = _____ mL; 500 mg = _____ mL

   Conversion factor: 1 g = 1000 mg

b. How many milliliters of Cefobid would you give? _____

37. **Order:** ceftriaxone 1000 mg, IM, daily.
    Drug available:

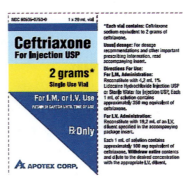

NDC 60505-0753-0   1 x 20 mL vial

Ceftriaxone
For Injection USP

2 grams*
Single Use Vial

For I.M. or I.V. Use
RETAIN IN CARTON UNTIL TIME OF USE

Rx Only

AX **APOTEX CORP.**

*Each vial contains: Ceftriaxone
sodium equivalent to 2 grams of
ceftriaxone.

Usual dosage: For dosage
recommendations and other important
prescribing information, read
accompanying insert.

Directions For Use:
For I.M. Administration:
Reconstitute with 4.2 mL 1%
Lidocaine Hydrochloride Injection USP
or Sterile Water for Injection USP. Each
1 mL of solution contains
approximately 350 mg equivalent of
ceftriaxone.

For I.V. Administration:
Reconstitute with 19.2 mL of an I.V.
diluent specified in the accompanying
package insert.

Each 1 mL of solution contains
approximately 100 mg equivalent of
ceftriaxone. Withdraw entire contents
and dilute to the desired concentration
with the appropriate I.V. diluent.

a. How many milliliters diluent would you add to the vial? _____

b. What is the reconstituted concentration for IM use? _____

c. How many milliliters of ceftriaxone would you give? _____

38. Order: cefazolin (Ancef) 0.25 g, IM, q12h.
Drug available: 2.0 mL of diluent = 2.2 mL

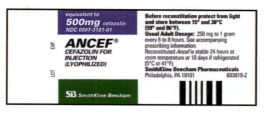

Note: Change grams to milligrams; drug label is in milligrams.

How many milliliters of Ancef would you give? _____

Questions 39 through 42 relate to drug dosage per body weight.

39. Order: amikacin (Amikin) 15 mg/kg/day, q8h, IM.
Drug available:

Patient weighs 140 pounds.

a. How many kilograms does the patient weigh? _____

b. How many milligrams should the patient receive daily? _____

c. How many milligrams should the patient receive q8h (three divided doses)?

_____

d. How many milliliters should the patient receive q8h? _____

40. Order: netilmicin sulfate (Netromycin) 2 mg/kg, q8h, IM.
Patient weighs 174 pounds.
Drug available: netilmicin 100 mg/mL.

a. How many kilograms does the patient weigh? _____

b. How many milligrams should the patient receive daily? _____

c. How many milligrams should the patient receive q8h? _____

d. How many milliliters should the patient receive q8h? _____

41. **Order:** midazolam HCl (Versed) 0.07 mg/kg, IM before general anesthesia.
    Patient weights: 156 pounds.
    Drug available:

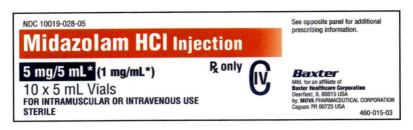

a. How many kilograms does the patient weigh? _____

b. How many milligrams should the patient receive? _____

c. How should midazolam be administered? _____

42. **Order:** Robinul 4 mcg/kg, IM × 1 dose.
    Drug available:

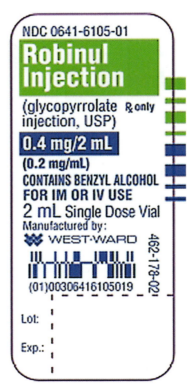

Patient weighs 72 kilograms.

a. How many milligrams should the patient receive? _____

b. How many milliliters should the patient receive? _____

43. Order: Lasix 0.5 mg/kg, IM, bid.
Drug available:

NDC 0517-5704-25
FUROSEMIDE
INJECTION, USP
40 mg/4 mL
(10 mg/mL)

4 mL SINGLE DOSE VIAL
FOR IV OR IM USE
Rx Only
AMERICAN REGENT, INC.
SHIRLEY, NY 11967

Each mL contains: Furosemide 10 mg,
Water for Injection q.s., Sodium Chloride
for isotonicity, Sodium Hydroxide and, if
necessary, Hydrochloric Acid to adjust pH
between 8.0 and 9.3.
WARNING: DISCARD UNUSED PORTION.
USE ONLY IF SOLUTION IS CLEAR AND
COLORLESS. PROTECT FROM LIGHT.
Store at 20° to 25°C (68° to 77°F) (See USP
Controlled Room Temperature).
Directions for Use: See Package Insert.
Rev. 10/10

Lot / Exp.

Patient weighs 130 pounds.

a. How many kilograms does the patient weigh? _____

b. How many milligrams should the patient receive per day? _____

c. How many milligrams should the patient receive every 12 hours? _____

d. How many milliliters per dose should the patient receive? _____

ANSWERS

I Needles

1. The 21-gauge needle because it is the smaller gauge number.
2. The 26-gauge needle because it is the larger gauge number.
3. The 20-gauge needle because it has the larger lumen (smaller gauge). A needle with a 20-gauge and 1½-inch length is used for IM injection.
4. The 25-gauge needle, because it has the smaller lumen (larger gauge). It is used for subcutaneous injections. The needle is not long enough for an IM injection.
5. The 21-gauge needle with 1½-inch length (21 g/1½ inch). Muscle is under subcutaneous or fatty tissue, so a longer needle is needed.

II Subcutaneous Injections

1. *Both* needle gauge and length combinations could be used.
2. **a.** 0.4 mL
   b. 45- to 90-degree angle. The angle depends on the amount of fatty tissue in the patient.
3. ¾ mL or 0.75 mL

4. BF: $\dfrac{D}{H} \times V = \dfrac{\overset{3}{\cancel{30}\ mg}}{\underset{4}{\cancel{40}\ mg}} \times 0.4\ mL = \dfrac{1.2}{4}$

   $= 0.3\ mL$ of Lovenox

   FE: $\dfrac{H}{V} = \dfrac{D}{X} = \dfrac{40\ mg}{0.4\ mg} = \dfrac{30}{X} =$

   (Cross multiply) $40\ X = 12$

   $X = 0.3\ mL$ of Lovenox

   or

   RP: H : V :: D : X
   $40\ mg : 0.4\ mL :: 30\ mg : X\ mL$
   $40\ X = 12$
   $X = 0.3\ mL$

   or

   DA mL $= \dfrac{0.4\ mL \times 30\ \cancel{mg}}{40\ \cancel{mg} \times 1} = \dfrac{12}{40} = 0.3\ mL$

5. BF: $\dfrac{D}{H} \times V = \dfrac{0.6 \text{ mg}}{0.4 \text{ mg}} \times 1 \text{ mL} = \dfrac{0.6}{0.4} = 1.5 \text{ mL}$

or

RP: H : V :: D : X
   0.4 mg : 1 mL :: 0.6 mg : X mL
   0.4 X = 0.6

   $X = \dfrac{0.6}{0.4} = 1.5 \text{ mL}$

or

DA: mL $= \dfrac{1 \text{ mL} \times 0.6 \text{ mg}}{0.4 \text{ mg} \times 1} = \dfrac{0.6}{0.4} = 1.5 \text{ mL}$

6. a. 50 units/kg $\times$ 65 kg = 3250 units

b. $\dfrac{D}{H} \times V = \dfrac{3250 \text{ units}}{10,000 \text{ units}} \times 1 = 0.325 \text{ mL}$

or

   H   : V ::   D   : X
10,000 units : 1 mL :: 3250 units : X
10,000 X = 3250
      X = 0.325 mL

Answer: Epogen 3250 units = 0.325 mL or
            0.33 mL

7. a. 198 lb ÷ 2.2 kg = 90 kg
   b. 90 kg $\times$ 6 mcg/kg = 540 mcg

c. $\dfrac{D}{H} \times V = \dfrac{540 \text{ mcg}}{300 \text{ mcg}} \times 1 \text{ mL} = 1.8 \text{ mL}$

Answer: Neupogen 540 mcg = 1.8 mL

d. Drug can be prepared in two syringes, one with 1 mL, and the other with 0.8 mL. With subcutaneous injections, one (1) mL is given per site unless the person weighs more than 200 lb or the dose has been approved by the health care provider.

8. a. Select 80 mg per 0.8 mL Lovenox.

b. BF: $\dfrac{D}{H} \times V = \dfrac{\overset{7}{\cancel{70}} \text{ mg}}{\underset{8}{\cancel{80}} \text{ mg}} \times 0.8 \text{ mL} = \dfrac{5.6}{8} = 0.7 \text{ mL of Lovenox}$

or

FE: $\dfrac{H}{V} = \dfrac{D}{X} = \dfrac{80 \text{ mg}}{0.8 \text{ mL}} = \dfrac{70 \text{ mg}}{X}$

(Cross multiply) 80 X = 56

   X = 0.7 mL of Lovenox

or

DA: mL $= \dfrac{0.8 \text{ mL} \times \overset{7}{\cancel{70}} \text{ mg}}{\underset{8}{\cancel{80}} \text{ mg} \times 1} = \dfrac{5.6}{8} = 0.7 \text{ mL of Lovenox}$

9. BF: $\dfrac{D}{H} \times V = \dfrac{8 \text{ mg}}{15 \text{ mg}} \times 1 \text{ mL} = 0.53 \text{ mL or } 0.5 \text{ mL}$

or

FE: $\dfrac{H}{V} = \dfrac{D}{X} = \dfrac{15 \text{ mg}}{1 \text{ mL}} = \dfrac{8 \text{ mg}}{X}$

(Cross multiply) 15 X = 8

   X = 0.53 mL or 0.5 mL

or

RP: H : V :: D : X
   15 mg : 1 mL :: 8 mg : X
         15 X = 8
         X = 0.53 mL or 0.5 mL

10. a. 120 units × 65 kilograms = 7800 units

b. BF: $\dfrac{D}{H} \times V = \dfrac{7800 \text{ Iunits}}{10,000 \text{ Iunits}} \times 0.4 \text{ mL} = \dfrac{3120}{10,000} = 0.3 \text{ mL subcut}$

or

RP: $\quad$ H $\quad$: $\quad$ V $\quad$ :: $\quad$ D $\quad$:X
$\quad$ 10,000 Iunits : 0.4 mL :: 7800 Iunits : X
$\qquad$ 10,000 X = 3120
$\qquad\qquad$ X = 0.3 mL

III Intramuscular Injections (Round off in tenths)

1. BF: $\dfrac{D}{H} \times V = \dfrac{50 \text{ mg}}{80 \text{ mg}} \times 2 \text{ mL} = \dfrac{100}{80} = 1.25 \text{ mL or } 1.3 \text{ mL}$

or

RP: $\quad$ H $\quad$: $\quad$ V $\quad$ :: $\quad$ D $\quad$: $\quad$ X
$\quad$ 80 mg : 2 mL :: 50 mg : X mL
$\qquad$ 80 X = 100
$\qquad\qquad$ X = $\dfrac{100}{80}$ = 1.25 mL or 1.3 mL

or

FE: $\dfrac{H}{V} = \dfrac{D}{X} = \dfrac{80 \text{ mg}}{2 \text{ mL}} = \dfrac{50 \text{ mg}}{X} = $

(Cross multiply) 80 X = 100
$\qquad\qquad$ X = 1.25 or 1.3 mL

or

DA: no conversion factor

$mL = \dfrac{2 \text{ mL} \times \overset{5}{\cancel{50} \text{ mg}}}{\underset{8}{\cancel{80} \text{ mg}} \times 1} = \dfrac{10}{8} = 1.25 \text{ mL or } 1.3 \text{ mL}$

Answer: tobramycin 50 mg = 1.25 mL or 1.3 mL

2. BF: $\dfrac{D}{H} \times V = \dfrac{\overset{3}{\cancel{75} \text{ mg}}}{\underset{5}{\cancel{125} \text{ mg}}} \times 2 \text{ mL} = \dfrac{6}{5} = 1.2 \text{ mL}$

or

RP: $\quad$ H $\quad$: $\quad$ V $\quad$ :: $\quad$ D $\quad$: $\quad$ X
$\quad$ 125 mg : 2 mL :: 75 mg : X mL
$\qquad$ 125 X = 150
$\qquad\qquad$ X = 1.2 mL

Answer: methylprednisolone 75 mg = 1.2 mL

3. 0.3 mL of vitamin B_{12} (cyanocobalamin)

4. 0.5 mL of naloxone (Narcan)

5. BF: $\dfrac{D}{H} \times V = \dfrac{4 \text{ mg}}{10 \text{ mg}} \times 2 \text{ mL} = \dfrac{8}{10} = 0.8 \text{ mL diazepam}$

RP: $\quad$ H $\quad$: $\quad$ V $\quad$ :: $\quad$ D $\quad$:X
$\quad$ 10 mg : 2 mL :: 4 mg : X
$\qquad$ 10 X = 8
$\qquad\qquad$ X = 0.8 mL of diazepam

or

FE: $\dfrac{H}{V} = \dfrac{D}{X} = \dfrac{10 \text{ mg}}{2 \text{ mL}} = \dfrac{4 \text{ mg}}{X}$

(Cross multiply) 10 X = 8
$\qquad\qquad$ X = 0.8 mL of diazepam

or

DA: no conversion factor

$mL = \dfrac{2 \text{ mL} \times \overset{2}{\cancel{4} \text{ mg}}}{\underset{5}{\cancel{10} \text{ mg}} \times 1} = \dfrac{4}{5} = 0.8 \text{ mL of diazepam}$

6. a. Select the Maxipime 1-g vial. The Maxipime 2-g vial is for intravenous use according to the drug label and cannot be used for intramuscular injection.

   b. Using 2.6 mL diluent = 3.0 mL of solution

   c. Change 500 mg to 0.5 g or 1 g to 1000 mg

$$BF: \frac{D}{H} \times V = \frac{0.5 \text{ g}}{1 \text{ g}} \times 3 \text{ mL} = 1.5 \text{ mL of cefepime twice a day}$$

7. $BF: \dfrac{D}{H} \times V = \dfrac{4 \text{ mg}}{5 \text{ mg}} \times 1 \text{ mL} = \dfrac{4}{5} = 0.8 \text{ mL of compazine}$

or

RP: H : V :: D :X
   5 mg : 1 mL :: 4 mg : X
           5 X = 4
           X = 0.8 mL

or

$FE: \dfrac{H}{V} = \dfrac{D}{X} = \dfrac{5 \text{ mg}}{1 \text{ mL}} = \dfrac{4 \text{ mg}}{X} = 5 \text{ X} = 4$

(Cross multiply) X = 0.8 mL

or

$DA: \text{mL} = \dfrac{1 \text{ mL} \times 4 \text{ mg}}{5 \text{ mg} \times 1} = \dfrac{4}{5} = 0.8 \text{ mL}$

8. 2.5 mL of secobarbital

9. a. 100-mg vial

   b. 0.75 mL of thiamine

10. ½ or 0.5 mL of hydroxyzine

11. 0.5 mL (½ mL) of Loxitane

12. a. 4.0 mL of diluent = 1,000,000 units (drug label)

   b. $BF: \dfrac{D}{H} \times V = \dfrac{\overset{1}{\cancel{250{,}000 \text{ units}}}}{\underset{4}{\cancel{1{,}000{,}000 \text{ units}}}} \times 4 \text{ mL} = \dfrac{4}{4} = 1 \text{ mL Pfizerpen}$

   DA: 1 million units = 1,000,000 units

$$\text{mL} = \dfrac{4 \text{ mL} \times \overset{1}{\cancel{250{,}000 \text{ units}}}}{\underset{4}{\cancel{1{,}000{,}000 \text{ units}}} \times 1} = \dfrac{4}{4} = 1 \text{ mL of Pfizerpen}$$

13. a. 750 mg of cefonicid (Monocid) is equivalent to 0.75 g.

   b. Drug label indicates that 2.5 mL of diluent should be added to the drug powder, which yields 3.1 mL of drug solution.

   c. $\dfrac{D}{H} \times V = \dfrac{0.75 \text{ g}}{1 \text{ g}} \times 3.1 \text{ mL}$

= 2.33 mL or 2.3 mL of cefonicid solution

14. a. meperidine 35 mg = 0.7 mL

   b. promethazine 10 mg = 0.4 mL

   c. Procedure: 1. Obtain 0.7 mL of meperidine from the ampule and 0.4 mL of promethazine from the ampule.
       2. Discard the remaining solutions within the ampules.

15. a. meperidine 50 mg = ½ or 0.5 mL

   b. atropine 0.3 mg = 0.75 or 0.8 mL (Round off in tenths)
   Atropine

$$BF: \frac{D}{H} \times V = \frac{0.3 \text{ mg}}{0.4 \text{ mg}} \times 1 \text{ mL} = 0.75 \text{ or } 0.8 \text{ mL}$$

or

Atropine

RP: H   :   V   ::   D   :   X

     0.4 mg : 1 mL :: 0.3 mg : X mL

       0.4 X = 0.3

$$X = \frac{0.3}{0.4} = 0.75 \text{ or } 0.8 \text{ mL}$$

or

Atropine

$$FE: \frac{H}{V} = \frac{D}{X} = \frac{0.4 \text{ mg}}{1 \text{ mL}} = \frac{0.3 \text{ mg}}{X} =$$

     0.4 X = 0.3

       X = 0.75 or 0.8 mL

Meperidine

$$DA: mL = \frac{1 \text{ mL} \times \overset{1}{\cancel{50 \text{ mg}}}}{\underset{2}{\cancel{100 \text{ mg}}} \times 1} = \frac{1}{2} \text{ or } 0.5 \text{ mL}$$

c. 1. The two drugs are compatible.
    2. Inject 0.75 (0.8) mL of air into the atropine vial.
    3. Inject 0.5 mL of air into the meperidine vial and withdraw 0.5 mL of meperidine.
    4. Withdraw 0.8 mL of atropine from the atropine vial. Discard both vials.

16. $BF: \dfrac{D}{H} \times V = \dfrac{20 \text{ mg}}{30 \text{ mg}} \times 1 \text{ mL} = 0.66 \text{ or } 0.7 \text{ mL}$

or

RP: H   :   V   ::   D   :   X

    30 mg : 1 mL :: 20 mg : X

      30 X = 20

        X = 0.66 or 0.7 mL

or

RP: H   :   V   ::   D   : X

    30 mg : 1 mL :: 20 mg : X

      30 X = 20

       X = 0.66 or 0.7 mL

17. **a.** Use either heparin vial; 5000 units/mL or 10,000 units/mL
    b. 0.5 mL of heparin (units 5000); 0.25 mL of heparin (units 10,000)

18. Librium 50 mg = 1 mL (100 mg = 2 mL)
After adding 2 mL of diluent, withdraw the entire drug solution to determine the total volume of drug solution. Expel half of the solution; the remaining drug solution is equivalent to chlordiazepoxide (Librium) 50 mg.

19. **a.** Change milligrams to grams by moving the decimal point three spaces to the *left:* 500. mg = 0.5 g.

Because the drug weight on the label is in grams, the conversion is to grams. However, the drug can be converted to milligrams by changing grams to milligrams (moving the decimal point three spaces to the *right*): 1 g = 1.000 mg = 1000 mg.

    b. Drug label states to add 3 mL of diluent and, after it is reconstituted, the drug solution will be 3.5 mL. Mandol 1 g = 3.5 mL.

    c. A 5-mL syringe is preferred: however, a 3-mL syringe can be used because less than 3 mL of the drug solution is needed.

    d. $BF: \dfrac{D}{H} \times V = \dfrac{0.5 \text{ g}}{1 \text{ g}} \times 3.5 \text{ mL} = 1.75 \text{ or } 1.8 \text{ mL}$

or

RP: H   :   V   ::   D   :   X

    1000 mg : 3.5 mL :: 500 mg : X mL

      1000 X = 1750

        X = 1.75 or 1.8 mL

or

$$DA: mL = \frac{3.5 \text{ mL} \times 0.5 \cancel{g}}{1 \cancel{g} \times 1} = 1.75 \text{ or } 1.8 \text{ mL}$$

Answer: cefamandole (Mandol) 500 mg = 1.8 mL

20. Change 400 milligrams to grams

400 mg = 0.400 g or 0.4 g

a. Total volume of drug solution is 2.6 mL; see drug label.

b. BF: $\dfrac{D}{H} \times V = \dfrac{0.4\,g}{1\,g} \times 2.6 = 1$ mL

or

RP: H : V :: D : X

1 g:2.6 mL::0.4 g:X mL

X = 2.6 × 0.4

X = 1 mL

ticarcillin 400 mg or 0.4 g = 1 mL

or

FE: $\dfrac{H}{V} = \dfrac{D}{X} = \dfrac{1\,g}{2.6\,mL} = \dfrac{0.4\,g}{X} =$

(Cross multiply) X = 1.04 mL or 1 mL

or

DA = $\dfrac{2.6\,mL \times 0.4\,\cancel{g}}{1\,\cancel{g} \times 1} = 1.04$ mL or 1 mL

21. BF: $\dfrac{D}{H} \times V = \dfrac{\overset{2}{\cancel{10}}\,mg}{\underset{3}{\cancel{15}}\,mg} \times 1\,mL = \dfrac{2}{3} = 0.66$ or 0.7 mL

or

FE: H : V :: D : X

15 mg:1 mL::10 mg:X mL

15 X = 10

X = 0.66 or 0.7 mL

22. 0.5 mL of Vistaril

23. a. Yes, 8 mg per day

b. BF: $\dfrac{D}{H} \times V = \dfrac{\overset{1}{\cancel{2}}\,mg}{\underset{2}{\cancel{4}}\,mg} \times 1\,mL = \dfrac{1}{2}$ or 0.5 mL

or

DA: mL = $\dfrac{1\,mL \times \overset{1}{\cancel{2}}\,mg}{\underset{2}{\cancel{4}}\,mg \times 1} = \dfrac{1}{2}$ or 0.5 mL

c. 3-mL syringe

d. Yes, the vial has a rubber top that is self-sealing.

24. a. Change milligrams to grams; move the decimal point three spaces to the *left:* 500. mg = 0.5 g

0.5 g × 3 (q8h) = 1.5 g per day

b. Add 2 mL of diluent to yield 2.6 mL (check drug information insert):

BF: $\dfrac{D}{H} \times V = \dfrac{0.5\,g}{1\,g} \times 2.6\,mL = 1.3$ mL per dose

25. a. Add 9 mL of diluent to yield 10 mL after dilution

b. BF: $\dfrac{D}{H} \times V = \dfrac{\overset{3}{\cancel{1500}}\,mg}{\underset{10}{\cancel{5000}}\,mg} \times 10\,mL = \dfrac{30}{10} = 3$ mL

or

FE: $\dfrac{H}{V} = \dfrac{D}{X} = \dfrac{5000\,mg}{10\,mL} = \dfrac{1500\,mg}{X}$

(Cross multiply) 5000 X = 15,000

X = 3 mL

26. a. Either the ampule or the vial could be used. The diazepam 5 mg/mL is a multiple-dose vial that contains 10 mL of drug solution.

b. BF: Ampule: $\dfrac{8\,mg}{10\,mg} \times 2\,mL = 1.6$ mL of diazepam

BF: Vial: $\dfrac{8\,mg}{5\,mg} \times 1\,mL = 1.6$ mL of diazepam

or

DA: Ampule: mL = $\dfrac{2\,mL \times \overset{4}{\cancel{8}}\,mg}{\underset{5}{\cancel{10}}\,mg \times 1} = \dfrac{8}{5} = 1.6$ mL

or

DA: Vial: mL = $\dfrac{1\,mL \times 8\,\cancel{mg}}{5\,\cancel{mg} \times 1} = \dfrac{8}{5} = 1.6$ mL

27. $\dfrac{\text{D}}{\text{H}} \times \text{V} = \dfrac{1.5 \text{ mg}}{\underset{1}{\cancel{2} \text{ mg}}} \times \overset{1}{\cancel{2}} \text{ mL} = 1.5 \text{ mL of Cogentin}$

28. a. 1 g = 1000 mg

b. 750 mg × 2 = 1500 mg of cefotaxime Na per day

c. BF: $\dfrac{\text{D}}{\text{H}} \times \text{V} = \dfrac{\overset{3}{\cancel{750}} \text{ mg}}{\underset{4}{\cancel{1000}} \text{ mg}} \times 3.4 \text{ mL} = \dfrac{10.2}{4} = 2.55 \text{ mL or } 2.6 \text{ mL of cefotazime Na (rounded off in tenths)}$

DA: mL $= \dfrac{3.4 \text{ mL} \times \overset{3}{\cancel{750}} \text{ mg}}{\underset{4}{\cancel{1000}} \text{ mg} \times \quad 1} = \dfrac{10.2}{4} = 2.55 \text{ mL or } 2.6 \text{ mL of cefotazime Na (rounded off in tenths)}$

29. RP: H : V :: D :X

$\qquad$ 50 mg : 1 mL :: 30 mg : X

$\qquad\qquad$ 50 X = 30

$\qquad\qquad\quad$ X = 0.6 mL of diphenhydramine HCl

FE: $\dfrac{\text{H}}{\text{V}} = \dfrac{\text{D}}{\text{X}} = \dfrac{50 \text{ mg}}{1 \text{ mL}} = \dfrac{30 \text{ mg}}{\text{X}}$

(Cross multiply) 50 X = 30

$\qquad\qquad$ X = 0.6 mL of diphenhydramine HCl

30. BF: $\dfrac{\text{D}}{\text{H}} \times \text{V} = \dfrac{10}{25} \times 5 = \dfrac{50}{25} = 2 \text{ mL}$ $\qquad$ **or** $\qquad$ RP: $\qquad$ H $\qquad$: V :: $\qquad$ D $\qquad$: X

$\qquad\qquad\qquad\qquad\qquad\qquad\qquad\qquad\qquad\qquad\qquad$ 25 million units : 5 mL :: 10 million units : X mL

$\qquad\qquad\qquad\qquad\qquad\qquad\qquad\qquad\qquad\qquad\qquad\qquad\qquad$ 25 X = 50

$\qquad\qquad\qquad\qquad\qquad\qquad\qquad\qquad\qquad\qquad\qquad\qquad\qquad\quad$ X = 2 mL

Answer: Intron A 2 mL three times a week

31. BF: $\dfrac{\text{D}}{\text{H}} \times \text{V} = \dfrac{2.5 \text{ mg}}{10 \text{ mg}} \times 1 \text{ mL} = 0.25 \text{ mL or } 0.3 \text{ mL}$

or
RP: H : V :: D :X $\qquad\qquad\qquad\qquad\qquad$ **or**
$\qquad$ 10 mg : 1 mL :: 2.5 mg : X $\qquad\qquad\qquad$ FE: $\dfrac{\text{H}}{\text{V}} = \dfrac{\text{D}}{\text{X}} = \dfrac{10 \text{ mg}}{1 \text{ mL}} = \dfrac{2.5 \text{ mg}}{\text{X}} =$
$\qquad\qquad$ 10 X = 2.5
$\qquad\qquad\quad$ X = 0.25 mL or 0.3 mL $\qquad\qquad\qquad\qquad\qquad$ 10 X = 2.5
$\qquad\qquad\qquad\qquad\qquad\qquad\qquad\qquad\qquad\qquad\qquad\qquad$ X = 0.25 mL or 0.3 mL
or
DA: no conversion factor

mL $= \dfrac{1 \text{ mL} \times \overset{1}{\cancel{2.5}} \text{ mg}}{\underset{4}{\cancel{10}} \text{ mg} \times \quad 1} = \dfrac{1}{4}$ or 0.25 mL

Answer: AquaMEPHYTON 2.5 mg = 0.25 mL or 0.3 mL

32. a. 4 mL = 3 g

b. BF: $\dfrac{\text{D}}{\text{H}} \times \text{V} = \dfrac{1 \text{ g}}{3 \text{ g}} \times 4 \text{ mL} = \dfrac{4}{3} = 1.3 \text{ mL of Unasyn}$ $\qquad$ **or**
$\qquad\qquad\qquad\qquad\qquad\qquad\qquad\qquad\qquad\qquad\qquad\qquad$ RP: H : V :: D : X
$\qquad\qquad\qquad\qquad\qquad\qquad\qquad\qquad\qquad\qquad\qquad\qquad\qquad$ 3 g : 4 mL :: 1 g : X mL
$\qquad\qquad\qquad\qquad\qquad\qquad\qquad\qquad\qquad\qquad\qquad\qquad\qquad\qquad$ 3 X = 4
$\qquad\qquad\qquad\qquad\qquad\qquad\qquad\qquad\qquad\qquad\qquad\qquad\qquad\qquad\quad$ X = 1.3 mL of Unasyn

33. DA: mL $= \dfrac{2 \text{ mL} \times 2 \text{ mg}}{5 \text{ mg} \times \quad 1} = \dfrac{4}{5} = 0.8 \text{ mL of droperidol}$

34. DA: mL $= \dfrac{1 \text{ mL} \times 5 \text{ mg}}{4 \text{ mg} \times \quad 1} = \dfrac{5}{4} = 1.25 \text{ mL or } 1.3 \text{ mL of dexamethasone (rounded off in tenths)}$

35. DA: **a:** $mL = \dfrac{1\ mL \quad \times \quad \overset{1}{\cancel{100}}\ \cancel{mcg}}{\underset{2}{\cancel{200}}\ \cancel{mcg} \quad \times \quad 1} = 0.5$ or ½ mL of levothyroxine

DA: **b:** Conversion factor: 1 mg = 1000 mcg

$$Tablet = \dfrac{1\ tablet \quad \times \quad \overset{80}{\cancel{1000}}\ \cancel{mcg} \times 0.025\ \cancel{mg}}{\underset{1}{\cancel{12.5}}\ \cancel{mcg} \times \quad 1\ \cancel{mg} \quad \times \quad 1} = 80 \times 0.025 = 2\ tablets\ of\ levothyroxine$$

36. **a.** 1 g = 2.4; 500 mg = 1.2 mL

b. DA: $mL = \dfrac{2.4\ mL \times \quad 1\ \cancel{g} \quad \times \overset{1}{\cancel{500}}\ \cancel{mg}}{1\ \cancel{g} \quad \times \underset{2}{\cancel{1000}}\ \cancel{mg} \times \quad 1} = \dfrac{2.4}{2} = 1.2\ mL$

Give 1.2 mL of Cefobid

37. **a.** 4.2 mL

b. 350 mg/mL

c. BF: $\dfrac{D}{H} \times V = \dfrac{1000\ mg}{350\ mg} \times 1\ mL = 2.85\ mL$ or 2.9 mL
     or RP: H : V ::   D   : X
          350 mg : 1 mL :: 1000 mg : X
                    350 X = 1000
                        X = 2.85 mL or 2.9 mL

or FE: $\dfrac{H}{V} = \dfrac{D}{X} = \dfrac{350\ mg}{1\ mL} = \dfrac{1000\ mg}{X}$
     (Cross multiply) 350 X = 1000
                        X = 2.85 mL or 2.9 mL

or DA: $mL = \dfrac{1\ mL \quad \times\ 1000\ mg}{350\ mg \times \quad 1} = 2.85\ mL$ or 2.9 mL

38. 0.25 g = 0.250 mg (250 mg)

a. Give 1.1 mL of Ancef.

39. **a.** 140 ÷ 2.2 = 63.6 kg

b. 15 mg × 63.6 × 1 = 954 mg daily

c. 954 ÷ 3 = 318 mg of amikacin q8h

d. BF: $\dfrac{D}{H} \times V = \dfrac{318\ mg}{500\ mg} \times 2 = \dfrac{636}{500} = 1.27$ or 1.3 mL

or FE: $\dfrac{H}{V} = \dfrac{D}{X} = \dfrac{500\ mg}{2\ mL} = \dfrac{318\ mg}{X\ mL} =$
     (Cross multiply) 500 X = 636
                        X = 1.27 or 1.3 mL

or RP: H : V ::   D   : X
          500 mg : 2 mL :: 318 mg : X mL
                500 X = 636
                    X = 1.27 or 1.3 mL (tenths)

or DA: $mL = \dfrac{2\ mL \quad \times\ 318\ \cancel{mg}}{500\ \cancel{mg} \times \quad 1} = \dfrac{636}{500} = 1.3\ mL$ per dose

Answer: give 1.27 or 1.3 mL of amikacin q8h (three times a day)

40. a. $174 \div 2.2 = 79.1$ kg

b. 2 mg $\times 79.1 = 158.2$ or 158 mg daily

c. $158 \div 3 = 52.6$ mg or 50 mg q8h (Round off to a number that can be administered; check with your institution)

d. BF: $\dfrac{D}{H} \times V = \dfrac{\overset{5}{\cancel{50}} \text{ mg}}{\underset{10}{\cancel{100}} \text{ mg}} \times 1 \text{ mL} = \dfrac{5}{10} = 0.5$ mL

or

RP: H : V :: D : X
$\qquad$ 100 mg : 1 mL :: 50 mg : X mL
$\qquad\qquad$ 100 X = 50
$\qquad\qquad\qquad$ X = 0.5 mL

or

FE: $\dfrac{H}{V} = \dfrac{D}{X} = \dfrac{100 \text{ mg}}{1 \text{ mL}} = \dfrac{50 \text{ mg}}{X \text{ mL}} =$
$\qquad\qquad\qquad$ 100 X = 50
$\qquad\qquad\qquad\qquad$ X = 0.5 mL

or

DA: mL $= \dfrac{1 \text{ mL} \times \overset{1}{\cancel{50}} \text{ mg}}{\underset{2}{\cancel{100}} \text{ mg} \times 1} = \dfrac{1}{2}$ or 0.5 mL

Answer: netilmicin 50 mg = 0.5 mL

41. a. 156 pounds = 70.9 or 71 kg

b. 0.07 mg $\times 71$ kg = 4.97 mg or 5 mg (rounded off)

c. Administered IM in two syringes at two sites, 2.5 mL in each syringe unless otherwise instructed

42. a. 4 mcg $\times 72$ kg = 288 mcg or 0.288 mg or 0.3 mg

Move the decimal place three places to the left to convert mcg to mg.

b. BF: $\dfrac{D}{H} \times V = \dfrac{0.3 \text{ mg}}{0.4 \text{ mg}} \times 2 \text{ mL} = \dfrac{0.6}{0.4} = 1.5$ mL of Robinul

or

FE: $\dfrac{H}{V} = \dfrac{D}{X} = \dfrac{0.4 \text{ mg}}{2 \text{ mL}} = \dfrac{0.3 \text{ mg}}{X}$
(Cross multiply) $0.4 X = 0.6$
$\qquad\qquad\qquad$ X = 1.5 mL

43. a. 130 lb = 59 kg

b. 59 milligrams per day

c. 29.5 milligrams per dose

d. BF: $\dfrac{D}{H} \times V = \dfrac{29.5 \text{ mg}}{40 \text{ mg}} \times 4 \text{ mL} = 2.95$ mL or 3 mL

or

RP: H : V :: D : X
$\qquad$ 350 mg : 4 mL :: 29.5 mg : X
$\qquad\qquad$ 40 X = 118
$\qquad\qquad\qquad$ X = 2.95 mL or 3 mL

or

FE: $\dfrac{H}{V} = \dfrac{D}{X} = \dfrac{40 \text{ mg}}{4 \text{ mL}} = \dfrac{29.5 \text{ mg}}{X}$
(Cross multiply) $40 X = 118$
$\qquad\qquad$ X = 2.95 mL or 3 mL

or

DA: mL $= \dfrac{4 \text{ mL} \times 29.5 \text{ mg}}{40 \text{ mg} \times 1} = 2.95$ mL or 3 mL

---

evolve   Additional practice problems are available in the Basic Calculations and Advanced Calculations sections of Drug Calculations Companion, version 5 on Evolve.

CHAPTER 10

Insulin Administration

Objectives
- Identify the different types of insulin.
- Determine prescribed insulin dosage in units using an insulin syringe.
- Describe the sites and angle for administering insulin.
- Explain the methods for mixing two insulin solutions in one insulin syringe.
- Explain the various methods of insulin administration, such as insulin pens, insulin pump.

Outline
INSULIN SYRINGES
INSULIN BOTTLES
SITES AND ANGLES FOR INSULIN INJECTIONS
TYPES OF INSULIN
MIXING INSULINS
INSULIN PEN DEVICES
INSULIN PUMPS

Insulin is secreted from pancreatic beta cells to help regulate blood glucose levels. Diabetes mellitus represents an insulin deficiency, and is characterized as either type 1 or type 2. The pancreatic beta cells in patients with type 1 do not secrete insulin, requiring patients to subcutaneously administer insulin to regulate glucose metabolism. Patients with type 2 secrete an insufficient amount of insulin to match glucose load, often necessitating the use of oral antidiabetic medications and/or subcutaneous insulin.

Insulin was obtained from beef and pork pancreases when it first became available in 1925. Synthetic human insulin (Humulin) first became available in the 1980s, and largely replaced beef and pork insulin in the United States. Beef insulin has not been available since 1998 due to allergy concerns. Although pork and human insulin are similar, pork insulin has not been available in the United States since December 2005 but may still be imported. The development of insulin analogs with different onsets and durations of action provides more options for patients today.

INSULIN SYRINGES

Insulin syringes have a capacity of 0.5 to 1 mL. Insulin is measured in *units,* using an insulin syringe. Insulin dosage must NOT be calculated in milliliters. The insulin syringe is calibrated as 2 units and 100 units equal 1 mL syringe. The insulin syringe is usually marked on one side in even units (10, 20, 30) and on the other side in odd units (5, 15, 25) (Figure 10-1).

Insulin syringes are available in $\frac{3}{10}$-, $\frac{1}{2}$-, and 1-mL sizes. The 1-mL insulin syringe may be purchased with a permanently attached needle or a detachable needle (Figure 10-2).

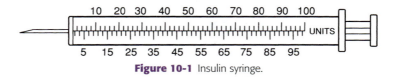

Figure 10-1 Insulin syringe.

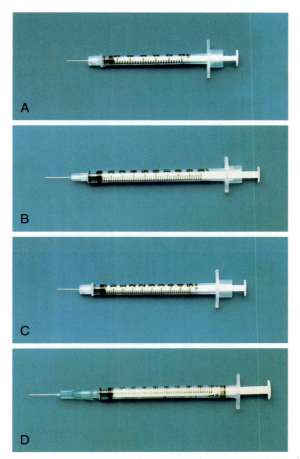

Figure 10-2 Four types of insulin syringes: **A,** ³/₁₀-mL insulin syringe with a permanently attached needle. **B,** ½-mL insulin syringe with a permanently attached needle. **C,** 1-mL insulin syringe with a permanently attached needle. **D,** 1-mL insulin syringe with a detachable needle. (From Becton, Dickinson and Company, Franklin Lakes, N.J.)

INSULIN BOTTLES

Insulin is prescribed and measured according to U.S. Pharmacopeia (USP) units. Most insulins are produced in concentrations of 100 units/mL. Insulin should be administered with an insulin syringe that is calibrated to correspond with the 100 units of insulin bottle. DO NOT use a tuberculin syringe. The insulin bottle and syringe are color-coded "orange" to avoid medication errors.

Insulin is ordered in units. For example, if the prescribed insulin dosage is 30 units, withdraw 30 units from the bottle of 100 units of insulin usig a 100-unit calibrated insulin syringe (Figure 10-3).

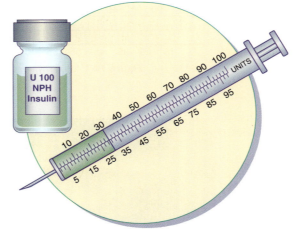

Figure 10-3 Unit-100 insulin bottle and unit-100 insulin syringe.

SITES AND ANGLES FOR INSULIN INJECTIONS

Insulin is a protein that can be given only by injection. Gastrointestinal (GI) secretions destroy the insulin structure. Figure 10-4 indicates the sites for insulin injection. People who inject their insulin usually use sites 3, 4, 5, or 6. Caregivers or health care workers who administer insulin usually use sites 1 or 2 (upper arm or the deltoid area).

> ! **CAUTION**
> • DO NOT administer insulin with a tuberculin syringe.

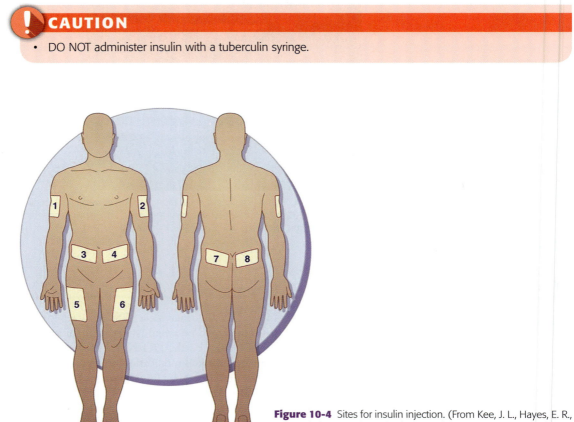

Figure 10-4 Sites for insulin injection. (From Kee, J. L., Hayes, E. R., & McCuistion, L. E. [2015]. *Pharmacology: a patient-centered nursing process approach.* 8th ed., Philadelphia: Elsevier.)

Insulin is administered at a 45- or 90-degree angle into the subcutaneous tissue. The subcutaneous absorption rate of insulin is slower because there are fewer blood vessels in the fatty tissue than in the muscular tissue. For an obese person, the angle may be 90 degrees, and for a very thin person the angle may be 45 degrees.

TYPES OF INSULIN

Insulin is categorized as rapid-acting, fast-acting, intermediate-acting, long-acting, and as commercial premixed insulin. The following drug labels (Figure 10-5) are arranged according to insulin action.

Rapid-Acting Insulins

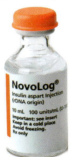
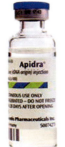
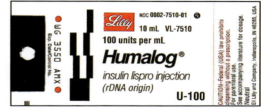

(From Novo Nordisk, Inc., Princeton, N.J.)

(Product images and trademarks are the property of and used with the permission of sanofi-aventis U.S. LLC, Bridgewater, N.J. as of September, 2015.)

Fast-Acting Insulins

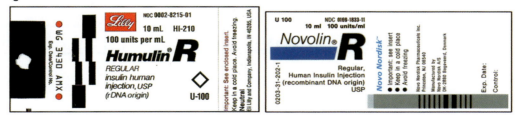

Intermediate-Acting Insulins

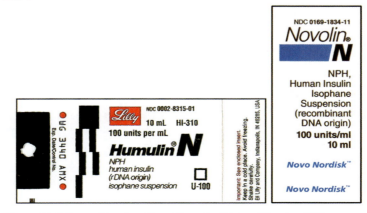

Figure 10-5 Types of insulins. (From Novo Nordisk Inc., Princeton, N.J.)

Long-Acting Insulins

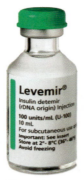

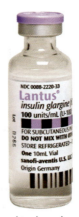

(From Novo
Nordisk, Inc.,
Princeton, N.J.)

(Product images and trademarks are the property
of and used with the permission of sanofi-aventis
U.S. LLC, Bridgewater, N.J. as of September, 2015.)

Combinations: Rapid- and Intermediate-Acting Insulins

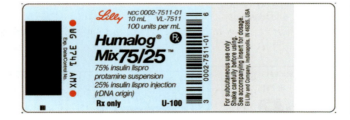

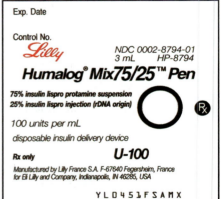

Fast- and Intermediate-Acting Insulins

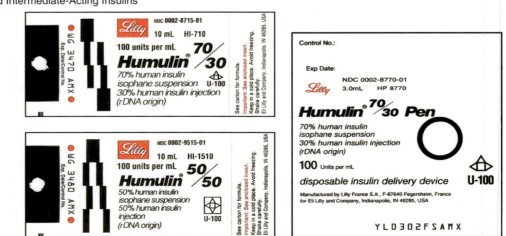

Figure 10-5 (cont'd) Types of insulins. (Lantus from sanofi-aventis U.S. Inc., Bridgewater, N.J.)

Insulins have various descriptions, including color, action, source, and manufacturer. They are either clear (regular or crystalline insulin) or cloudy (NPH) because of the substance, protamine, used to prolong the action of insulin in the body. Only clear (regular) insulin can be given IV as well as subcutaneously.

Insulin action is broken down into onset, peak, and duration. *Onset* is how long it takes the insulin to begin working. *Peak* is when the insulin is working most effectively, and *duration* is how long the insulin remains effective. Additionally, insulins are either DNA recombinant or analogs. Since 2005 only human insulin has been available in the United States. *Human insulin* is DNA recombinant and is manufactured; it does not come from cadavers. *Analog insulin* is human insulin that has been manipulated to change the action. The three insulin manufacturers are Eli Lilly, NovoNordisk, and Sanofi-Aventis. Humulin and Novolin are examples of brand names of insulins.

Insulin is categorized as rapid-acting, fast-acting, intermediate-acting, long-acting, and commercial premixed insulin (see Figure 10-5). Insulin is prescribed in units and administered in units. The first rapid-acting insulin, Humalog (lispro insulin), was approved for use in 1996. Lispro (Humalog) and the new rapid-acting insulins, aspart and glulisine, act faster than regular insulin and thus can be administered 5 to 15 minutes before mealtime, whereas regular insulin is given 30 minutes before meals. Rapid-acting insulins can become effective within 5 to 15 minutes of injection and last 3 to 5 hours. Lispro insulin (Humalog) is formed by reversing two amino acids in human regular insulin (Humulin R). Aspart insulin (NovoLog) is an analog of human insulin with a rapid onset. It is structured identically to human insulin except for one amino acid. Glulisine insulin (Apidra), like aspart insulin, is a synthetic analog of natural human insulin (see Table 10-1 and Figure 10-5). **Rapid-acting (Aspart, Apidra, and Humalog) and fast-acting (regular) insulins can be given intravenously as well as subcutaneously. Intermediate-acting and long-acting insulins can ONLY be administered subcutaneously.**

Fast-acting insulin (regular insulin) is also clear but takes longer to start working compared with rapid-acting insulins. It is administered 30 minutes before meals and is effective for 6 to 8 hours. If it is given during or after the meal, the patient may experience low blood sugars. Fast-acting insulin is known as regular or R insulin. Humulin R and Novolin R are brand names of fast-acting human insulin.

Intermediate-acting insulin (NPH, Humulin N, Novolin N) is administered 30 minutes before meals (breakfast) and becomes effective in 1 to 2 hours. Its duration of action in the body is 12 to 18 hours. This type of insulin contains protamine, which prolongs the action in the body. It is cloudy because of the protamine added to the regular insulin. It can ONLY be given subcutaneously. Humulin N can be mixed with Humulin R (regular insulin) or rapid-acting insulin in the same syringe.

The long-acting insulins are insulin detemir (Levemir), an analog of human insulin, and insulin glargine (Lantus). Lantus is the first long-acting recombinant DNA (rDNA) human insulin for patients with type 1 and 2 diabetes mellitus. Lantus and Levemir are clear, colorless insulins that are to be given ONLY subcutaneously and NOT intravenously. **Lantus and Levemir CANNOT be mixed with other insulins or given intravenously.** The long-acting insulin acts within 1 to 2 hours and lasts in the body for 18 to 24 hours. The Levemir vial is tall and has a green top. The Lantus vial is taller and narrower than the other types of insulin. It has a purple top and purple print on the label. Levemir is usually administered in the evening or at bedtime; however, it can be administered once or twice a day subcutaneously. Lantus is usually administered at bedtime; thus, the incidence of nocturnal hypoglycemia is not common. Some patients report more pain at the injection site with long-acting insulins than with Humulin N (NPH).

The use of commercially premixed combination insulins has become popular for patients with diabetes mellitus who mix fast-acting and intermediate-acting insulins. Examples are two groups: the rapid- and intermediate-acting insulin and the fast- and intermediate-acting insulins. The two rapid- and intermediate-acting insulins are Novolog mix 70/30 and Humalog mix 75/25. The fast- and intermediate-acting insulins are Humulin 70/30, Novolin 70/30, and Humulin 50/50 (see Table 10-1). They are available in vials or pens that resemble a fountain pen. Some patients need less than 30% Humulin R and more Humulin N, so these combinations of insulins cannot be used. They must mix their insulins according to the prescribed units of insulin.

The onset, peak, and duration times are given in Table 10-1 for four groups of insulins: rapid-acting, fast-acting, intermediate-acting, and long-acting. The table includes the peak and return times after the insulins are administered.

TABLE 10-1 Types of Insulin

| | | | | | ACTION | | |
Generic (Brand)	Route	Color	Pregnancy Category	Time to Administer	Onset	Peak	Duration (Dose-Related)
Rapid-Acting Insulin (Short Duration)							
aspart (NovoLog)	A: subcut, IV	Clear	B	5-15 min before meals	5-15 min	1-3 h	3-5 h
glulisine (Apidra)	A: subcut, IV	Clear	B	5-15 min before meals	5-15 min	1-2 h	3-4.5 h
lispro (Humalog)	A: subcut, IV	Clear	B	5-15 min before meals	5-15 min	0.5-2 h	3-5 h
Fast-Acting Insulin (Slower Duration)							
regular insulin (Humulin R, Novolin R)	A,C: subcut, IV	Clear	B	15-30 min before meals	0.5-1 h	2-4 h	6-8 h
Intermediate-Acting Insulin							
NPH Insulin, Humulin N, Novolin N	A,C: subcut	Cloudy	B	30 min before meals	1-2 h	6-12 h	12-18 h
Long-Acting Insulin							
determir (Levemir)	A: subcut	Clear	C	Dinner or bedtime	1-2 h	6-8 h	14-24 h (dose related)
glargine (Lantus)	A: subcut	Clear	C	Bedtime	1.5-2 h	No peak	24 h
COMBINATIONS							
Rapid- and Intermediate-Acting Insulin							
70% aspart protamine/ 30% aspart insulin (NovoLog mix 70/30)	A: subcut	Cloudy	B	15 min before meals	15 min	1-4 h	12-18 h
75% lispro protamine/ 25% lispro insulin (Humalog mix 75/25)	A: subcut	Cloudy	B	15 min before meals	15 min-2h	2-6 h	14-18 h
Fast- and Intermediate-Acting Insulin							
70% NPH/30% regular insulin (Humulin 70/30, Novolin 70/30)	A: subcut	Cloudy	B	15 min before meals	30-60 min	2-8 h	10-18 h
50% NPH/50% regular insulin (Humulin 50/50)	A: subcut	Cloudy	B	15 min before meals	15-60 min	2-6 h	10-18 h

A, adult; *C,* child; *h,* hour; *min,* minute; *subcut;* subcutaneous; *IV,* intravenous, <, less than.
CAUTION: Levemir and Lantus should NOT be mixed with other insulins and should NEVER be given intravenously.

With severe hyperglycemia (high blood sugar), Humulin R units 500 may be ordered. This unit type of insulin is of high potency and **NOT** for ordinary use. It is a high-risk drug. It is given with caution.

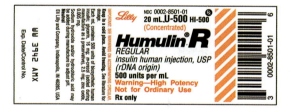

When the blood sugar level becomes extremely low (less than 40 mg/mL) and/or the patient is unconscious, glucagon injection is given. It increases the blood sugar level. Many diabetic patients have glucagon emergency kits in their homes for use if this occurs (Figure 10-6).

Figure 10-7 compares the action-time and rapid-acting, fast-acting, intermediate-acting, and long-acting insulins.

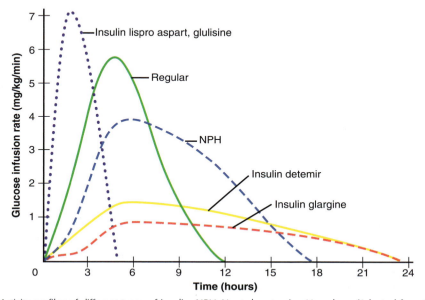

Figure 10-6 Glucagon emergency kit for home use. (From Eli Lilly and Company. All rights reserved. Used with permission.)

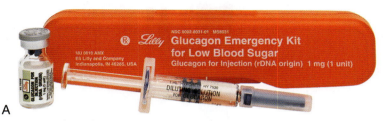

Figure 10-7 Activity profiles of different types of insulin. *NPH,* Neutral protamine Hagedorn. (Adapted from Rosenstock, J., Wyne, K. [2003]. Insulin treatment in type 2 diabetes. In Goldstein BJ, Müller-Wieland D, editors: *Textbook of type 2 diabetes,* London, Martin Dunitz, Ltd.; Plank J, Bodenlenz, M., Sinner, F., et al. [2005]. A double-blind, randomized, dose-response study investigating the pharmacodynamic and pharmacokinetic properties of the long-acting insulin analog detemir, *Diabetes Care* 28:1107-1112. Rave, K., Bott, S., Heinemann, L., et al. [2005]. Time-action profile of inhaled insulin in comparison with subcutaneously injected insulin lispro and regular human insulin, *Diabetes Care* 28:1077-1082.)

MIXING INSULINS

Regular insulin is frequently mixed with insulins containing protamine, such as Humulin N. REMEMBER: Insulin is prescribed in units and administered in units. Lantus and Levemir insulins can **NOT** be mixed with regular (rapid- or fast-acting) insulin.

EXAMPLE Problem and method for mixing insulin.

PROBLEM: **Order:** Humulin R insulin units 10 and Humulin N insulin units 40, subcut.
Drug available: Humulin R insulin units 100 and Humulin N insulin units 100, both in multidose vials. The insulin syringe is marked units 100.

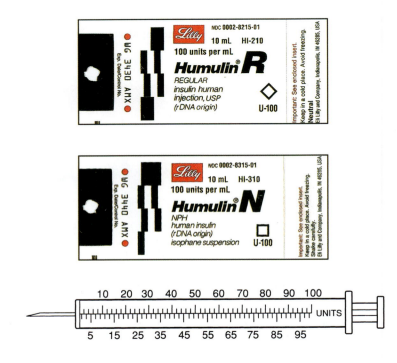

Method:

1. Gently roll insulin bottles between palms to evenly distribute the insulin solution. DO NOT shake insulin. Cleanse the rubber tops with alcohol.
2. Draw up 40 units of air* and inject into the Humulin N insulin bottle. Do not allow the needle to come into contact with the Humulin N insulin solution. Withdraw the needle.
3. Draw up 10 units of air and inject into the Humulin R insulin bottle.
4. Withdraw 10 units of Humulin R insulin. **Humulin R insulin is withdrawn before Humulin N insulin.**
5. Withdraw 40 units of Humulin N insulin.
6. Administer the two insulins immediately after mixing. Do not allow the insulin mixture to stand, because unpredicted physical changes might occur.

---

*You may draw up 50 units of air; inject 40 units into the NPH bottle and 10 units into the regular insulin bottle.

PRACTICE PROBLEMS ▶ I INSULIN

Answers can be found on pages 202 to 203.

1. **Order:** Humulin N insulin 35 units, subcut.
   Drug available: Humulin N insulin units 100 and units 100 insulin syringe.
   Indicate on the insulin syringe the amount of insulin that should be withdrawn.

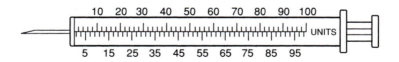

2. **Order:** Apidra (insulin glulisine) 10 units, subcut, STAT.
   Drug available: The syringe is units-100 insulin syringe.

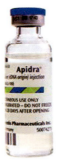

(Product images and trademarks are the property
of and used with the permission of sanofi-aventis
U.S. LLC, Bridgewater, N.J. as of September, 2015.)

Indicate on the insulin syringe the amount of insulin that should be withdrawn.

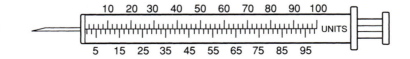

3. **Order:** Humalog insulin units 8 and Humulin N insulin units 52.
   Drug available: Humalog insulin units 100 and Humulin N insulin units 100.
   The insulin syringe is units 100.
   Explain the method for mixing the two insulins.

   _____

Indicate on the units-100 insulin syringe how much Humalog insulin should be withdrawn and
how much Humulin N insulin should be withdrawn.

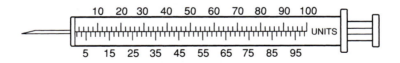

4. Order: Humulin R insulin units 15 and Humulin N insulin units 45.
   Drug available: Humulin R insulin units-100 and Humulin N insulin units 100.
   The insulin syringe is units 100.
   Explain the method for mixing the two insulins.

   _____

   Indicate on the units-100 insulin syringe how much Humulin R insulin and how much Humulin N insulin should be withdrawn.

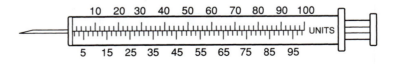

5. Order: Insulin detemir (Levemir) 40 units, subcut, at bedtime/hour of sleep.
   Drug available: The syringe is units-100 insulin syringe.

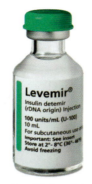

(From Norvo Nordisk, Inc., Princeton, N.J.)

Indicate on the insulin syringe the amount of insulin that should be given.

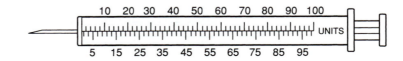

a. Can Levemir be mixed with regular insulin? _____

6. Order: Novolin N insulin, 38 units, subcut, 30 minutes before breakfast.
Drug available: The insulin syringe is 100 units.

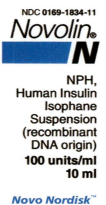

NDC 0169-1834-11

Novolin®

N

NPH,
Human Insulin
Isophane
Suspension
(recombinant
DNA origin)
100 units/ml
10 ml

Novo Nordisk™

Novo Nordisk™

Indicate on the insulin syringe the amount of Novolin N insulin that should be given.

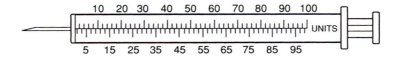

7. Order: Lantus insulin, 35 units, subcut, at bedtime.
Drug available: The insulin syringe is 100 units.

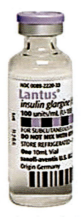

(Product images and trademarks are the property
of and used with the permission of sanofi-aventis
U.S. LLC, Bridgewater, N.J. as of September, 2015.)

Indicate on the insulin syringe the amount of Lantus insulin that should be given.

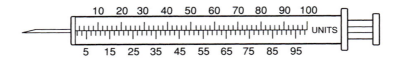

INSULIN PEN DEVICES

There are two types of insulin pen devices: pre-filled and reusable. Both types require insulin pen needles to dispense the insulin.

Pre-filled insulin pen devices are filled with 300 units or 3 mL of units-100 insulin. Before each insulin dose, a small disposable needle is placed on the end of the insulin pen device and then the insulin dose is dialed in. As the dose is dialed in, the plunger comes out. After the dose is dialed, the needle is placed subcutaneously and the plunger pushed down.

In some hospitals or medical institutions, the insulin pen is primed with 2 units of insulin before administration. Check with the institution's policy for priming the insulin pen with 2 units of insulin before administering the insulin dose. After the insulin is delivered, the dose indicator returns to zero and the needle is removed from the skin. The needle is discarded. A new needle is placed on the prefilled pen before each injection. The pre-filled pen device is reused for multiple injections until all the insulin is dispensed. Once the insulin is completely dispensed, the pen is thrown away (Figure 10-8).

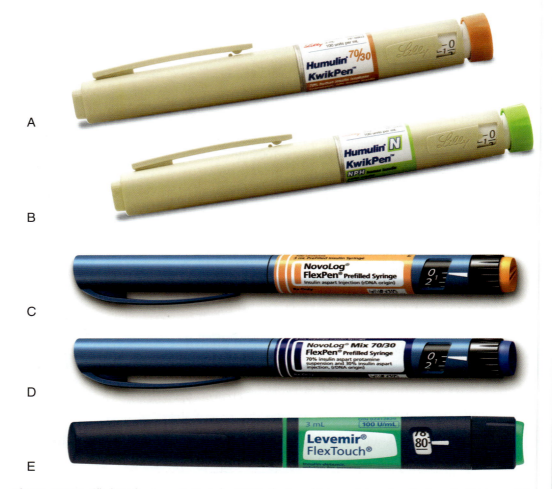

Figure 10-8 Prefilled insulin pens. **A,** Humulin 70/30 short- and intermediate-acting. **B,** Humulin N intermediate-acting. **C,** Novolog® rapid-acting. **D,** Novolog® 70/30 short- and intermediate-acting. **E,** Levemir® long-acting. (**A** and **B,** Copyright Eli Lilly and Company. All rights reserved. Used with permission. **C** to **E,** From Novo Nordisk Inc., Princeton, N.J.)

Reusable insulin pen devices are filled with disposable insulin cartridges. The cartridges are filled with 150 units (1.5 mL) or 300 units (3 mL) of units-100 insulin. The cartridge is placed in the pen device. Before each insulin dose, a small disposable needle is placed on the end of the insulin pen device and then the insulin dose is dialed in. As the dose is dialed in, the plunger comes out. After the dose is dialed, the needle is placed subcutaneously and the plunger pushed down. Following the insulin delivery, the dose indicator returns to zero and the needle is removed from the skin. The needle is removed from the pen device. The pre-filled pen device is reused for multiple injections until all the insulin is dispensed from the cartridge. Once the cartridge is empty, the cartridge is thrown away and a new cartridge placed in the reusable pen device.

PRACTICE PROBLEMS ▶ II INSULIN PEN DEVICES

Answers can be found on page 204.

1. Your patient receives 25 units of units-100 Levemir insulin by FlexPen twice a day. The pen holds 300 units. How many days will one pen last?

_____

2. Lantus SoloStar Pens are dispensed in boxes of five pens. Each pen holds 300 units. If your patient receives 75 units of units-100 Lantus insulin once a day at bedtime, how many doses can the patient get from the box of five pens?

_____

INSULIN PUMPS

There are two types of insulin pumps—the implantable and the external (portable). The implantable insulin pump is surgically implanted in the abdomen and delivers a basal insulin infusion and bolus doses with meals either intravenously or intraperitoneally. With implantable insulin pumps, there are fewer hypoglycemic reactions, and blood glucose levels are mostly controlled.

External (portable) insulin pumps, also called *continuous subcutaneous insulin infusion* or CSII, have been available since 1983. CSII mimics the body's normal delivery of insulin. The external insulin pump keeps blood glucose (sugar) levels as close to normal as possible. The continuous delivery of insulin is called the *basal rate* and the larger pre-meal doses are called *bolus doses*. The insulin delivery setting is programmed by a diabetes expert and adjusted by the patient. Before the patient eats, the pump is programmed to dispense a large dose through the catheter. The patient then (1) programs insulin infusion at a basal rate of units per hour (a rate that can be adjusted), (2) delivers bolus infusions to cover meals (the patient pushes a button to deliver a bolus dose during meals), (3) changes delivery rates at specific times of the day (e.g., from 3 AM to 9 AM) to avoid early-morning hyperglycemia, and (4) overrides the set basal rate to allow for unexpected changes in activity such as early-morning exercise.

Most insulin pump systems consist of the insulin pump, an insulin reservoir, plastic tubing, and insertion set. The insulin reservoir holds 150 to 300 units of rapid- or fast-acting insulin, which is held in the insulin pump. The plastic tubing is attached to a metal or plastic needle and placed subcutaneously by the patient. The needle can be inserted into the abdomen, upper thigh, or upper arm. Only regular insulin is used because protamine insulin, such as Humulin N, can cause unpredictable blood glucose levels. The pump can deliver small amounts of insulin such as 0.1 or 0.2 units much more accurately than a traditional insulin syringe. Again, these pumps used a remote control to program the basal rates and bolus doses. The patient usually changes the insertion site every 3 days.

A glucose sensor device is available to check the fluid glucose level. The sensor is separate from the insulin pump and is attached to the body surface area. Radio-like wave sounds are transmitted to the pump, which records the glucose level on the pump every 5 minutes. An alarm warns of low or high glucose levels.

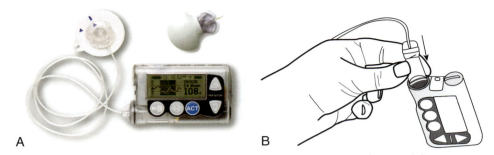

A   B

Figure 10-9 A, Medtronic Paradigm REAL-Time System. **B,** Insert the reservoir into the top of the pump case. (From Medtronic, Inc., Minneapolis, Minn.)

The use of the insulin pump helps to decrease the risk of severe hypoglycemic reactions and maintains glucose control. However, glucose levels should still be monitored at least daily with or without an insulin pump. The person with type 1 diabetes mellitus has the greatest benefit from use of an insulin pump. This method should reduce the number of long-term diabetic complications compared with the use of multiple injections of regular and modified types of insulins. Figure 10-9 shows an example of an insulin pump.

PRACTICE PROBLEMS ▶ III INSULIN PUMP

Answers can be found on page 204.

1. Your patient receives 50 units of basal insulin in a 24-hour period. His basal rate is the same for all 24 hours. How much insulin does your patient receive each hour?

    _____ unit/hour/24 hours

2. Your patient's pump setting are:

    Midnight to 3 AM   1.4 units/hr = _____ units for 3 hours

    3 AM to 7 AM   2.6 units/hr = _____ units for 4 hours

    7 AM to 5 PM   1.2 units/hr = _____ units for 10 hours

    5 PM to midnight   1.4 units/hr = _____ units for 7 hours

    How much basal insulin would your patient receive in 24 hours? _____

3. Your patient's insulin reservoir holds 180 units of insulin. The patient uses 2.5 units per hour. How often does the patient need to refill the insulin reservoir? _____

ANSWERS

I Insulin

1. Withdraw 35 units of Humulin N insulin to the 35 mark on the insulin syringe. Both the insulin and the syringe have the same concentration: units 100.

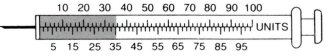

2. Withdraw 10 units of Apidra insulin.

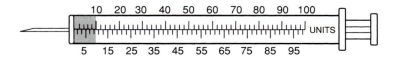

3. Inject 52 units of air into the Humulin N insulin bottle. Do not allow the needle to touch the insulin solution. Inject 8 units of air into the Humalog insulin bottle and withdraw 8 units of Humalog insulin. Withdraw 52 units of Humulin N insulin. Total amount of insulin should be 60 units. Do *not* allow the insulin mixture to stand. Administer immediately because Humulin N contains protamine, and unpredicted physical changes could occur with a delay in administration.

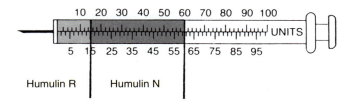

4. Inject 45 units of air into the Humulin N insulin bottle. Inject 15 units of air into the Humulin R insulin bottle and withdraw 15 units of Humulin R insulin. Withdraw 45 units of Humulin N insulin. Total amount of insulin should be 60 units.

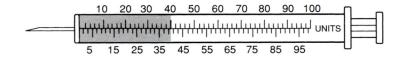

5. Withdraw 40 units of Levemir insulin.

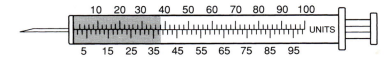

   a. No. CANNOT BE MIXED WITH REGULAR INSULIN.
6. Withdraw 38 units of Novolin N insulin.

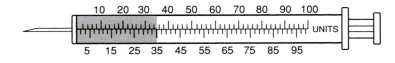

7. Withdraw 35 units of Lantus insulin.

II Insulin Pen Devices

1. 300 units per pen ÷ by 25 units = 12 doses per pen
   12 ÷ 2 doses per day = 6 days
2. 300 units per pen × 5 pens = 1500 units per box
   1500 units (5 pens) ÷ 75 units per day = 20 doses per box

III Insulin Pumps

1. 50 units per 24 hours ÷ 24 hours per day = 2.08 units of basal insulin per hour
2. Patient receives 36.4 units of insulin (basal) in 24 hours

   Midnight to 3 AM: 1.4 units/hr, 3 hours × 1.4 units = 4.2 units in 3 hours
   3 AM to 7 AM: 2.6 units/hr, 4 hours × 2.6 units = 10.4 units in 4 hours
   7 AM to 5 PM: 1.2 units/hr, 10 hours × 1.2 units = 12.0 units in 10 hours
   5 PM to midnight: 1.4 units/hr, 7 hours × 1.4 units = 9.8 units in 7 hours

3. 2.5 units per hours × 24 hours = 60 units per 24 hours or per day
   180 units per reservoir ÷ 60 units per day = 3 days
   Patient must refill insulin reservoir every 3 days.

evolve   Additional practice problems are available in the Basic Calculations and Advanced Calculations sections of Drug Calculations Companion, version 5 on Evolve.

CHAPTER 11

Intravenous Preparations With Clinical Applications

Objectives
- Identify catheter types and sites for intravenous (IV) access.
- Examine the three methods for calculating IV flow rate and select one of the methods for IV calculation.
- Calculate drops per minute of prescribed IV solutions for IV therapy.
- Determine the drop factor according to the manufacturer's product specification.
- Calculate the drug dosage for IV medications.
- Calculate the flow rate for IV drugs being administered in a prescribed amount of solution.
- Explain the types and uses of electronic IV infusion devices.
- Calculate the rate of direct IV injection.

Intravenous (IV) therapy is used for administering fluids containing water, dextrose, fat emulsions, vitamins, electrolytes, and drugs. Approximately 90% of all hospitalized patients, some outpatients, and some home-care patients receive IV therapy. Many drugs cannot be absorbed through the gastrointestinal tract and must be administered intravenously to provide bioavailability with direct absorption and fast action. Certain drugs that need to be absorbed immediately are administered by direct IV injection, sometimes over several minutes. However, many drugs administered intravenously are irritating to the veins because of the drug's pH or osmolality and must be diluted and administered slowly.

Advantages of IV drug therapy are (1) rapid drug distribution into the bloodstream, (2) rapid onset of action, and (3) no drug loss to tissues. There are many complications of IV therapy, some of which are sepsis, thrombosis, phlebitis, air emboli, infiltration, and extravasation. The nurse must monitor for signs of these complications during the course of IV therapy.

Three methods are used to administer IV fluid and drugs: (1) direct IV drug injection, (2) continuous IV infusion, and (3) intermittent IV infusion. Continuous IV administration replaces fluid loss, maintains fluid balance, and is a vehicle for drug administration. Intermittent IV administration is primarily used for giving IV drugs at prescribed intervals.

Nurses play an important role in preparing and administering IV solutions and drugs. Nursing functions and responsibilities include (1) knowledge of IV sets and their drop factors, (2) calculating IV flow rates, (3) verifying compatibility of the IV solution and the drug, (4) mixing and diluting drugs in IV solution, (5) regulating IV infusion devices, (6) maintaining patency of IV accesses, and (7) monitoring for signs and symptoms of infiltration or other potential complications.

INTRAVENOUS SITES AND DEVICES

The successful administration of IV drugs and fluids depends on patent vascular access. The most common site for short-term (less than 1 week) IV therapy is the peripheral short site, which uses the dorsal and ventral surfaces of the upper extremities. Catheter length is normally 1 to 3 inches (Figure 11-1, *A* and *B*).

The peripheral midline site for IV therapy uses the veins in the area of the antecubital fossa—the basilic, brachial, cephalic, cubital, or medial. Midline peripheral catheters are between 3 and 8 inches in length and can stay in place 2 to 4 weeks.

The peripherally inserted central catheter (PICC) (Figure 11-2) can be used for IV therapy for up to 1 year. The catheter length is 21 inches. The insertion site is the region of the antecubital fossa that uses the same veins as the peripheral midline. The catheter is advanced through the vein in the upper arm until the tip rests in the lower third of the superior vena cava. Because the tip of the PICC line rests in the superior vena cava, it is considered a central line. Compared to other types of access, the multilumen PICC is more dependable and cost-effective. It is also versatile because it can be used for medication, IV fluids, blood products, total parenteral nutrition (TPN), and blood sampling. Infection rates are also very low with PICC lines. Another benefit of the PICC line is that it can be maintained on an outpatient basis, therefore patients can be discharged earlier from the hospital. In some states registered nurses certified in IV therapy can insert PICC lines.

Central venous access is used for patients who need long-term continuous infusions of fluids, medication, or nutritional support that cannot be sustained with a peripheral site. Central venous access is also used for patients who have poor peripheral veins, require a large amount of IV fluid or blood products in a short amount of time, or are receiving medication that is known to be too caustic for peripheral vessels. Central venous catheters (CVC) provide access to the superior vena cava and the inferior vena cava. A CVC placed in the internal jugular vein or the right or left subclavian vein is commonly used to access the superior vena cava. The inferior vena cava can be accessed through the femoral vein (Figure 11-3). Length of the CVC can vary from 6 to 28 inches. Insertion requires a competent provider to perform a sterile procedure involving the cannulation of the selected percutaneous vein with a single- or multilumen catheter. An x-ray is taken at the end of the procedure to confirm placement of the tip of the catheter in the superior vena cava just above the right atrium.

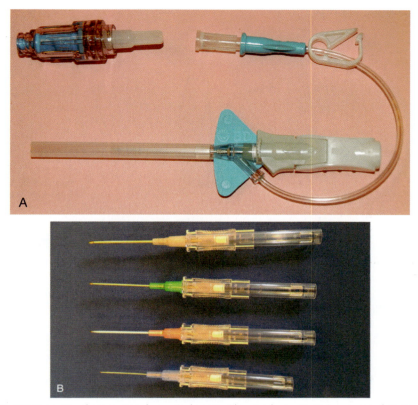

Figure 11-1 A, BD Nexiva IV catheter system has a single port with cap adapter. **B,** Various types of Becton Dickinson (BD) catheters.

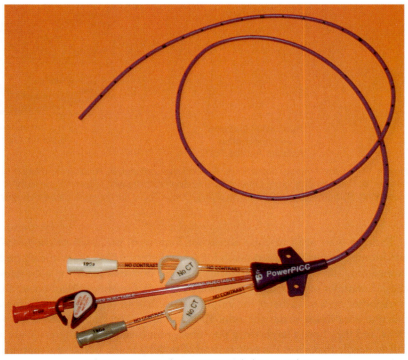

Figure 11-2 Bard PowerPICC triple-lumen catheter.

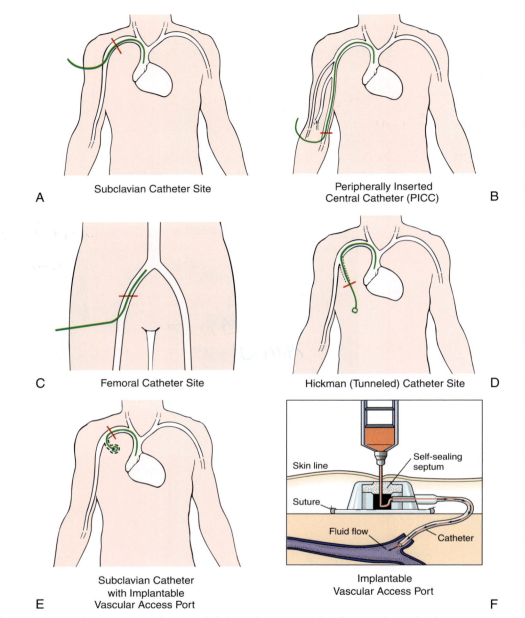

Figure 11-3 Central venous access sites. **A,** Subclavian catheter. **B,** Peripherally inserted central catheter (PICC). **C,** Femoral catheter. **D,** Hickman (tunneled) catheter. **E,** Subclavian catheter with implantable vascular access port. **F,** Implantable vascular access port. (**F,** from Perry, A. G., & Potter, P. A. [2006]. *Clinical nursing skills and techniques.* 6th ed. St. Louis: Mosby.)

Patients who need vascular access for long-term use, such as chemotherapy, antibiotic therapy, or nutritional support, are given much longer catheters, which are tunneled under the skin after the vein is cannulated. The catheter and its drug infusion port exit from the subcutaneous tissue to a site on the chest. Examples of these devices are the Hickman, Groshong, NeoStar, and Cook catheters.

Another type of catheter for long-term use has an implantable infusion port that is inserted in the subcutaneous tissue under the skin. These devices are called *vascular access ports,* also known as Port-a-caths, and they have a larger drug port or septum than other catheters. Care must be taken to use a non-coring needle that slices the port instead of making holes, so that the septum will close instead of leaking after the needle has been removed (Figure 11-3).

Intermittent Infusion Add-On Devices

When IV access sites are used for intermittent therapy instead of continuous infusion, they must be flushed periodically to maintain patency. An intermittent infusion add-on device can be attached to the end of the vascular access device, catheter, or needle to close the connection that was attached to the IV tubing. There are many types of add-on devices, such as extension loops, solid cannula caps, and injection access caps. All add-on devices should use a needleless Luer-Lok design as a safety measure. Use of add-on devices should be included as part of the protocol of the institution (Figure 11-4). These devices have ports (stoppers) where needleless syringes can be inserted when drug therapy is resumed. This practice can eliminate the need for a constant low-rate infusion to keep the vein open (KVO) and reduce excessive fluid intake. The use of intermittent infusion devices can allow the patient greater mobility and can be cost-effective because less IV tubing, IV solution, and regulating equipment are needed.

IV sites should be flushed every 8 to 12 hours or before and after each drug infusion, depending on institutional policy, to maintain patency. Table 11-1 gives suggested flushing times. Prefilled single-use syringes of saline solution are available to flush infusion devices (Figure 11-5, *A* and *B*). The intent of prefilled single-use syringes is to prevent the cross-contamination that can occur with a multidose vial. The volume of the flush used for vascular access devices is twice the volume of the catheter plus any connected devices such as a three-way stopcock or an extension set.

TABLE 11-1 Venous Access Devices: Flushing for Peripheral and Central Venous Catheters*				
Catheter Type	**Length (inches)**	**Flush Before Drug Use**	**Flush After Drug Use**	**Volume/mL**
Peripheral	1-2	NS	NS	1-3
Central venous				
Single-lumen	8	NS	HS	1-3
Multilumen	8	NS	HS	1-3
External tunneled Hickman, Cook, or Groshong	35	NS	HS or NS Flush q12h if not used	10
Peripherally inserted central catheter (PICC)	20	NS	NS Flush q12h if not used	10
Implanted vascular access device	35	NS	HS or NS Flush q12h if not used	10

*If the adapter/cap is pressurized, then normal saline is used, not a heparin solution. Follow the institution policy procedure and manufacturer's guidelines.
HS, Heparinized saline; *NS,* normal saline.

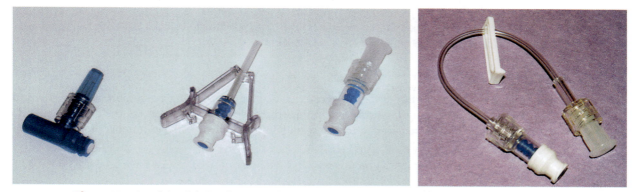

Figure 11-4 Needleless infusion devices. Medication in a needleless syringe can be inserted into a needleless infusion device.

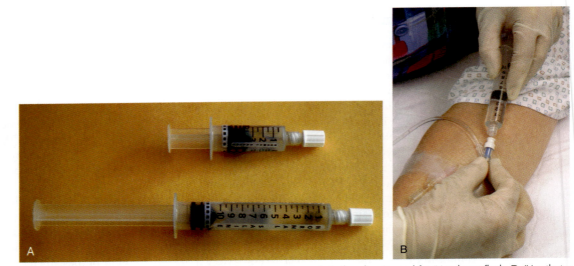

Figure 11-5 A, BD 3-mL and 10-mL prefilled, single-use syringe of sterile saline is used for IV catheter flush. **B,** IV catheter flush. The prefilled, single-use syringe is attached to the port of the IV tubing. (**B,** From Perry, A. G., & Potter, P. A. [2010]. *Clinical nursing skills and techniques.* 7th ed. St Louis: Mosby.)

DIRECT INTRAVENOUS INJECTIONS

Medications that are given by the IV injection route are calculated in the same manner as medications for intramuscular (IM) injection. This route is often referred to as *IV push.* Clinically, it is the preferred route for patients with poor muscle mass or decreased circulation, or for a drug that is poorly absorbed from the tissues. Medications administered by this route have a rapid onset of action, and calculation errors can have serious, even fatal, consequences. Drug information inserts must be read carefully, and attention must be paid to the amount of drug that can be given per minute. If the drug is pushed into the bloodstream at a faster rate than is specified in the drug literature, adverse reactions to the medication are likely to occur.

Calculating the amount of time needed to infuse a drug given by direct IV infusion can be done using the ratio and proportion method.

YOU MUST REMEMBER

When giving drugs by direct IV infusion, always verify the compatibility of the IV solution and the drug, or precipitation may result. Precipitation is a crystallization or suspension of particles in a solution, causing an occlusion of the intravenous line. Incompatibility can be avoided if the IV tubing is flushed with a compatible solution of normal saline before and after administration.

EXAMPLES Set up a ratio and proportion using the recommended amount of drug per minute on one side of the equation; these are the known variables. On the other side of the equation are the desired amount of the drug and the unknown desired minutes: a. amount in milliliters (mL); b. number of minutes.

PROBLEM 1:   Order: Dilantin 200 mg, IV, STAT.

Drug available: Dilantin 250 mg/5 mL. IV infusion not to exceed 50 mg/min.

a.   BF: $\dfrac{D}{H} \times V = \dfrac{\overset{4}{\cancel{200}} \text{ mg}}{\underset{5}{\cancel{250}} \text{ mg}} \times 5 \text{ mL} = \dfrac{20}{5} = 4 \text{ mL}$

or

RP: H : V ::   D   : X
250 mg : 5 mL :: 200 mg : X mL
250 X = 1000
X = 4 mL

or

FE: $\dfrac{H}{V} = \dfrac{D}{X} = \dfrac{250 \text{ mg}}{5 \text{ mL}} = \dfrac{200 \text{ mg}}{X}$

(Cross multiply)   250 X = 1000
X = 4 mL

or

DA: $\text{mL} = \dfrac{5 \text{ mL} \times \overset{4}{\cancel{200}} \text{ mg}}{\underset{5}{\cancel{250}} \text{ mg} \times 1} = \dfrac{20}{5} = 4 \text{ mL}$

200 mg = 4 mL (discard 1 mL of the 5 mL)

b.   known drug : known minutes :: desired drug : desired minutes
50 mg   :   1 min   ::   200 mg   :   X min
50 X = 200
X = 4 min

PROBLEM 2:   Order: Lasix 120 mg, IV, STAT.

Drug available: Lasix 10 mg/mL. IV infusion not to exceed 40 mg/min.

a.   RP: H : V ::   D : X
10 mg : 1 mL :: 120 mg : X mL
10 X = 120
X = 12 mL of Lasix

or

DA: $\text{mL} = \dfrac{1 \text{ mL} \times \overset{12}{\cancel{120}} \text{ mg}}{\underset{1}{\cancel{10}} \text{ mg} \times 1} = 12 \text{ mL of Lasix}$

b.   known drug : known minutes :: desired drug : desired minutes
40 mg   :   1 min   ::   120 mg   :   X min
40 X = 120
X = 3 min

When dosing instructions give the amount of drug and specify infusion time, the amount of drug can be divided by the number of minutes to attain the per-minute amount to be infused.

PROBLEM 3:   Order: inamrinone (Inocor) 65 mg, IV bolus over 3 minutes.

Drug available: Inocor 100 mg/20 mL.

a.   RP: H : V :: D : X
100 mg : 20 mL :: 65 mg : X mL
100 X = 1300
X = 13 mL

or

DA: $\text{mL} = \dfrac{\overset{1}{\cancel{20}} \text{ mL} \times 65 \text{ mg}}{\underset{5}{\cancel{100}} \text{ mg} \times 1} = \dfrac{65}{5} = 13 \text{ mL}$

b. $\dfrac{13 \text{ mL}}{3 \text{ min}} = 4.3 \text{ mL/min}$

PRACTICE PROBLEMS ▶ I DIRECT IV INJECTION

Answers can be found on pages 239 to 240.

A. Determine the amount in milliliters of drug solution to administer.

B. Determine the number of minutes that is required for the direct IV drug dose to be administered for each of the practice problems.

1. Order: protamine sulfate 50 mg, IV, STAT.
   Drug available:

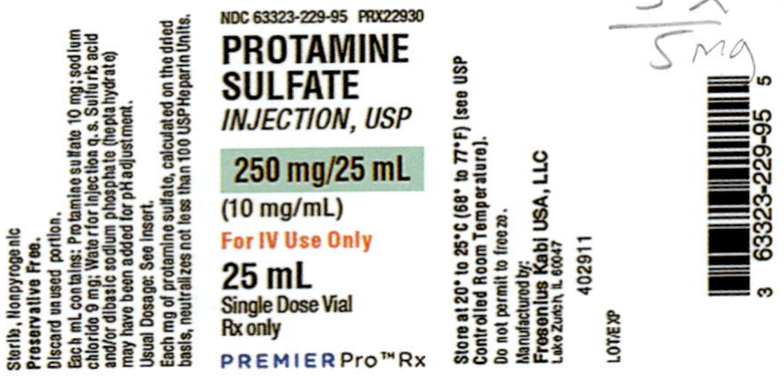

[Handwritten annotations:]

Known drug : Known min : dd : dm
   5mg   1min   50mg   X

$$\frac{5X}{5mg} = \frac{50mg/min}{5mg}$$

$$X = 10 \text{ min}$$

$$\frac{D}{H} \times V$$

$$\frac{50mg}{250mg} \times 25mL = 5mL$$

0.2

[Drug label:]

NDC 63323-229-95 PRX22930
PROTAMINE SULFATE
INJECTION, USP
250 mg/25 mL
(10 mg/mL)
For IV Use Only
25 mL
Single Dose Vial
Rx only
PREMIER Pro™ Rx

Sterile, Nonpyrogenic. Preservative Free. Discard unused portion.
Each mL contains: Protamine sulfate 10 mg; sodium chloride 9 mg; Water for Injection q.s. Sulfuric acid and/or dibasic sodium phosphate (heptahydrate) may have been added for pH adjustment.
Usual Dosage: See insert.
Each mg of protamine sulfate, calculated on the dried basis, neutralizes not less than 100 USP Heparin Units.

Store at 20° to 25°C (68° to 77°F) [see USP Controlled Room Temperature].
Do not permit to freeze.
Manufactured by:
Fresenius Kabi USA, LLC
Lake Zurich, IL 60047
402911
LOT/EXP

3 63323-229-95 5

IV infusion not to exceed 5 mg/min.

a. Amount in milliliters ___5 mL___

b. Number of minutes to administer ___10 min___

2. Order: dextrose 50% in 50 mL, IV, STAT.
   Drug available: dextrose 50% in 50 mL.
   IV infusion not to exceed 10 mL/min.

   Number of minutes to administer 50% of 50 mL _____

3. Order: calcium gluconate 4.65 mEq, IV, STAT.
   Drug available:

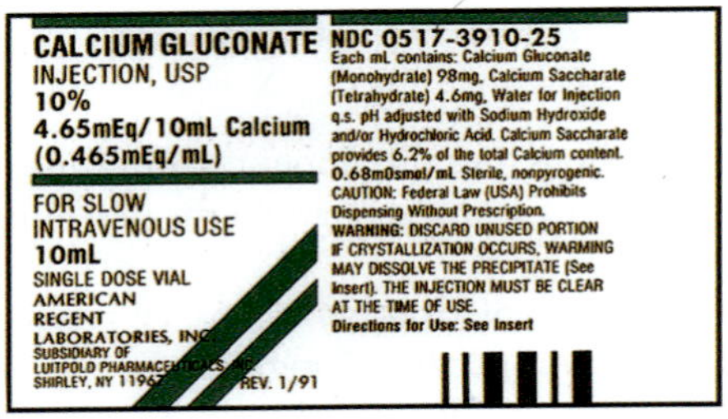

[Drug label:]

CALCIUM GLUCONATE
INJECTION, USP
10%
4.65mEq/10mL Calcium
(0.465mEq/mL)

FOR SLOW
INTRAVENOUS USE
10mL
SINGLE DOSE VIAL
AMERICAN
REGENT
LABORATORIES, INC.
SUBSIDIARY OF
LUITPOLD PHARMACEUTICALS, INC.
SHIRLEY, NY 11967   REV. 1/91

NDC 0517-3910-25
Each mL contains: Calcium Gluconate (Monohydrate) 98mg, Calcium Saccharate (Tetrahydrate) 4.6mg, Water for Injection q.s. pH adjusted with Sodium Hydroxide and/or Hydrochloric Acid. Calcium Saccharate provides 6.2% of the total Calcium content. 0.68mOsmol/mL Sterile, nonpyrogenic.
CAUTION: Federal Law (USA) Prohibits Dispensing Without Prescription.
WARNING: DISCARD UNUSED PORTION IF CRYSTALLIZATION OCCURS, WARMING MAY DISSOLVE THE PRECIPITATE (See Insert). THE INJECTION MUST BE CLEAR AT THE TIME OF USE.
Directions for Use: See Insert

IV infusion not to exceed 1.5 mL/min. Note: 4.65 mEq/10 mL.

a. Amount in milliliters _____

b. Number of minutes _____

4. Order: fentanyl 12.5 mcg, IV, q4h, PRN for pain.
   Drug available: fentanyl 100 mcg in 2 mL.
   IV infusion not to exceed 10 mcg/min.

   a. Amount in milliliters _____

   b. Number of minutes _____

5. Order: morphine sulfate 6 mg, IV, q3h, PRN.
    Drug available:

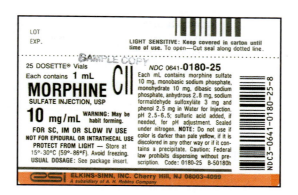

Infusion not to exceed 10 mg/4 min.

a. Amount in milliliters _____

b. Number of minutes _____

6. Order: digoxin 0.25 mg, IV, daily.
    Drug available:

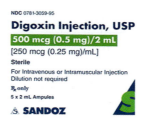

Infuse slowly over 5 minutes.

a. Amount in milliliters _____

b. How many mL/min should be infused? _____

7. Order: Haldol 2 mg, IV, q4h, PRN.
    Drug available: Haldol 5 mg/mL.
    IV infusion not to exceed 1 mg/min.

a. Amount in milliliters _____

b. Number of minutes _____

8. Order: Ativan 6 mg, IV, q6h, PRN.
    Drug available: Ativan 4 mg/mL.
    IV infusion not to exceed 2 mg/min.

a. Amount in milliliters _____

b. Number of minutes _____

9. **Order:** diltiazem (Cardizem) 20 mg IV over 2 minutes.
Drug available:

NDC 0088-1790-32

CARDIZEM® Injectable
(diltiazem HCl Injection)

25 mg (5 mg/mL) FOR DIRECT INTRAVENOUS BOLUS
INJECTION AND CONTINUOUS
INTRAVENOUS INFUSION

Sterile 5-mL Vial

SINGLE-USE CONTAINER. DISCARD UNUSED PORTION. Mfd. for
Date Removed From Refrigeration _____ Hoechst Marion Roussel, Inc.
Kansas City, MO 64137 USA
Date To Be Discarded _____ 50007742   C6

a. How many milliliters (mL) would you give? _____

b. How many milliliters (mL) would you infuse per minute? _____

10. **Order:** granisetron (Kytril) 10 mcg/kg, 30 minutes before chemotherapy.
Infuse 1 mg over 60 seconds.
Patient weighs 140 pounds.
Drug available:

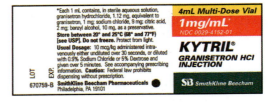

a. How many kilograms (kg) does the patient weigh? _____

b. How many milligrams (mg) should the patient receive? _____

c. For how many seconds should the drug dose be infused? _____

YOU MUST REMEMBER

Consider the length of the injection port on the tubing from the patient's IV site. If the IV rate is very low, (e.g., 30 mL/hr), the IV medication may take a long time to reach the patient. The drug dose is not complete until all of the drug has entered the patient. Therefore, the tubing will have to be flushed to ensure that the dose reaches the patient in a timely manner.

CONTINUOUS INTRAVENOUS ADMINISTRATION

When IV fluids are required, the health care provider orders the amount of solution per liter or milliliter to be administered for a specific time, such as for 24 hours. The nurse calculates the IV flow rate according to the drop factor, the amount of fluid to be administered, and the infusion time.

Intravenous Infusion Sets

All infusion sets have the same components: a sterile spike for entry into the IV bag or bottle, a drip chamber for counting drops and managing flow, a roller clamp that controls flow through the tubing, tubing length from drip chamber to IV site, Y-site for adding a secondary set or giving IV drugs, and the needleless adapter (which attaches to the IV catheter in the vessel) (Figure 11-6). Often a filter is added to the IV line to remove bacteria, particles, and air. Figure 11-7 shows two types of IV containers.

IV sets are either vented or unvented. Vented sets are used for IV bottles that have no vents and need a vent for air to enter the bottle so that the fluid will flow out. Unvented sets are for bottles or bags that either have their own venting system or do not need a venting system. Glass bottles are primarily used when the medication is not compatible with plastic because the drug either adheres to the plastic or is absorbed by the plastic.

If the IV infusion is not placed on a flow control device but instead is delivered by gravity, then the hourly rate will have to be adjusted manually. It is necessary to know the drop factor of the IV set to calculate the hourly infusion rate. The drop factor, or the number of drops per milliliter (mL), is printed on the package of the infusion set and found on top of the drip chamber. Sets that deliver large drops per milliliter (10, 15, or 20 gtt/mL) are referred to as *macrodrip sets,* and those that deliver small drops per milliliter (60 gtt/mL) are called *microdrip* or *minidrip* sets (Figure 11-8).

Drip rates are adjusted by counting the drops coming into the drip chamber. While looking at the second hand of your watch, adjust the roller clamp to determine the correct number of drops in one minute. It is more difficult to count when the drops are smaller and the drop rate is faster. One advantage of the microdrip set is that the number of milliliters per hour is the same as the drops per minute (e.g., if the infusion rate is 50 mL/hr, the drip rate is 50 gtt/min). When the IV rate is 100 mL/hr or higher, the macrodrip set generally is used. Slow drip rates (less than 100 mL/hr) make macrodrip adjustments too difficult (e.g., at 50 mL/hr, the macrodrip rate would be 8 gtt/min). Therefore if the IV rate is 100 mL/hr or lower, the microdrip is preferred.

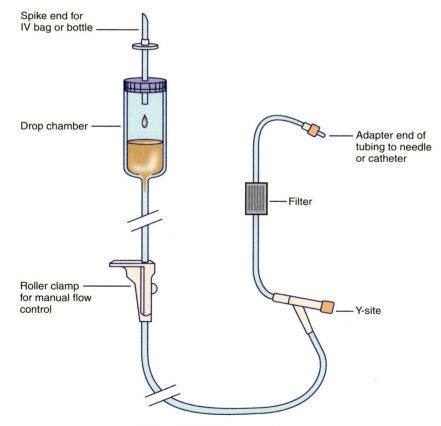

Figure 11-6 Intravenous tubing set.

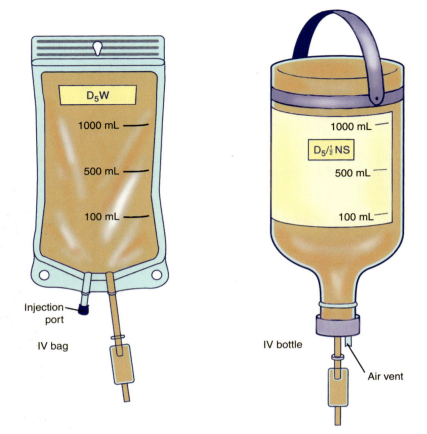

Figure 11-7 Intravenous bag and bottle.

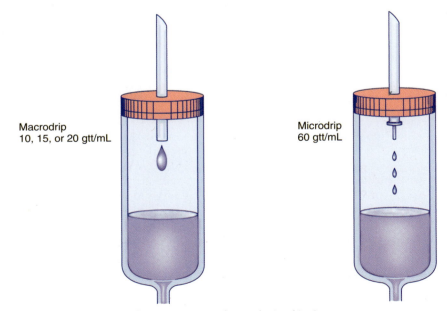

Figure 11-8 Macrodrop and microdrip sizes.

At times, IV fluids are given at a slow rate to *keep vein open* (KVO), also called *to keep open* (TKO). Reasons for ordering KVO include (1) a suspected or potential emergency situation requiring rapid administration of fluids and drugs, and (2) the need to maintain an open line to give IV drugs at specified hours. For KVO, a microdrip set (60 gtt/mL) and a 250-mL IV bag can be used. KVO should have a specific infusion rate, such as 10 to 20 mL/hr, or should be given according to the institution's protocol.

CALCULATION OF INTRAVENOUS FLOW RATE

Three different methods can be used to calculate IV flow rate (drops per minute or gtt/min). The nurse should select one of these methods, memorize it, and use it to calculate dosages.*

▶ **THREE-STEP METHOD**

a. $\dfrac{\text{Amount of solution}}{\text{Hours to administer}} = \text{mL/hr}$

b. $\dfrac{\text{mL per hour}}{60 \text{ minutes}} = \text{mL/min}$

c. mL per minute × gtt per mL of IV set = gtt/min

▶ **TWO-STEP METHOD**

a. Amount of fluid ÷ Hours to administer = mL/hr

b. $\dfrac{\text{mL per hour} \times \text{gtt/mL (IV set)}}{60 \text{ minutes}} = \text{gtt/min}$

▶ **ONE-STEP METHOD**

$$\dfrac{\text{Amount of fluid} \times \text{gtt/mL (IV set)}}{\text{Hours to administer} \times \text{Minutes per hour (60)}} = \text{gtt/min}$$

Safety Considerations

All IV infusions should be checked every half-hour or hour, according to the policy of the institution, to ensure the appropriate rate of infusion and to assess for potential problems, especially when manual flow control is used. Common problems associated with IV infusions are kinked tubing, infiltration, and "free-flow" IV rates. If IV tubing kinks and the flow is interrupted, the prescribed amount of fluid will not be given, and the access site can clot. When IV infiltration occurs, fluid leaks into the tissues around the IV site, causing redness, swelling, and discomfort. A more serious complication is extravasation, which occurs when the infiltrated medication damages the tissues at the IV site, resulting in sloughing and necrosis of exposed tissue.

Again, in this situation the prescribed amount of IV fluid is not infused. Free-flow IV rate refers to a rapid infusion of IV fluids, faster than prescribed, causing fluid overload, or too much fluid in the intravascular space, which can cause hypertension, pulmonary edema, and/or dyspnea. Medications that are administered faster than prescribed also can result in toxicity. A free-flow IV rate is the most prevalent drug error and has led to the use of electronic infusion devices.

Electronic infusion devices are not without flaws; mechanical problems occur and these devices can be incorrectly programmed, resulting in the wrong infusion rate. Fluid overload, thrombus formation, infiltration, and extravasation are complications of IV therapy that can be avoided with frequent monitoring of IV infusions. See Appendix A for more detailed information on safe practice for IV drug administration.

---

*The two-step method is the most commonly used method of calculating IV flow rate.

Adding Drugs Used for Continuous Intravenous Administration

Nurses may need to prepare medications from vials and add the medication into the patient's IV solution bag for some continuous infusions. This process of mixing or compounding an IV solution should be completed before the IV bag or bottle is hung. The medication is prepared using sterile technique and is added through the injection port to the bag or bottle that is to be rotated, or gently agitated, to ensure that the drug is dispersed. Failure to adequately disperse the medication can result in a higher concentration of medication close to the bottom of the bag or bottle. This would deliver a higher concentration of the added medication, potentially causing harm to the patient. Medication labels must be placed on the IV bag or bottle, clearly stating the patient's name and any other identifiers as specified by policy, such as name of the drug, amount, concentration, and strength of all ingredients without abbreviation; also, date, nurse's initials, time, and the time the IV should be completed should be provided. It is important to follow institutional policies and procedures when adding medication to continuous IV fluid.

NOTE

DO NOT add the drug while the infusion is running unless the bag is rotated. A drug solution injected into an upright infusing IV solution causes the drug to concentrate into the lower portion of the IV bag and not be dispersed. The patient will receive a concentrated drug solution, and this can be harmful (e.g., if the drug is potassium chloride).

Types of Solutions

All IV solutions contain various solutes and electrolytes that are added for specific therapies. Common solutes include dextrose (D) and sodium chloride (NaCl). The strength of the solution is expressed in percent (%), such as 0.45%, which means 0.45 g in 100 mL. Common commercially prepared IV solutions are dextrose in water (D_5W), dextrose with one-half normal saline solution (D_5 0.45%), normal saline solution (0.9% NaCl), one-half normal saline solution (0.45% NaCl), and lactated Ringer's solution (LR). Lactated Ringer's solution contains sodium, chloride, potassium, calcium, and lactate.

Tonicity of IV Solutions

The terms *tonicity* and *osmolality* have been used interchangeably, but *tonicity* refers to the concentration of IV solution, whereas *osmolality* is the concentration of body fluids (e.g., blood, serum). IV solutions produce tonicity in the cells of the body; this is the movement of water molecules into and out of the cells because of their surrounding aqueous environment. IV solutions are divided into three categories: hypertonic, hypotonic, and isotonic. The range of tonicity is measured in milliosmoles, and the normal range is 240 to 340 mOsm: +50 mOsm and/or −50 mOsm of 290 mOsm. Hypertonic solutions cause water molecules to diffuse out of the cells and exert a hyperosmolar effect. For example, a hypertonic solution is D_5 0.9% normal saline (NaCl) because it has an osmolarity of 560 mOsm. Hypotonic solutions cause water molecules to diffuse into the cells and exert a hypo-osmolar effect. A solution of 0.45% normal saline (NaCl) is hypo-osmolar and has an osmolarity of 154 mOsm. D_5W is iso-osmolar with an osmolality of 250 mOsm; however, the dextrose is metabolized quickly, leaving only water, thus making the solution hypotonic. Isotonic solutions maintain the same concentration of water molecules on both sides of the cell, so no net movement occurs. The osmolarity of isotonic solutions is 240 to 340 mOsm, similar to blood, lactated Ringer's (LR), and 0.9% normal saline (NaCl) solution. Table 11-2 lists the names of selected IV solutions, their tonicity, and their osmolarity, as well as the abbreviations for these solutions.

TABLE 11-2 Abbreviations for IV Solutions with Tonicity and Osmolarity

IV Solution	Tonicity	mOsm	Abbreviation(s)
5% dextrose in water	Iso	250	D_5W, 5% D/W
10% dextrose in water	Hyper	500	$D_{10}W$, 10% D/W
0.9% sodium chloride, normal saline solution	Iso	310	0.9% NaCl, NS
0.45% sodium chloride, ½ normal saline solution	Hypo	154	0.45% NaCl, ½ NS
5% dextrose in 0.9% sodium chloride	Hyper	560	D_5NS, 5% D/NS, 5% D/0.9% NaCl, D_5 PSS
Dextrose 5%/0.2% sodium chloride	Iso	326	D_5/0.2% NaCl
5% dextrose in 0.45% sodium chloride, 5% dextrose in ½ normal saline solution	Hyper	410	D_5½ NS, 5% D/½, NSS
Lactated Ringer's solution	Iso	274	LR

EXAMPLES Two problems in determining IV flow rate are given. Each problem is solved with each of the three methods for calculating IV flow rate.

PROBLEM 1: Order: 1000 mL of D_5½ NS (5% dextrose in ½ normal saline solution) in 6 hours. Available: 1 L (1000 mL) of D_5½ NS solution bag: IV set labeled 10 gtt/mL. How many drops per minute (gtt/min) should the patient receive?

Three-Step Method: **a.** $\dfrac{1000 \text{ mL}}{6 \text{ hr}}$ = 166.6 or 167 mL/hr

b. $\dfrac{167 \text{ mL}}{60 \text{ min}}$ = 2.7 or 2.8 mL/min

c. 2.8 mL/min × 10 gtt/mL = 28 gtt/min

Two-Step Method: **a.** 1000 mL ÷ 6 hr = 167 mL/hr

b. $\dfrac{167 \text{ mL/hr} \times \overset{1}{\cancel{10}} \text{ gtt/mL}}{\underset{6}{\cancel{60}} \text{ min}} = \dfrac{167}{6}$ = 28 gtt/min

10 and 60 cancel to 1 and 6.

If mL/hr is given, use only part **b** of the two-step method for calculating IV flow rate.

One-Step Method: $\dfrac{1000 \text{ mL} \times \overset{1}{\cancel{10}} \text{ gtt/mL}}{6 \text{ hr} \quad \times \quad \underset{6}{\cancel{60}} \text{ min}} = \dfrac{1000}{36}$ = 28 gtt/min

10 and 60 cancel to 1 and 6.

For the purpose of avoiding errors, the use of a hand calculator is strongly suggested.

Answer: 28 gtt/min.

PROBLEM 2: Order: 1000 mL of D_5W (5% dextrose in water), 1 vial of MVI (multiple vitamin), and 20 mEq of KCl (potassium chloride) every 8 hours.
Available: 1000 mL D_5W solution bag
   1 vial of MVI = 5 mL
   40 mEq/20 mL of KCl in an ampule
   IV set labeled 15 gtt/mL
How many milliliters (mL) of KCl would you withdraw as equivalent to 20 mEq of KCl?
How would you mix KCl in the IV bag?
How many drops per minute should the patient receive?

Procedure: MVI: Inject 5 mL of MVI into the rubber stopper on the IV bag.
   KCl: Calculate the prescribed dosage for KCl by using the basic formula, ratio and proportion, fractional equation (FE) method, or dimensional analysis.

$$\text{BF:}\ \frac{D}{H} \times V = \frac{20\ \text{mEq}}{40\ \text{mEq}} \times 20\ \text{mL} = \frac{400}{40} = 10\ \text{mL}$$

or
$$\text{RP:}\quad H\ :\ V\ ::\ D\ :\ X$$
$$40\ \text{mEq} : 20\ \text{mL} :: 20\ \text{mEq} : X\ \text{mL}$$
$$40\,X = 400$$
$$X = 10\ \text{mL}$$

or
$$\text{FE:}\ \frac{H}{V} = \frac{D}{X} = \frac{40\ \text{mEq}}{20\ \text{mL}} = \frac{20\ \text{mEq}}{X}$$
$$(\text{Cross multiply})\quad 40\,X = 400$$
$$X = 10\ \text{mL}$$

or
$$\text{DA:}\ \text{mL} = \frac{V \times D}{H \times 1}$$

$$\text{mL} = \frac{20\ \text{mL} \times \overset{1}{20\ \text{mEq}}}{\underset{2}{40\ \text{mEq}} \times 1} = \frac{20}{2} = 10\ \text{mL}$$

Withdraw 10 mL of KCl and inject it into the rubber stopper on the IV bag. Make sure the KCl solution and MVI additives are dispersed throughout the IV solution by rotating the IV bag.

Three-Step Method: **a.** $\dfrac{1000\ \text{mL}}{8\ \text{hr}} = 125\ \text{mL/hr}$

   b. $\dfrac{125\ \text{mL}}{60\ \text{min}} = 2.0\text{–}2.1\ \text{mL/min}$

   c. $2.1 \times 15 = 31\ (31.25\ \text{gtt/min})$

Two-Step Method: **a.** $1000 \div 8 = 125\ \text{mL/hr}$

   b. $\dfrac{125\ \text{mL/hr} \times \overset{1}{15}\ \text{gtt/mL}}{\underset{4}{60}\ \text{min}} = \dfrac{125}{4} = 31\ (31.25\ \text{gtt/min})$

   15 and 60 cancel to 1 and 4.
   IV flow rate should be 31.

One-Step Method: $\dfrac{1000\ \text{mL} \times \overset{1}{15}\ \text{gtt/mL}}{8\ \text{hr} \times \underset{4}{60}\ \text{min}} = \dfrac{1000}{32} = 31\ \text{gtt/min}\ (31.25\ \text{gtt/min})$

   15 and 60 cancel to 1 and 4.
   IV flow rate should be 31 gtt/min.

NOTE

Medication volume can be added to the total volume if strict intake and output are recorded. In general, an IV bag contains more fluid than is labeled on the bag; some estimates are as high as 50 mL. Count all volume added to bag, 1 mL or greater. If an electronic infusion device is used, the patient will receive the amount programmed into the device.

PRACTICE PROBLEMS ▶ **II CONTINUOUS INTRAVENOUS ADMINISTRATION**

Answers can be found on pages 240 and 241.

Select *one* of the three methods for calculating IV flow rate. The two-step method is preferred by most nurses.

1. Order: 1000 mL of D_5W to run for 12 hours. $\dfrac{1000mL}{12hrs}$ 83.3 micro drip <100ml

   a. Would you use a macrodrip or microdrip IV set? _____

   b. Calculate the drops per minute (gtt/min) using one of the three methods.

   __83.3 / 60 min = 1.4 mL X 60 gtt = 84 gtt/min__

2. Order: 3 L of IV solutions for 24 hours: 2 L of 5% D/½ NS and 1 L of D_5W.

   a. One liter is equal to ___1000___ mL.

   b. Each liter should run for ___8___ hours.

   c. The institution uses an IV set with a drop factor of 15 gtt/mL. How many drops per minute

      (gtt/min) should the patient receive? _____

3. Order: 250 mL of D_5W for KVO.

   a. What type of IV set would you use? _____

      Why? _____

   b. How many drops per minute should the patient receive? _____

4. Order: 1000 mL of 5% D/0.2% NaCl with 10 mEq of KCl for 10 hours.
   Available: Macrodrip IV set with a drop factor of 20 gtt/mL and microdrip set;
   KCl 20 mEq/20 mL vial.

   a. How many milliliters (mL) of KCl should be injected into the IV bag?

      _____

   b. How is KCl mixed in the IV solution? _____

   c. How many drops per minute (gtt/min) should the patient receive with both the macrodrip set

      and the microdrip set? _____

5. A liter (1000 mL) of IV fluid was started at 9 AM and was to run for 8 hours. The IV set delivers
   15 gtt/mL. Four hours later, only 300 mL has been absorbed.

   a. How much IV fluid is left? _____

   b. Recalculate the flow rate for the remaining IV fluids. _____

6. The patient is to receive D₅W, 100 mL/hr.
   Available: Microdrip set (60 gtt/mL).
   How many drops per minute should the patient receive? _____

7. Order: 1000 D₅W with 40 mEq KCl at 125 mL/hr.
   Drug available:

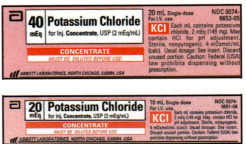

   a. Which concentration of KCl would you choose? _____
   b. How many milliliters of KCl should be injected into the IV bag?

   _____

   c. How many hours will the IV infusion last? _____

8. Order: 1000 D₅/½ NS with 20 mEq KCl at 100 mL/hr.
   Available: Macrodrip set (10 gtt/mL).
   Drug available:

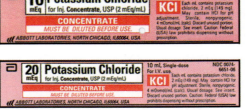

   a. Which concentration of KCl would you choose? _____
   b. How many milliliters of KCl should be injected into the IV bag? _____
   c. How many hours will the IV infusion last? _____
   d. How many drops per minute should the patient receive? _____

INTERMITTENT INTRAVENOUS ADMINISTRATION

Giving drugs via the intermittent IV route has many advantages. The IV route allows for rapid therapeutic concentration of the drug and control over the onset of action and peak concentrations. Blood serum concentrations can be achieved via the IV route if the oral route is unavailable because of the patient's condition, such as gastrointestinal malabsorption or neurological deficits that prevent swallowing. The intermittent IV route can be used on an outpatient basis and can ensure compliance with drug therapy. The IV route also allows for the rapid correction of electrolyte imbalances. IV medications can be given at intervals within a 24-hour period for days or weeks. These medications are administered in a small volume of fluid (50 to 250 mL of D₅W or saline solution). The drug solution usually is delivered to the patient in 15 minutes to

2 hours, depending on the medication. A separate delivery set or secondary set is used for intermittent therapy if the patient is also receiving continuous infusion through the same IV site.

Secondary Intravenous Sets

Secondary IV sets are used to infuse small fluid volumes such as, 50, 100, 250, and 500 mL in bags or bottles. Three types of tubing can be used. The first is similar to a regular IV set but with shorter tubing that is inserted or piggybacked into the primary IV line port. The second is a calibrated cylinder or chamber, which holds 150 mL, with brand names such as Buretrol, Volutrol, and SoluSet, also inserted into the primary set port. The third type is the regular set used with the infusion pump and piggybacked into the primary set at a port closer to the patient (Figure 11-9).

Medication is prepared and injected into a bag or a cylinder. If the cylinder is used, the drug is diluted with a measured amount of IV solution. After infusion, the cylinder is rinsed with 15 to 30 mL of the IV solution to clear the medication from the tubing. If the bag is used, the infusion runs until the bag is emptied.

If the fluid is delivered by gravity flow, the medication bag or cylinder needs to be raised higher than the primary set for the medication to infuse. Be aware that the drip chamber of the primary set must be observed to see that the medication is infusing properly from the secondary set and is not flowing into the primary set instead of the patient. If the secondary set is not flowing properly, then the IV site must be checked for patency.

Adding Drugs Used for Intermittent Intravenous Administration

Drugs that are given by intermittent infusion must be diluted and infused over a specific period of time. The pH and the osmolarity determine the dilution. A slower infusion time allows for the medication to be diluted in the blood vessel, thereby preventing phlebitis and high concentrations in the plasma and

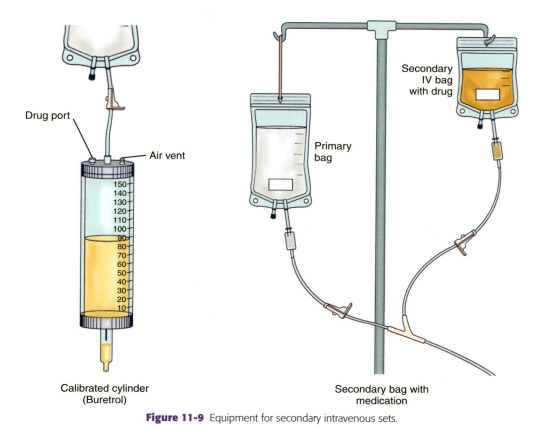

Figure 11-9 Equipment for secondary intravenous sets.

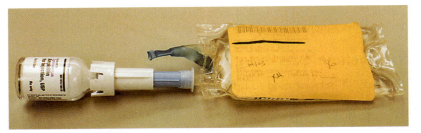

Figure 11-10 Medication mixed and attached to an IV bag.

tissues, which might cause time-related overdose, toxic effects, or allergic reaction. Drug-dosing instructions indicate the amount and type of solution and the length of infusion time. If the medication is not premixed from the pharmacy, the nurse must calculate the drug dose from the physician's order, then calculate the flow rate from the drug-dosing information.

Clinical agencies frequently have their own protocols for dilutions; if not, the drug information insert should provide infusion guidelines. If the information is not available, the hospital's pharmacy should be contacted. It is recommended that one set be used for the same drug to prevent admixture. Every set should be dated and labeled because one set can be used multiple times for the same drug in a 24-hour period. Guidelines and protocols help prevent drug and fluid incompatibilities.

Drugs administered by Buretrol, Volutrol, or SoluSet may be prepared by the nurse. Powdered drugs must be reconstituted with sterile water or normal saline solution following manufacturers' guidelines. Once the medication is added to the Buretrol, then the appropriate amount and type of IV fluid is added to the medication, and the infusion rate is adjusted. For medication diluted in bags or bottles, the powdered drug can be reconstituted the same way, or a spike adaptor can be used that can be attached to the vial and the bag. Fluid from the IV bag is flushed into the vial, reconstituting the powder, and then is flushed back into the bag. This process decreases contamination and is cost-effective. Mixing may be done by either the pharmacy or by the nurse (Figure 11-10).

The current trend in IV administration is the use of premixed or "ready to use" IV drugs in 50-mL to 1000-mL bags. These premixed IV medications can be prepared by the manufacturer or by the hospital's pharmacy. Problems of contamination and drug errors are decreased with the use of premixed IV medication. Each IV drug bag has separate tubing to prevent admixture. The actual cost of premixed medication is lower because there is less risk and less waste; it also saves nurses time. Because not all hospitals have admixture pharmacy systems in place, nurses will continue to prepare some drugs for IV administration.

NOTE

Sometimes the medication volume that is added to a bag or bottle adds a significant amount of volume. In those situations the 10% guideline applies. If the volume of medication for IV infusion exceeds 10% of the IV solution volume in the bag or bottle, then the amount of the medication volume should be withdrawn from the IV bag/bottle and replaced with the medication. For example, if the medication volume is 10 mL and a 100-mL bag is used, 10 mL should be aspirated from the IV bag injection port and replaced with the medication so that the total volume will still be 100 mL. If the medication's volume is less than 10%, then add the volume of medication to the volume of the bag or bottle. For example, 7 mL of medication is less than 10% of a 100-mL bag, so the total volume will be 107 mL. Follow your institution's protocol.

ADD-Vantage System

This system is similar to a secondary IV infusion or a piggyback system in which the nurse or pharmacist prepares the IV drugs. Figure 11-11 shows steps that the nurse takes in preparing the ADD-Vantage drug for IV administration.

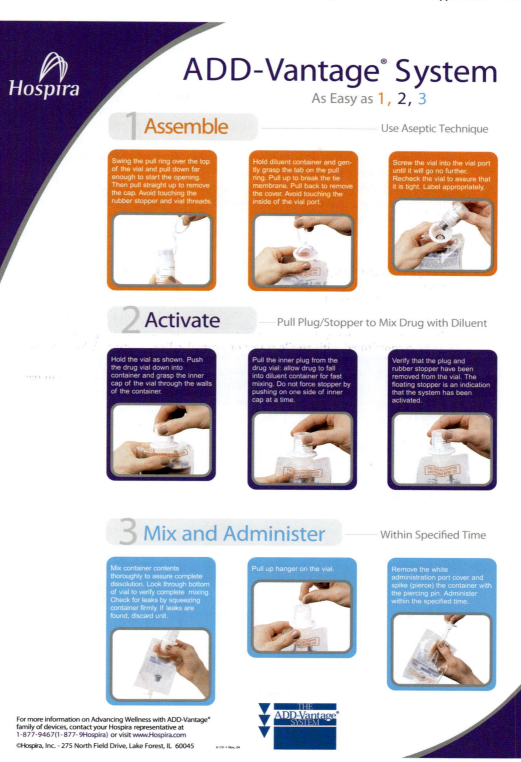

Figure 11-11 Hospira ADD-Vantage system. (From Hospira, Inc., Lake Forest, Ill.)

Electronic Intravenous Infusion Pumps

Infusion pumps are used for accurate fluid and drug administration (Figure 11-12). The peristaltic, volumetric, and syringe are three basic types of infusion pumps and all use a motor mechanism to create positive pressure to infuse fluid. The first is the linear peristaltic pump that uses a specially designed IV administration set that when placed in the pump, allows for ridges in the pump to move in a wavelike motion against the tubing to propel fluid along. The volumetric pump also has a specifically designed administration set with a reservoir that fills and empties every cycle to deliver the programmed fluid rate. The increments of fluid delivered with volumetric pumps can be as small as one tenth to one hundredth of a milliliter. The volumetric pump is considered more accurate than the peristaltic pump and the volumetric design is more widely manufactured.

The syringe pump uses a gear and screw mechanism to push fluid through IV tubing. One advantage of the syringe pump is that it does not require special tubing. A major disadvantage is that the syringe pump can hold only 2-mL to 100-mL syringes. The syringe pump is ideal for infusion of very small increments and some brands of pumps can infuse in nanograms. Syringe pumps are commonly used in pediatrics, oncology, obstetrics, and anesthesia (Figure 11-13, *A*).

The general-purpose pumps have safety features such as air-in-line, occlusion and infusion-complete alarms, as well as low-battery or low-power alerts (Figure 11-13, *B* and *C*). Pumps deliver a specific volume of fluid at a specific rate, measured in milliliters per hour (mL/hr). The general-purpose pump delivers at the rate of 0.1 to 999.9 mL/hr. The tubing for infusion pumps includes a safety feature called a flow regulator to prevent "free flow" when the tubing is removed from the pump. These regulators can be adjusted similarly to the roller clamp but are to be used only temporarily until the tubing can be placed back in the pump. Sensors in the pumps detect full or partial occlusion, especially at low flow rates. Another design feature is an alarm that notifies the nurse of an empty fluid container or any upstream occlusion, such as a clamp, that has not been released.

Programmable infusion pumps are now available that have important safety features that help in preventing IV drug errors. Programmable pumps, often referred to as "smart" pumps, have customized software that contains a library of medications and the maximum and minimum rates, known as guardrail limit, at which the medications should safely infuse (Figure 11-13, *E*). Hospitals can develop dosing parameters for each IV drug used in each patient area and update as needed. Once the IV medication solution is prepared, the nurse chooses the drug from the pump's library, then selects the dose to be given, the amount of solution in which the drug is diluted, and the time of the infusion. The pump calculates the infusion rate and will

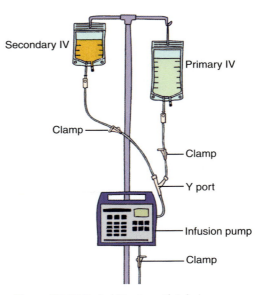

Figure 11-12 Typical IV setup with infusion pump.

infuse the drug at the correct rate. If the software recognizes an incorrect concentration or infusion time, the pump will alarm to alert the nurse so that the problem can be evaluated and corrected.

Multichannel Pumps

Multichannel smart pumps have a main software module or platform that houses the drug library. The infusion channel where the IV tubing is placed is docked or added to the platform. The platform controls infusion rates through the channel, and extra channels (up to four) can be added to handle multiple drug infusions at different infusion rates (Figure 11-13, *F*).

Ambulatory Pumps

Ambulatory pumps are volumetric and used primarily for outpatients because of their small size and light weight. This type of programmable pump is used for intermittent and continuous infusion or demand dosing. Ambulatory pumps can accommodate high volume rates, such as 125 mL/hr, and low dosing rates, such as 0.02 to 1 mL.

Patient-Controlled Analgesia

Patient-controlled analgesia (PCA) pumps are computerized devices that are programmed so patients can self-administer IV analgesics (Figure 11-13, *D*). These battery-operated infuser pumps latch onto a cassette or bag of a narcotic that can be infused into a patient with the use of PCA-compatible tubing. A continuous rate, demand dose, and frequency of administration can be programmed into the pump. These

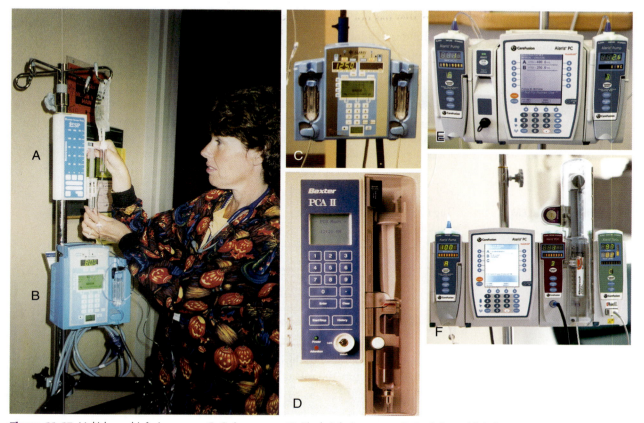

Figure 11-13 Multichannel infusion pump. **A,** Syringe pump. **B,** Single-infusion pump. **C,** Dual-channel infusion pump. **D,** Patient-controlled analgesia (PCA) pump. **E,** Alaris System Large Volume Pump with PCA. **F,** Example of the Medley pump module attached to the Medley programming module. (From ALARIS Medical Systems, Inc., San Diego, Calif. **E** and **F,** Copyright 2011 CareFusion Corporation; used with permission.)

set limits are ordered by the prescriber and prevent overdosage. The patient is able to administer a dose of pain medication using a control button attached to the PCA pump. The pump keeps a record of how much pain medication was delivered and how frequently the pain button was used. Each patient's pain should be assessed and PCA therapy should be documented per your institution's policy. Commonly used narcotics administered on a PCA pump are morphine, fentanyl, and hydromorphone.

The use of infusion pumps is becoming the standard of care for IV medication delivery. IV pumps with programmable software allow for the precise and accurate delivery of medication, especially compared to the roller clamp adjustment and visual drop counting method. Remember, every model of pump has different features and capabilities. It is essential that the nurse has a working knowledge and understanding of the equipment to deliver safe patient care.

FLOW RATES FOR INFUSION PUMPS AND SECONDARY SETS

When medication is given via the infusion pump, the primary IV flow is halted while the medication is infused. Once the secondary infusion is complete, the primary IV fluid can be restarted (see Figure 11-12). If a smart pump is used, the drug is selected from the library with the prescribed concentration, and the rate per hour is determined by the calculations from the pump. However, if a general-purpose pump is used, the nurse must calculate the rate per hour. If pumps are not available for infusion, then the nurse must calculate the secondary set IV rate in drops per minute.

▶ ONE-STEP METHOD FOR IV DRUG CALCULATION WITH SECONDARY SET

$$\frac{\text{Amount of solution} \times \text{gtt/mL of the set}}{\text{Minutes to administer}} = \text{gtt/minute}$$

$$\text{Amount of solution} \div \frac{\text{Minutes to administer}}{60 \text{ minutes/hour}} = \text{mL/hour}$$

NOTE

Medication volume that exceeds 1 mL should be added to the dilution volume in intermittent drug therapy. Because smaller volumes of fluid are used for IV infusion, drug dosage may be decreased if the volume of medication is not included in the dilution volume. The amount of solution in the formula should include both volumes.

EXAMPLES **PROBLEM 1:** Order: Tagamet 200 mg, IV, q6h.
Drug available:

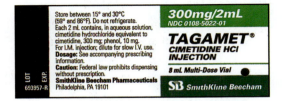

Set and solution: Buretrol set with drop factor of 60 gtt/mL; 500 mL of D_5W.
Instructions: Dilute drug in 100 mL of D_5W and infuse over 20 minutes.

Drug calculation:

$$\text{BF:} \frac{\text{D}}{\text{H}} \times \text{V} = \frac{200 \text{ mg}}{300 \text{ mg}} \times 2 \text{ mL} = \frac{400}{300} = 1.3 \text{ mL of Tagamet}$$

or

RP: H : V :: D : X

300 mg : 2 mL :: 200 mg : X mL

$$300\,X = 400$$

$$X = \frac{400}{300}$$

$$X = 1.3\ \text{mL of Tagamet}$$

or

FE: $\dfrac{H}{V} = \dfrac{D}{X} = \dfrac{300\ \text{mg}}{2\ \text{mL}} = \dfrac{200\ \text{mg}}{X} =$

(Cross multiply) $300\,X = 400$

$$X = 1.3\ \text{mL}$$

or

DA: $\text{mL} = \dfrac{2\ \text{mL} \times \overset{2}{\cancel{200}}\ \text{mg}}{\underset{3}{\cancel{300}}\ \text{mg} \times 1} = \dfrac{4}{3} = 1.3\ \text{mL}$

Flow rate calculation: 100 mL + 1.3 mL = 101.3 mL or 101 mL

$$\frac{\text{Amount of solution} \times \text{gtt/mL}}{\text{Minutes to administer}} = \frac{101\ \text{mL} \times \overset{3}{\cancel{60}}\ \text{gtt}}{\underset{1}{\cancel{20}}\ \text{min}} = 303\ \text{gtt/min}$$

Answer: Inject 1.3 mL of Tagamet into 100 mL of D_5W in the Buretrol chamber.
Regulate IV flow rate to 303 gtt/min.
It would be impossible to count 303 gtt/min. Instead of using the Buretrol, the nurse could use a secondary set with a larger drop factor or a regulator.

PROBLEM 2:   Order: Mandol 500 mg, IV, q6h.
Drug available:

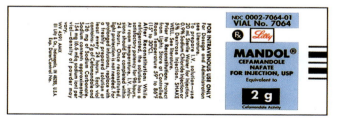

Label: Add 20 mL of diluent.
Set and solution: Secondary set with 100 mL D_5W and a drop factor of 15 gtt/mL.

Instructions: Dilute in 100 mL of D_5W and infuse over 30 minutes.

Drug calculation: (2.0 g = 2.000 mg).

BF: $\dfrac{D}{H} \times V = \dfrac{500\ \text{mg}}{2000\ \text{mg}} \times 20\ \text{mL} = \dfrac{10,000}{2000} = 5\ \text{mL of Mandol}$

or

RP: H : V :: D : X

2000 mg : 20 mL :: 500 mg : X mL

$$2000\,X = 10,000$$

$$X = 5\ \text{mL of Mandol}$$

or

FE: $\dfrac{H}{V} = \dfrac{D}{X} = \dfrac{2000\ \text{mg}}{20\ \text{mL}} = \dfrac{500\ \text{mg}}{X} =$

(Cross multiply) $2000\,X = 10,000$

$$X = 5\ \text{mL of Mandol}$$

or

DA: $\text{mL} = \dfrac{\overset{10}{\cancel{20}}\ \text{mL} \times 1\ \cancel{g} \times \overset{1}{\cancel{500}}\ \text{mg}}{\underset{1}{\cancel{2}}\ \cancel{g} \times \underset{2}{\cancel{1000}}\ \text{mg} \times 1} = \dfrac{10}{2} = 5\ \text{mL of Mandol}$

Flow rate calculation: 100 mL + 5 mL = 105 mL

$$\frac{\text{Amount of solution} \times \text{gtt/mL}}{\text{Minutes to administer}} = \frac{105 \text{ mL} \times \overset{1}{\cancel{15}} \text{ gtt/mL}}{\underset{2}{\cancel{30}} \text{ min}} = \frac{105}{2} = 52.5 \text{ or } 53 \text{ gtt/min}$$

Answer: Inject 5 mL of Mandol into the 100 mL D$_5$W bag.
Regulate IV flow rate to 53 gtt/min.

PROBLEM 3: Order: Zithromax 500 mg IV daily for 2 days.
Drug available:

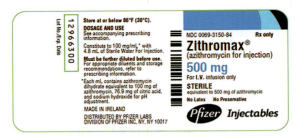

Label: Add 4.8 mL of sterile water to reconstitute to 100 mg/mL = 5 mL
Set and solution: Use an infusion pump.

Instructions: Dilute in 250 mL D$_5$W and infuse over 3 hours.

Flow rate calculation: 250 mL D$_5$W + 5 mL of medication = 255 mL

$$\text{Amount of solution} \div \frac{\text{Minutes to administer}}{60 \text{ minutes/hr}} = 255 \text{ mL} \div \frac{\overset{3}{\cancel{180}} \text{ min}}{\underset{1}{\cancel{60}} \text{ min/hr}} = 255 \times \frac{1}{3} = 85 \text{ mL/hr}$$

Answer: Infusion rate should be set at 85 mL/hr.

PROBLEM 4: Order: albumin 25 g, IV, now.
Available: albumin 25 g in 50 mL.
Set: Use an infusion pump.

Instructions: Administer over 25 minutes, or 2 mL/min.

Drug calculation: Not applicable.

Infusion pump rate:

$$50 \text{ mL} \div \frac{25 \text{ min}}{60 \text{ min}} = 50 \times \frac{60}{25} = \frac{3000}{25} = 120 \text{ mL/hr}$$

Answer: Infusion rate should be set at 120 mL/hr.

PROBLEM 5: Order: potassium phosphate 10 mM IV in 100 mL NS over 90 minutes.
Drug available:

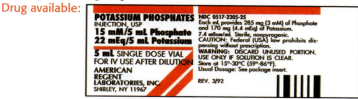

Set: Use an infusion pump.

Drug calculation:

$$\text{BF:} \frac{D}{H} \times V = \frac{10 \text{ mM}}{15 \text{ mM}} \times 5 \text{ mL} = \frac{50}{15} = 3.3 \text{ mL of potassium phosphate}$$

or
RP: H : V :: D : X
   15 mM : 5 mL :: 10 mM : X mL
      15 X = 50
         X = 3.3 mL of potassium phosphate

or
FE: $\frac{H}{V} = \frac{D}{X} = \frac{15 \text{ mM}}{5 \text{ mL}} = \frac{10 \text{ mM}}{X \text{ mL}}$

(Cross multiply) 15 X = 50
            X = 3.3 mL of
               potassium
               phosphate

or
$$\text{DA: mL} = \frac{5 \text{ mL} \times \overset{2}{\cancel{10}} \text{ mM}}{\underset{3}{\cancel{15}} \text{ mM} \times 1} = \frac{10}{3} = 3.3 \text{ mL}$$

Infusion pump rate: Amount of solution ÷ $\dfrac{\text{Minutes to administer}}{60 \text{ minutes}}$ = mL/hr

$$103 \text{ mL} \div \frac{90 \text{ min}}{60 \text{ min}} = 103 \times \frac{60}{90} = 68.6 \text{ or } 69 \text{ mL/hr}$$

Answer: Rate on the infusion pump should be 69 mL/hr to deliver potassium phosphate 10 mM in 90 minutes.

> ### NOTE
> When the electrolyte potassium is administered peripherally, the maximum infusion rate is 10 mEq/hr.

PRACTICE PROBLEMS ▶ III INTERMITTENT INTRAVENOUS ADMINISTRATION

Answers can be found on pages 241 to 245.

Calculate the fluid rate by using a calibrated cylinder (Buretrol), a secondary set, or an infusion pump, as indicated in each question.

1. Order: Cefazolin 250 mg, IV, q6h.
   Drug available: Cefazolin 1 g vial to be diluted with 2.5 mL.

   Set solution: Set Buretrol for a drop factor of 60 gtt/mL.

   Instructions: Dilute drug in 75 mL of NS and infuse over 30 minutes in Buretrol.

   a. 250 mg = _____ grams

   b. *Drug calculation:* _____

   c. *Flow rate calculation:* _____

2. Order: acetaminophen 500 mg, IV, q6h PRN for fever >38° C.
Patient's temperature is currently 38.5° C.
Drug available: Ofirmev 1000 mg/100 mL.

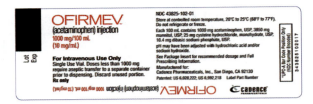

Set: secondary set with a drop factor of 6 gtt/mL.

Instructions: Infuse over 15 minutes.

a. *Drug calculation:*

_____

b. *Flow rate calculation:*

_____

3. Order: ticarcillin (Ticar) 500 mg, IV, q6h.
Drug available:

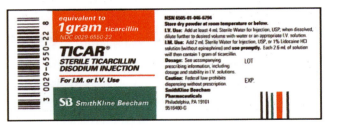

Set and solution: Buretrol set with a drop factor of 60 gtt/mL; infusion pump; 500 mL of D₅W.

Instructions: Dilute drug in 75 mL of D₅W and infuse over 40 minutes.

a. *Drug calculation:* Add _____ mL to ticarcillin vial (see drug label).

_____

b. *Flow rate calculation (gtt/min):*
How many drops per minute should the patient receive with use of the Buretrol set?

_____

c. *Infusion pump rate calculation (mL/hr):*
With an infusion pump, how many mL/hr should be administered?

_____

4. **Order:** piperacillin 2.5 g, IV, q6h.
   Drug available: piperacillin 4 g vial in powdered form; add 7.8 mL of diluent to yield 10 mL of drug solution (4 g = 10 mL).

   Set and solution: Buretrol set with a drop factor of 60 gtt/mL; infusion pump; 500 mL of D_5W.

   Instructions: Dilute drug in 100 mL of D_5W and infuse over 30 minutes.

   a. *Drug calculation:*

   _____

   b. *Flow rate calculation (gtt/min):*
      How many drops per minute should the patient receive with use of the Buretrol set?

   _____

   c. *Infusion pump rate calculation (mL/hr):*
      With an infusion pump, how many mL/hr should be administered?

   _____

5. **Order:** methicillin (Staphcillin) 1 g, IV, q6h.
   Drug available: Staphcillin 4 g in powdered form in vial; add 5.7 mL of diluent to yield 8 mL (1 g = 2 mL).

   Set and solution: secondary set with a drop factor of 15 gtt/mL; 100-mL bag of D_5W; infusion pump.

   Instructions: Dilute drug in 100 mL of D_5W and infuse over 40 minutes.

   a. *Drug calculation:* _____
      Explain the procedure for diluting the drug and adding it to the IV bag.

   _____

   b. *Flow rate calculation (gtt/min):*
      How many drops per minute should the patient receive with use of a secondary set?

   _____

   c. *Infusion pump rate calculation (mL/hr):*
      With an infusion pump, how many mL/hr should be administered?

   _____

6. **Order:** ciprofloxacin 250 mg, IV, q12h.
   Drug available:

Set and solution: Secondary set with drip factor 15 gtt/mL; 250 mL of D₅W.

Instructions: Add ciprofloxin 250 mg to 250 mL D₅W and infuse over 60 minutes.

a. *Drug calculation:*

_____

b. *Flow rate calculation (gtt/min):*
   How many drops per minute should the patient receive?

_____

7. **Order:** doxycycline (Vibramycin), 100 mg, IV, q12h.
   Drug available:

Set and solution: 100 mL of D₅W; secondary set with drop factor 15 gtt/mL; infusion pump.

Instructions: Mix Vibramycin vial with 10 mL of diluent; dilute in 100 mL of D₅W and infuse in 40 minutes.

a. *Flow rate calculation (gtt/min):*

_____

b. *Infusion pump rate calculation (mL/hr):*

_____

8. **Order:** ranitidine (Zantac) 50 mg, IV, q6h.
   Set: infusion pump.
   Drug available: premixed drug in bag (Zantac 50 mg in 0.45% NaCl [½ NSS]).

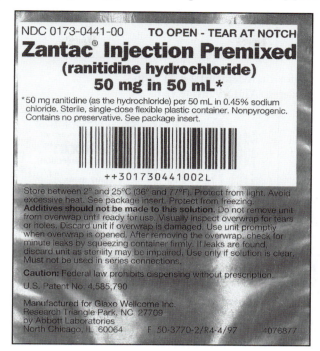

Instructions: Infuse over 15 minutes.

   a. *Infusion pump rate calculation:* _____

9. **Order:** cefepime (Maxipime) 750 mg, IV, q12h.
   Set and solution: infusion pump; 100 mL D_5W.
   Drug available:

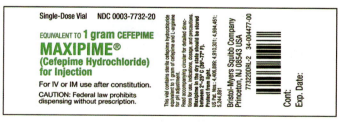

Instructions: Add 8.7 mL of diluent to Maxipime to yield 10 mL of drug solution. Dilute in 100 mL of D_5W; infuse over 30 minutes.

   a. *Drug calculation:*

   _____

   b. *Infusion pump rate calculation (mL/hr):* _____

10. **Order:** rifampin (Rifadin) 600 mg, IV, daily.
    Set and solution: infusion pump; 500 mL D_5W.
    Drug available: Rifadin, 600 mg sterile powder.

    Instructions: Add 10 mL of diluent to the rifampin vial. Dilute rifampin in 500 mL of D_5W; infuse over 3 hours.

    a. *Infusion pump rate calculation (mL/hr):* _____

11. **Order:** cefoxitin (Mefoxin) 2 g, IV, q8h.
    Drug available: ADD-Vantage vial.

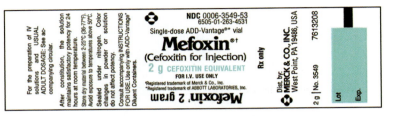

    Set and solution: 100 mL of 0.9% NaCl diluent bag for ADD-Vantage; Mefoxin vial for ADD-Vantage.

    Instructions: Dilute Mefoxin in 100 mL of NS (0.9% NaCl) and infuse in 30 minutes.

    a. How would you prepare Mefoxin 2 g powdered vial with the diluent bag? (See page 225 as

    needed.) _____

    b. *Infusion pump rate calculation (mL/hr):* _____

12. **Order:** Hycamtin (topotecan HCl) 1.5 mg/m²/day, IV, daily for 5 days.
    Adult weight and height: 140 lb, 66 inches.
    Drug available:

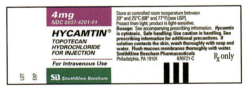

    Set and solution: 100 mL of D_5W; infusion pump.

    Instructions: Mix Hycamtin with 5.6 mL of diluent, equals 6 mL of Hycamtin; dilute in 100 mL of D_5W and infuse over 30 minutes.

    a. What is the patient's m² (BSA)? See Figure 7-1 on page 100.

    b. *Drug calculation:* _____

    c. *Infusion pump rate calculation (mL/hr):* _____

13. Order: Velban (vinblastine): initially 3.7 mg/m^2 as a single dose.
    Adult weight and height: 180 lb, 70 inches.
    Drug available:

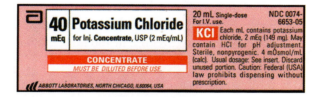

Set and solution: 250 mL of D$_5$W; infusion pump.

Instructions: Mix vinblastine powdered vial with 10 mL of diluent and inject solution into 250 mL of D$_5$W. Infuse over 1 hour.

a. What is the patient's m^2 (BSA)? _____

b. *Drug calculation:* _____

c. *Infusion pump rate calculation (mL/hr):* _____

14. Order: potassium chloride 20 mEq in 150 mL D$_5$W infused over 2 hours.
    Drug available:

![Potassium Chloride 40 mEq for Inj. Concentrate, USP (2 mEq/mL). 20 mL Single-dose. For I.V. use. NDC 0074-6653-05. KCl Each mL contains potassium chloride, 2 mEq (149 mg). May contain HCl for pH adjustment. Sterile, nonpyrogenic. 4 mOsmol/mL (calc). Usual dosage: See insert. Discard unused portion. Caution: Federal (USA) law prohibits dispensing without prescription. CONCENTRATE MUST BE DILUTED BEFORE USE. ABBOTT LABORATORIES, NORTH CHICAGO, IL60064, USA]

Set and solution: secondary set with drop factor of 15 gtt/mL; 150-mL bottle D$_5$W; infusion pump.

a. *Drug calculation:*

_____

b. *Infusion pump rate calculation (mL/hr):* _____

15. **Order:** magnesium sulfate 5 g in 100 mL D_5W infused over 3 hours.
    Drug available:

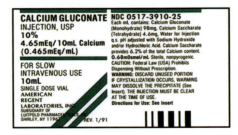

Set and solution: secondary set with drip factor of 15 gtt/mL; 100-mL bag D_5W; infusion pump.

Drug calculation:

a. 1 mL = _____ mg (see drug label)

b. 5 g = _____ mL

c. *Infusion pump rate calculation (mL/hr):*

_____

16. **Order:** calcium gluconate 10%, 16 mEq in 100 mL D_5W, infused over 30 minutes.
    Drug available:

Set and solution: secondary set with a drip factor of 15 gtt/mL; 100-mL bag D_5W; infusion pump.

a. *Drug calculation:*

_____

b. *Infusion pump rate calculation (mL/hr):*

_____

ANSWERS

I Direct IV Injection

1. a. 5-mL drug solution

  b. known drug : known minutes :: desired drug : desired minutes

      5 mg   :   1 min   ::   50 mg   :   X min

                    5 X = 50

                      X = 10 minutes

2. known drug : known minutes :: desired drug : desired minutes

     10 mL   :   1 min   ::   50 mL   :   X min

                    10 X = 50

                     X = 5 minutes

3. a. 10 mL

  b. known drug : known minutes :: desired drug : desired minutes

     1.5 mL   :   1 min   ::   10 mL   :   X min

                 1.5 X = 10

                   X = 6.6 minutes or 7 minutes

4. a. 0.25 mL fentanyl

  b. known drug : known minutes :: desired drug : desired minutes

     10 mcg   :   1 min   :: 12.5 mcg :   X min

                  10 X = 12.5

                    X = 1.25 minutes

5. a. RP: H : V :: D :X

       10 mg : 1 mL :: 6 mg : X

            10 X = 6

              X = 0.6 mL morphine

  or

  FE: $\dfrac{H}{V} = \dfrac{D}{X} = \dfrac{10 \text{ mg}}{1 \text{ mL}} = \dfrac{6 \text{ mg}}{X}$

              10 X = 6

              X = 0.6 mL

  b. known drug : known minutes :: desired drug : desired minutes

     10 mg   :   4 min   ::   6 mg   :   X min

                  10 X = 24

                    X = 2.4 minutes

6. a. 1 mL

  b. known drug : known minutes :: desired drug : desired minutes

     1 mL   :   5 min   ::   X mL   :   1 min

                    5 X = 1

                    X = 0.2 mL/minute

7. a. DA: $\text{mL} = \dfrac{1 \text{ mL} \times 2 \text{ mg}}{5 \text{ mg} \times 1} = \dfrac{2}{5} = 0.4 \text{ mL of Haldol}$

  b. known drug : known minutes :: desired drug : desired minutes

     1 mg   :   1 min   ::   2 mg   :   X min

                    X = 2 minutes

8. a. BF: $\dfrac{D}{H} \times V = \dfrac{6 \text{ mg}}{4 \text{ mg}} \times 1 = 1.5 \text{ mL of Ativan}$

  b. known drug : known minutes :: desired drug : desired minutes

     2 mg   :   1 min   ::   6 mg   :   X min

                  2 X = 6

                    X = 3 minutes

9. a. RP: H : V :: D : V

25 mg : 5 mL :: 20 mg : X mL

25 X = 100

X = 4 mL

or

FE: $\dfrac{H}{V} = \dfrac{D}{X} = \dfrac{25\ mg}{5\ mL} = \dfrac{20\ mg}{X\ mL}$

(Cross multiply) 25 X = 100

X = 4 mL

or

DA: $V = \dfrac{V \times D}{H \times 1}$

$mL = \dfrac{5\ mL \times \overset{4}{\cancel{20\ mg}}}{\underset{5}{\cancel{25\ mg}} \times 1} = \dfrac{20}{5} = 4\ mL$

b. $\dfrac{\text{Amount of drug}}{\text{Number of minutes}} = \dfrac{4\ mL}{2\ min} = 2\ mL/min$

Answer: Infuse 2 mL of cardizem per minute.

10. a. 140 lb ÷ 2.2 = 64 kg

b. 10 mcg × 64 kg = 640 mcg

Change micrograms (mcg) to milligrams by moving the decimal point three spaces to the *left:* 640 mcg = 0.640 mg or 0.6 mg.

c. Known drug : known seconds :: desired drug : desired seconds

1 mg : 60 seconds :: 0.6 mg : X sec

X = 36 seconds

Answer: Infuse 0.6 mg of granisetron (Kytril) over 36 seconds.

II Continuous Intravenous Administration

1. a. Microdrip set because the patient is to receive 83 mL/hr

b. Three-step method: (a) $\dfrac{1000\ mL}{12\ hr} = 83\ mL/hr$

(b) $\dfrac{83\ mL/hr}{60\ min} = 1.38\ mL/min\ or\ 1.4\ mL$

(c) 1.4 mL/min × 60 gtt/mL = 84 gtt/min

Using a microdrip set (60 gtt/mL), IV should run at 84 gtt/min.

2. a. 1 L = 1000 mL

b. Each liter should run for 8 hours.

c. Two-step method: 1000 ÷ 8 = 125 mL/hr

$\dfrac{125\ mL \times \overset{1}{\cancel{15}}\ gtt/min}{\underset{4}{\cancel{60}}\ min} = \dfrac{125}{4} = 31\text{--}32\ gtt/min$

With a 15-gtt/mL drop set, IV should run at 31 to 32 gtt/min.

3. a. Microdrip set with drop factor of 60 gtt/mL is used because the hourly rate is low and would make drops easier to count.

b. One-step method: $\dfrac{250\ mL \times \overset{1}{\cancel{60}}\ gtt/min}{24\ hr \times \underset{1}{\cancel{60}}\ min/hr} = 10\ gtt/min$

With a microdrip set, IV should run at 10 gtt/min. KVO usually means 24 hours.

4. a. 10 mL of KCl

b. Use a 10-mL syringe; withdraw 10 mL of KCl and inject into the rubber stopper part of the IV bag.

c. Microdrip set: 100 gtt/min

Macrodrip set: drop factor of 20 gtt/mL; 33 gtt/min (33.3 gtt/min)

5. **a.** 700 mL of IV fluid is left and 4 hours are left.
   b. Recalculate using 700 mL and 4 hours to run.

   Three-step method: (a) $\dfrac{700 \text{ mL}}{4 \text{ hr}} = 175 \text{ mL/hr}$

   (b) $\dfrac{175 \text{ mL/hr}}{60 \text{ min}} = 2.9 \text{ mL/min}$

   (c) $2.9 \text{ mL/min} \times 15 \text{ gtt/mL} = 43.5 \text{ gtt/min or } 44 \text{ gtt/min}$

6. 100 gtt/min

   Two-step method: $\dfrac{100 \times \overset{1}{\cancel{60}} \text{ gtt/mL}}{\underset{1}{\cancel{60}} \text{ min}} = 100 \text{ gtt/min}$

7. **a.** KCl 40 mEq/20 mL
   b. 20 mL

   c. $\dfrac{1000 \text{ mL}}{125 \text{ mL/hr}} = 8 \text{ hours}$

8. **a.** KCl 20 mEq/10 mL
   b. 10 mL

   c. $\dfrac{1000 \text{ mL}}{100 \text{ mL/hr}} = 10 \text{ hours}$

   d. $\dfrac{100 \text{ mL} \times \overset{1}{\cancel{10}} \text{ gtt/mL}}{\underset{6}{\cancel{60}} \text{ min}} = \dfrac{100}{6} = 16.6 \text{ gtt/min or } 17 \text{ gtt/min}$

   or

   $\dfrac{1000 \text{ mL} \times \overset{1}{\cancel{10}} \text{ gtt/mL}}{\underset{1}{\cancel{10}} \text{ hr} \times 60 \text{ min}} = \dfrac{1000}{60} = 16.6 \text{ gtt/min or } 17 \text{ gtt/min}$

III Intermittent Intravenous Administration

1. **a.** 250 mg = 0.25 g
   b. *Drug calculation:*

   BF: $\dfrac{D}{H} \times V = \dfrac{0.25 \text{ g}}{1 \text{ g}} \times 2.5 \text{ mL} = 0.6 \text{ mL}$

   or

   RP: H :   V :: D : X
   1 g : 2.5 mL :: 0.25 g : X mL
   1 X = 2.5 × 0.25
   X = 0.6 mL

   or

   DA: mL $= \dfrac{2.5 \text{ mL} \times 1 \text{ g} \times 250 \text{ mg}}{1 \text{ g} \times 1000 \text{ mg} \times 1} = 0.6 \text{ mL}$

   or

   FE: $\dfrac{H}{V} = \dfrac{D}{X} = \dfrac{1 \text{ g}}{2.5 \text{ mL}} = \dfrac{0.25 \text{ g}}{X} = X = 0.6 \text{ mL}$

   c. *Flow rate calculation:* Amount of solution: 75 mL + 0.6 mL = 75.6 or 76 mL

   $\dfrac{\text{Amount of solution} \times \text{gtt/mL}}{\text{Minutes to administer}} = \dfrac{76 \text{ mL} \times 60 \text{ gtt/mL}}{30 \text{ min}} = 152 \text{ gtt/min}$

   Regulate flow rate for 152 gtt/min.

2. a. *Drug calculation:*

$$BF: \frac{D}{H} \times V = \frac{500 \text{ g}}{1000 \text{ mg}} \times 100 \text{ mL} = 50 \text{ mL}$$

or

$$RP: \quad H \quad : \quad V \quad :: \quad D \quad : \quad X$$
$$1000 \text{ g}: 100 \text{ mL} :: 500 \text{ mg} : X \text{ mL}$$
$$1000 \, X = 50{,}000$$
$$X = 50 \text{ mL}$$

or

$$DA: mL = \frac{100 \text{ mL} \times 500 \text{ mg}}{1000 \text{ mg} \times 1} = 50 \text{ mL}$$

or

$$FE: \frac{H}{V} = \frac{D}{X} = \frac{1000 \text{ mg}}{100 \text{ mL}} = \frac{500 \text{ mg}}{X}$$

$$1000 \, X = 50{,}000$$
$$(\text{Cross multiply}) \, X = 50 \text{ mL}$$

b. *Flow rate calculation:*

$$\frac{\text{Amount of solution} \times \text{gtt/mL}}{\text{Minutes to administer}} = \frac{100 \text{ mL} \times 6 \text{ gtt/mL}}{15 \text{ minutes}} = 40 \text{ gtt/min}$$

Regulate flow rate of secondary tubing for 40 gtt/min.

3. a. *Drug calculation:*

$$BF: \frac{D}{H} \times V = \frac{500 \text{ mg}}{1000 \text{ mg}} \times 4 \text{ mL} = \frac{2000}{1000} = 2 \text{ mL is the dose for 500 mg of ticarcillin.}$$

b. *Flow rate calculation:* Amount of solution: 75 mL D$_5$W + 2 mL of drug solution = 77 mL
For Buretrol set:

$$\frac{77 \text{ mL} \times \overset{3}{\cancel{60}} \text{ gtt/mL (set)}}{\underset{2}{\cancel{40}} \text{ minutes}} = \frac{231}{2} = 115.5 \text{ or } 116 \text{ gtt/min}$$

c. *Infusion pump rate calculation:*

$$\text{Amount of solution} \div \frac{\text{Minutes to administer}}{60 \text{ min/hr}} = \text{mL/hr}$$

$$77 \text{ mL} \div \frac{\overset{2}{\cancel{40}} \text{ min to administer}}{\underset{3}{\cancel{60}} \text{ min/hr}} = 77 \times \frac{3}{2} = \frac{231}{2} = 116 \text{ mL/hr}$$

Set pump rate at 116 mL/hr to deliver Ticar 500 mg in 40 minutes.

4. a. *Drug calculation:*

$$BF: \frac{D}{H} \times V = \frac{2.5 \text{ g}}{\underset{2}{\cancel{4} \text{ g}}} \times \overset{5}{\cancel{10}} \text{ mL} = \frac{12.5}{2} = 6.25 \text{ mL}$$

or

$$FE: \frac{H}{V} = \frac{D}{X} = \frac{4 \text{ g}}{10 \text{ mL}} = \frac{2.5 \text{ g}}{X \text{ mL}}$$

$$(\text{Cross multiply}) \, 4 \, X = 25$$
$$X = 6.25 \text{ mL}$$

or

$$RP: \; H : \; V \; :: \; D \; : \; X$$
$$4 \text{ g} : 10 \text{ mL} :: 2.5 \text{ g} : X \text{ mL}$$
$$4 \, X = 25$$
$$X = 6.25 \text{ mL}$$
piperacillin 2.5 g = 6.25 mL

or

$$DA: mL = \frac{10 \text{ mL} \times 2.5 \cancel{\text{g}}}{4 \cancel{\text{g}} \times 1} = \frac{25}{4} = 6.25 \text{ mL}$$

b. *Flow rate calculation for Buretrol set:* amount of solution: 6.25 mL + 100 mL = 106.25 mL

$$\frac{106 \text{ mL} \times \overset{2}{\cancel{60}} \text{ gtt/mL}}{\underset{1}{\cancel{30}} \text{ min/hr}} = 212 \text{ gtt/min}$$

c. *Infusion pump rate calculation:* 100 mL + 6 mL medication = 106 mL

$$106 \text{ mL} \div \frac{\overset{1}{\cancel{30}} \text{ min to administer}}{\underset{2}{\cancel{60}} \text{ min/hr}} = 106 \times \frac{2}{1} = 212 \text{ mL/hr}$$

Set pump rate at 212 mL/hr to deliver piperacillin 2.5 g in 30 minutes.

5. a. *Drug calculation:* Staphcillin 4 g = 8 mL

$$\text{BF:} \frac{D}{H} \times V = \frac{1\,g}{4\,g} \times 8\,\text{mL} = \frac{8}{4} = 2\,\text{mL dose of Staphcillin}$$

Amount of solution: 2 mL + 100 mL = 102 mL

b. *Flow rate calculation for secondary set:*

$$\frac{102\,\text{mL} \times 15\,\text{gtt/mL (set)}}{40\,\text{minutes}} = \frac{1530}{40} = 38.25\text{ or }38\,\text{gtt/min}$$

c. *Infusion pump rate calculation:* amount of solution: 100 mL + 2 mL = 102 mL

$$102\,\text{mL} \times \frac{\overset{2}{\cancel{40}}\text{ min to administer}}{\underset{3}{\cancel{60}}\text{ min/hr}} = 102 \times \frac{3}{2} = \frac{306}{2} = 153\,\text{mL/hr}$$

Set pump rate at 153 mL/hr to deliver Staphcillin 1 g in 40 minutes.

6. a. *Drug calculation:*

$$\text{BF:} \frac{D}{H} \times V = \frac{250\,\text{mg}}{\underset{10}{\cancel{400}}\,\text{mg}} \times \overset{1}{\cancel{40}}\,\text{mL} = \frac{250}{10} = 25\,\text{mL}$$

or

$$\text{RP:}\quad H\ :\ V\ ::\ D\ :\ X$$
$$400\,\text{mg}:40\,\text{mL}::250\,\text{mg}:X\,\text{mL}$$
$$400\,X = 10{,}000$$
$$X = 25\,\text{mL}$$

or

$$\text{FE:} \frac{H}{V} = \frac{D}{X} = \frac{400}{40} = \frac{250}{X} =$$

(Cross multiply) 400 X = 10,000
$$X = 25\,\text{mL of ciprofloxacin}$$

or

$$\text{DA: mL} = \frac{\overset{1}{\cancel{40}}\,\text{mL} \times 250\,\cancel{\text{mg}}}{\underset{10}{\cancel{400}}\,\cancel{\text{mg}} \times 1} =$$

25 mL of ciprofloxacin

b. *Flow rate calculation (gtt/min):*
Amount of solution: 25 mL + 250 mL = 275 mL

$$\frac{275\,\text{mL} \times 15\,\text{gtt/mL}}{60\,\text{min/hr}} = \frac{4125}{60} = 68.75\text{ or }69\,\text{gtt/min}$$

7. a. *Flow rate calculation (gtt/min):*
Amount of solution: 10 mL + 100 mL = 110 mL

$$\frac{110\,\text{mL} \times \overset{3}{\cancel{15}}\,\text{gtt/mL}}{\underset{8}{\cancel{40}}\text{ min to admin}} = \frac{330}{8} = 41.25\text{ or }41\,\text{gtt/min}$$

b. *Infusion pump rate calculation (mL/hr):*

$$110\,\text{mL} \div \frac{40\,\text{min}}{60\,\text{min}} = 110\,\text{mL} \times \frac{\overset{6}{\cancel{60}}}{\underset{4}{\cancel{40}}} = \frac{660}{4} = 165\,\text{mL/hr}$$

8. a. *Amount of solution:*

$$\frac{\text{Min to administer}}{60\,\text{mL/hr}} = 50\,\text{mL} \div \frac{15\,\text{min}}{60\,\text{min}} = 50\,\text{mL} \times \frac{\overset{4}{\cancel{60}}\text{ min}}{\underset{1}{\cancel{15}}\text{ min}} = 200\,\text{mL/hr}$$

Infusion pump rate calculation: 200 mL/hr

9. 1 g = 1000 mg (use conversion table as needed) of Maxipime

a. *Drug calculation:*

$$\frac{D}{H} \times V = \frac{\overset{3}{\cancel{750}}\,\text{mg}}{\underset{4}{\cancel{1000}}\,\text{mg}} \times 10\,\text{mL} = \frac{30}{4} = 7.5\,\text{mL drug solution}$$

Amount of solution: 7.5 mL + 100 mL = 107.5 mL

b. *Infusion pump rate calculation:*

$$107.5 \text{ mL} \div \frac{30 \text{ min to administer}}{60 \text{ min/hr}} = 107.5 \text{ mL} \times \frac{\overset{2}{\cancel{60}}}{\underset{1}{\cancel{30}}} = 215 \text{ mL/hr pump rate}$$

10. *Amount of solution:* 10 mL + 500 mL = 510 mL

   a. *Infusion pump rate calculation:* $510 \text{ mL} \div \dfrac{180 \text{ min}}{60 \text{ min/hr}} = 510 \text{ mL} \times \dfrac{\overset{1}{\cancel{60}}}{\underset{3}{\cancel{180}}} = \dfrac{510}{3} = 170 \text{ mL/hr}$

11. **a.** See page 225 for mixing ADD-Vantage drugs. Mix 2 g of cefoxitin (Mefoxin) using ADD-Vantage vial with ADD-Vantage 100 mL diluent bag.

   b. *Infusion pump rate calculation (mL/hr):*

$$100 \text{ mL} \div \frac{30 \text{ min to administer}}{60 \text{ min/hr}} =$$

$$100 \text{ mL} \times \frac{\overset{2}{\cancel{60}}}{\underset{1}{\cancel{30}}} = 200 \text{ mL/hr}$$

12. **a.** BSA: 1.74 m^2; see Figure 7-1, page 100.

   b. *Drug calculation:*
   1.5 mg × 1.74 m^2 = 2.61 or 2.6 mg/m^2/day

$$\text{BF:} \frac{D}{H} \times V = \frac{2.6 \text{ mg}}{\underset{2}{\cancel{4}} \text{ mg}} \times \overset{3}{\cancel{6}} \text{ mL} = \frac{7.8}{2} = 3.9 \text{ mL or 4 mL}$$

   Amount of solution: 4 mL + 100 mL = 104 mL

   c. *Infusion pump rate calculation (mL/hr):*

$$104 \text{ mL} \div \frac{30 \text{ min to administer}}{60 \text{ min/hr}} = 104 \times \frac{\overset{2}{\cancel{60}}}{\underset{1}{\cancel{30}}} = 208 \text{ mL/hr}$$

13. **a.** 2.05 m^2 (BSA)

   b. *Drug calculation:*
   3.7 mg × 2.05 m^2 = 7.58 or 7.6 mg/m^2
   Velban 10 mg diluted in 10 mL
   Each mg = 1 mL; 7.6 mg = 7.6 mL
   Amount of solution: 7.6 mL + 250 mL = 257.6 mL

   c. *Infusion pump rate calculation (mL/hr):*

$$257.6 \text{ mL} \div \frac{60}{60} = 257.6 \times \frac{\overset{1}{\cancel{60}}}{\underset{1}{\cancel{60}}} = 257.6 \text{ or } 258 \text{ mL/hr}$$

14. **a.** *Drug calculation:*

$$\text{BF:} \frac{D}{H} \times V = \frac{20 \text{ mEq}}{40 \text{ mEq}} \times 20 \text{ mL} = \frac{400}{40} = 10 \text{ mL KCl}$$

or
$$\text{RP:} \quad H \ : \ V \ :: \ D \ :X$$
$$40 \text{ mEq} : 20 \text{ mL} :: 20 \text{ mEq} : X$$
$$40\,X = 400$$
$$X = 10 \text{ mL KCl}$$

or
$$\text{FE:} \frac{H}{V} = \frac{D}{X} = \frac{40 \text{ mEq}}{20 \text{ mL}} = \frac{20 \text{ mEq}}{X \text{ mL}}$$

(Cross multiply) $40\,X = 400$
$X = 10 \text{ mL}$

or
$$\text{DA: mL} = \frac{20 \text{ mL} \times \overset{1}{\cancel{20}} \text{ mEq}}{\underset{2}{\cancel{40}} \text{ mEq} \times 1} = \frac{20}{2} = 10 \text{ mL}$$

Amount of solution: 150 mL + 10 mL = 160 mL

b. *Infusion pump rate calculation:*

$$160 \text{ mL} \div \frac{120 \text{ min to administer}}{60 \text{ min/hr}} = 160 \times \frac{1}{2} = 80 \text{ mL/hr}$$

Set pump rate at 80 mL/hr to deliver KCl 20 mEq in 2 hours.

15. *Drug calculation:*

a. 1 mL = 500 mg and 2 mL = 1 g

b. BF: $\dfrac{D}{H} \times V = \dfrac{5 \text{ g}}{1 \text{ g}} \times 2 = 10 \text{ mL}$

or
RP: H : V :: D : X
   1 : 2 :: 5 : X
   X = 10
   X = 10 mL KCl magnesium sulfate

or
FE: $\dfrac{H}{V} = \dfrac{D}{X} = \dfrac{1 \text{ g}}{2 \text{ mL}} = \dfrac{5 \text{ g}}{X \text{ mL}}$

or
DA: mL = $\dfrac{1 \text{ mL} \times \overset{2}{\cancel{1000}} \text{ mg} \times 5 \cancel{\text{ g}}}{\underset{1}{\cancel{500}} \cancel{\text{ mg}} \times \quad 1 \cancel{\text{ g}} \quad \times 1} = 10 \text{ mL}$

(Cross multiply) X = 10 mL of magnesium sulfate

Amount of solution: 10 mL + 100 mL = 110 mL

c. *Infusion pump rate calculation:*

$$110 \text{ mL} \div \frac{\overset{3}{\cancel{180}} \text{ min to administer}}{\underset{1}{\cancel{60}} \text{ min/hr}} = 110 \times \frac{1}{3} = 36.6 \text{ or } 37 \text{ mL/hr}$$

Set pump rate at 37 mL/hr to deliver magnesium sulfate 5 g in 3 hours.

16. a. *Drug calculation:*

BF: $\dfrac{D}{H} \times V = \dfrac{16 \text{ mEq}}{4.65 \text{ mEq}} \times 10 \text{ mL} = 34.4 \text{ mL}$

or
RP: H : V :: D : X
   4.65 mEq : 10 mL :: 16 mEq : X mL
      4.65 X = 160
         X = 34.4 mL

or
FE: $\dfrac{H}{V} = \dfrac{D}{X} = \dfrac{4.65}{10} = \dfrac{16}{X}$
   4.65 X = 160
      X = 34.4 mL

or
DA: mL = $\dfrac{10 \text{ mL} \times 16 \cancel{\text{ mEq}}}{4.65 \cancel{\text{ mEq}} \times 1} = 34.4 \text{ mL}$

Amount of solution: 34.4 mL + 100 mL = 134.4 mL

b. *Infusion pump rate calculation:*

$$134.4 \text{ mL} \div \frac{\overset{1}{\cancel{30}} \text{ min to administer}}{\underset{2}{\cancel{60}} \text{ min/hr}} = 134.4 \times \frac{2}{1} = 268.8 \text{ or } 269 \text{ mL/hr}$$

---

evolve   Additional practice problems are available in the Intravenous Calculations and Advanced Calculations sections of Drug Calculations Companion, version 5, on Evolve.

ANSWERS

I Direct IV Injection

1. **a.** 5-mL drug solution
   b. known drug : known minutes :: desired drug : desired minutes
   $$5 \text{ mg} : 1 \text{ min} :: 50 \text{ mg} : X \text{ min}$$
   $$5X = 50$$
   $$X = 10 \text{ minutes}$$

2. known drug : known minutes :: desired drug : desired minutes
   $$10 \text{ mL} : 1 \text{ min} :: 50 \text{ mL} : X \text{ min}$$
   $$10X = 50$$
   $$X = 5 \text{ minutes}$$

3. **a.** 10 mL
   b. known drug : known minutes :: desired drug : desired minutes
   $$1.5 \text{ mL} : 1 \text{ min} :: 10 \text{ mL} : X \text{ min}$$
   $$1.5X = 10$$
   $$X = 6.6 \text{ minutes or 7 minutes}$$

4. **a.** 0.25 mL fentanyl
   b. known drug : known minutes :: desired drug : desired minutes
   $$10 \text{ mcg} : 1 \text{ min} :: 12.5 \text{ mcg} : X \text{ min}$$
   $$10X = 12.5$$
   $$X = 1.25 \text{ minutes}$$

5. **a.** RP: $\quad$ H : V :: D : X
   $$10 \text{ mg} : 1 \text{ mL} :: 6 \text{ mg} : X$$
   $$10X = 6$$
   $$X = 0.6 \text{ mL morphine}$$

   or
   FE: $\dfrac{H}{V} = \dfrac{D}{X} = \dfrac{10 \text{ mg}}{1 \text{ mL}} = \dfrac{6 \text{ mg}}{X}$
   $$10X = 6$$
   $$X = 0.6 \text{ mL}$$

   b. known drug : known minutes :: desired drug : desired minutes
   $$10 \text{ mg} : 4 \text{ min} :: 6 \text{ mg} : X \text{ min}$$
   $$10X = 24$$
   $$X = 2.4 \text{ minutes}$$

6. **a.** 1 mL
   b. known drug : known minutes :: desired drug : desired minutes
   $$1 \text{ mL} : 5 \text{ min} :: X \text{ mL} : 1 \text{ min}$$
   $$5X = 1$$
   $$X = 0.2 \text{ mL/minute}$$

7. **a.** DA: $mL = \dfrac{1 \text{ mL} \times 2 \text{ mg}}{5 \text{ mg} \times 1} = \dfrac{2}{5} = 0.4$ mL of Haldol
   b. known drug : known minutes :: desired drug : desired minutes
   $$1 \text{ mg} : 1 \text{ min} :: 2 \text{ mg} : X \text{ min}$$
   $$X = 2 \text{ minutes}$$

8. **a.** BF: $\dfrac{D}{H} \times V = \dfrac{6 \text{ mg}}{4 \text{ mg}} \times 1 = 1.5$ mL of Ativan
   b. known drug : known minutes :: desired drug : desired minutes
   $$2 \text{ mg} : 1 \text{ min} :: 6 \text{ mg} : X \text{ min}$$
   $$2X = 6$$
   $$X = 3 \text{ minutes}$$

9. a. RP: $\text{H} \ : \ \text{V} \ :: \ \text{D} \ : \ \text{V}$

 $25 \text{ mg} : 5 \text{ mL} :: 20 \text{ mg} : \text{X mL}$

 $25 \text{ X} = 100$

 $\text{X} = 4 \text{ mL}$

or

FE: $\dfrac{\text{H}}{\text{V}} = \dfrac{\text{D}}{\text{X}} = \dfrac{25 \text{ mg}}{5 \text{ mL}} = \dfrac{20 \text{ mg}}{\text{X mL}}$

(Cross multiply) $25 \text{ X} = 100$

 $\text{X} = 4 \text{ mL}$

or

DA: $\text{V} = \dfrac{\text{V} \times \text{D}}{\text{H} \times 1}$

$$\text{mL} = \dfrac{5 \text{ mL} \times \overset{4}{\cancel{20}} \text{ mg}}{\underset{5}{\cancel{25}} \text{ mg} \times 1} = \dfrac{20}{5} = 4 \text{ mL}$$

b. $\dfrac{\text{Amount of drug}}{\text{Number of minutes}} = \dfrac{4 \text{ mL}}{2 \text{ min}} = 2 \text{ mL/min}$

Answer: Infuse 2 mL of cardizem per minute.

10. a. 140 lb ÷ 2.2 = 64 kg

b. 10 mcg × 64 kg = 640 mcg

Change micrograms (mcg) to milligrams by moving the decimal point three spaces to the *left:* 640 mcg = 0.640 mg or 0.6 mg.

c. Known drug : known seconds :: desired drug : desired seconds

 1 mg   : 60 seconds   ::   0.6 mg   :   X sec

 X = 36 seconds

Answer: Infuse 0.6 mg of granisetron (Kytril) over 36 seconds.

II Continuous Intravenous Administration

1. a. Microdrip set because the patient is to receive 83 mL/hr

b. Three-step method: (a) $\dfrac{1000 \text{ mL}}{12 \text{ hr}} = 83 \text{ mL/hr}$

 (b) $\dfrac{83 \text{ mL/hr}}{60 \text{ min}} = 1.38 \text{ mL/min or } 1.4 \text{ mL}$

 (c) 1.4 mL/min × 60 gtt/mL = 84 gtt/min

Using a microdrip set (60 gtt/mL), IV should run at 84 gtt/min.

2. a. 1 L = 1000 mL

b. Each liter should run for 8 hours.

c. Two-step method: 1000 ÷ 8 = 125 mL/hr

$$\dfrac{125 \text{ mL} \times \overset{1}{\cancel{15}} \text{ gtt/min}}{\underset{4}{\cancel{60}} \text{ min}} = \dfrac{125}{4} = 31\text{–}32 \text{ gtt/min}$$

With a 15-gtt/mL drop set, IV should run at 31 to 32 gtt/min.

3. a. Microdrip set with drop factor of 60 gtt/mL is used because the hourly rate is low and would make drops easier to count.

b. One-step method: $\dfrac{250 \text{ mL} \times \overset{1}{\cancel{60}} \text{ gtt/min}}{24 \text{ hr} \times \underset{1}{\cancel{60}} \text{ min/hr}} = 10 \text{ gtt/min}$

With a microdrip set, IV should run at 10 gtt/min. KVO usually means 24 hours.

4. a. 10 mL of KCl

b. Use a 10-mL syringe; withdraw 10 mL of KCl and inject into the rubber stopper part of the IV bag.

c. Microdrip set: 100 gtt/min

Macrodrip set: drop factor of 20 gtt/mL; 33 gtt/min (33.3 gtt/min)

5. **a.** 700 mL of IV fluid is left and 4 hours are left.
   b. Recalculate using 700 mL and 4 hours to run.

   Three-step method: (a) $\dfrac{700 \text{ mL}}{4 \text{ hr}} = 175 \text{ mL/hr}$

   (b) $\dfrac{175 \text{ mL/hr}}{60 \text{ min}} = 2.9 \text{ mL/min}$

   (c) $2.9 \text{ mL/min} \times 15 \text{ gtt/mL} = 43.5 \text{ gtt/min or } 44 \text{ gtt/min}$

6. 100 gtt/min

   Two-step method: $\dfrac{100 \times \overset{1}{\cancel{60}} \text{ gtt/mL}}{\underset{1}{\cancel{60}} \text{ min}} = 100 \text{ gtt/min}$

7. **a.** KCl 40 mEq/20 mL
   b. 20 mL

   c. $\dfrac{1000 \text{ mL}}{125 \text{ mL/hr}} = 8 \text{ hours}$

8. **a.** KCl 20 mEq/10 mL
   b. 10 mL

   c. $\dfrac{1000 \text{ mL}}{100 \text{ mL/hr}} = 10 \text{ hours}$

   d. $\dfrac{100 \text{ mL} \times \overset{1}{\cancel{10}} \text{ gtt/mL}}{\underset{6}{\cancel{60}} \text{ min}} = \dfrac{100}{6} = 16.6 \text{ gtt/min or } 17 \text{ gtt/min}$

   or

   $\dfrac{1000 \text{ mL} \times \overset{1}{\cancel{10}} \text{ gtt/mL}}{\underset{1}{\cancel{10}} \text{ hr} \times 60 \text{ min}} = \dfrac{1000}{60} = 16.6 \text{ gtt/min or } 17 \text{ gtt/min}$

III Intermittent Intravenous Administration

1. **a.** 250 mg = 0.25 g
   b. *Drug calculation:*

   BF: $\dfrac{D}{H} \times V = \dfrac{0.25 \text{ g}}{1 \text{ g}} \times 2.5 \text{ mL} = 0.6 \text{ mL}$

   or

   RP: H : V :: D : X
   $1 \text{ g} : 2.5 \text{ mL} :: 0.25 \text{ g} : X \text{ mL}$
   $1 X = 2.5 \times 0.25$
   $X = 0.6 \text{ mL}$

   or

   DA: $\text{mL} = \dfrac{2.5 \text{ mL} \times 1 \text{ g} \times 250 \text{ mg}}{1 \text{ g} \times 1000 \text{ mg} \times 1} = 0.6 \text{ mL}$

   or

   FE: $\dfrac{H}{V} = \dfrac{D}{X} = \dfrac{1 \text{ g}}{2.5 \text{ mL}} = \dfrac{0.25 \text{ g}}{X} = X = 0.6 \text{ mL}$

   c. *Flow rate calculation:* Amount of solution: 75 mL + 0.6 mL = 75.6 or 76 mL

   $\dfrac{\text{Amount of solution} \times \text{gtt/mL}}{\text{Minutes to administer}} = \dfrac{76 \text{ mL} \times 60 \text{ gtt/mL}}{30 \text{ min}} = 152 \text{ gtt/min}$

   Regulate flow rate for 152 gtt/min.

2. a. *Drug calculation:*

$$\text{BF: } \frac{D}{H} \times V = \frac{500 \text{ g}}{1000 \text{ mg}} \times 100 \text{ mL} = 50 \text{ mL}$$

or

$$\text{RP: } \quad H \quad : \quad V \quad :: \quad D \quad : \quad X$$
$$1000 \text{ g} : 100 \text{ mL} :: 500 \text{ mg} : X \text{ mL}$$
$$1000 \text{ X} = 50,000$$
$$X = 50 \text{ mL}$$

or

$$\text{DA: mL} = \frac{100 \text{ mL} \times 500 \text{ mg}}{1000 \text{ mg} \times 1} = 50 \text{ mL}$$

or

$$\text{FE: } \frac{H}{V} = \frac{D}{X} = \frac{1000 \text{ mg}}{100 \text{ mL}} = \frac{500 \text{ mg}}{X}$$
$$1000 \text{ X} = 50,000$$
$$(\text{Cross multiply}) \text{ X} = 50 \text{ mL}$$

b. *Flow rate calculation:*

$$\frac{\text{Amount of solution} \times \text{gtt/mL}}{\text{Minutes to administer}} = \frac{100 \text{ mL} \times 6 \text{ gtt/mL}}{15 \text{ minutes}} = 40 \text{ gtt/min}$$

Regulate flow rate of secondary tubing for 40 gtt/min.

3. a. *Drug calculation:*

$$\text{BF: } \frac{D}{H} \times V = \frac{500 \text{ mg}}{1000 \text{ mg}} \times 4 \text{ mL} = \frac{2000}{1000} = 2 \text{ mL is the dose for 500 mg of ticarcillin.}$$

b. *Flow rate calculation:* Amount of solution: 75 mL D_5W + 2 mL of drug solution = 77 mL
For Buretrol set:

$$\frac{77 \text{ mL} \times \overset{3}{\cancel{60}} \text{ gtt/mL (set)}}{\underset{2}{\cancel{40}} \text{ minutes}} = \frac{231}{2} = 115.5 \text{ or } 116 \text{ gtt/min}$$

c. *Infusion pump rate calculation:*

$$\text{Amount of solution} \div \frac{\text{Minutes to administer}}{60 \text{ min/hr}} = \text{mL/hr}$$

$$77 \text{ mL} \div \frac{\overset{2}{\cancel{40}} \text{ min to administer}}{\underset{3}{\cancel{60}} \text{ min/hr}} = 77 \times \frac{3}{2} = \frac{231}{2} = 116 \text{ mL/hr}$$

Set pump rate at 116 mL/hr to deliver Ticar 500 mg in 40 minutes.

4. a. *Drug calculation:*

$$\text{BF: } \frac{D}{H} \times V = \frac{2.5 \text{ g}}{\underset{2}{\cancel{4}} \text{ g}} \times \overset{5}{\cancel{10}} \text{ mL} = \frac{12.5}{2} = 6.25 \text{ mL}$$

or

$$\text{FE: } \frac{H}{V} = \frac{D}{X} = \frac{4 \text{ g}}{10 \text{ mL}} = \frac{2.5 \text{ g}}{X \text{ mL}}$$
$$(\text{Cross multiply}) \text{ } 4 \text{ X} = 25$$
$$X = 6.25 \text{ mL}$$

or

$$\text{RP: } H : \quad V \quad :: \quad D : X$$
$$4 \text{ g} : 10 \text{ mL} :: 2.5 \text{ g} : X \text{ mL}$$
$$4 \text{ X} = 25$$
$$X = 6.25 \text{ mL}$$
piperacillin 2.5 g = 6.25 mL

or

$$\text{DA: mL} = \frac{10 \text{ mL} \times 2.5 \text{ g}}{4 \text{ g} \times 1} = \frac{25}{4} = 6.25 \text{ mL}$$

b. *Flow rate calculation for Buretrol set:* amount of solution: 6.25 mL + 100 mL = 106.25 mL

$$\frac{106 \text{ mL} \times \overset{2}{\cancel{60}} \text{ gtt/mL}}{\underset{1}{\cancel{30}} \text{ min/hr}} = 212 \text{ gtt/min}$$

c. *Infusion pump rate calculation:* 100 mL + 6 mL medication = 106 mL

$$106 \text{ mL} \div \frac{\overset{1}{\cancel{30}} \text{ min to administer}}{\underset{2}{\cancel{60}} \text{ min/hr}} = 106 \times \frac{2}{1} = 212 \text{ mL/hr}$$

Set pump rate at 212 mL/hr to deliver piperacillin 2.5 g in 30 minutes.

5. a. *Drug calculation:* Staphcillin 4 g = 8 mL

$$\text{BF:} \frac{D}{H} \times V = \frac{1\,g}{4\,g} \times 8\,mL = \frac{8}{4} = 2\,mL \text{ dose of Staphcillin}$$

Amount of solution: 2 mL + 100 mL = 102 mL

b. *Flow rate calculation for secondary set:*

$$\frac{102\,mL \times 15\,gtt/mL\,(set)}{40\,minutes} = \frac{1530}{40} = 38.25 \text{ or } 38\,gtt/min$$

c. *Infusion pump rate calculation:* amount of solution: 100 mL + 2 mL = 102 mL

$$102\,mL \times \frac{\overset{2}{40}\,min\,to\,administer}{\underset{3}{60}\,min/hr} = 102 \times \frac{3}{2} = \frac{306}{2} = 153\,mL/hr$$

Set pump rate at 153 mL/hr to deliver Staphcillin 1 g in 40 minutes.

6. a. *Drug calculation:*

$$\text{BF:} \frac{D}{H} \times V = \frac{250\,mg}{\underset{10}{400}\,mg} \times \overset{1}{40}\,mL = \frac{250}{10} = 25\,mL$$

or

$$\text{RP:} \quad H \quad : \quad V \quad :: \quad D \quad : \quad X$$
$$400\,mg : 40\,mL :: 250\,mg : X\,mL$$
$$400\,X = 10,000$$
$$X = 25\,mL$$

or

$$\text{FE:} \frac{H}{V} = \frac{D}{X} = \frac{400}{40} = \frac{250}{X} =$$

(Cross multiply) 400 X = 10,000
X = 25 mL of ciprofloxacin

or

$$\text{DA: mL} = \frac{\overset{1}{40}\,mL \times 250\,mg}{\underset{10}{400}\,mg \times 1} =$$

25 mL of ciprofloxacin

b. *Flow rate calculation (gtt/min):*
Amount of solution: 25 mL + 250 mL = 275 mL

$$\frac{275\,mL \times 15\,gtt/mL}{60\,min/hr} = \frac{4125}{60} = 68.75 \text{ or } 69\,gtt/min$$

7. a. *Flow rate calculation (gtt/min):*
Amount of solution: 10 mL + 100 mL = 110 mL

$$\frac{110\,mL \times \overset{3}{15}\,gtt/mL}{\underset{8}{40}\,min\,to\,admin} = \frac{330}{8} = 41.25 \text{ or } 41\,gtt/min$$

b. *Infusion pump rate calculation (mL/hr):*

$$110\,mL \div \frac{40\,min}{60\,min} = 110\,mL \times \frac{\overset{6}{60}}{\underset{4}{40}} = \frac{660}{4} = 165\,mL/hr$$

8. a. *Amount of solution:*

$$\frac{\text{Min to administer}}{60\,mL/hr} = 50\,mL \div \frac{15\,min}{60\,min} = 50\,mL \times \frac{\overset{4}{60}\,min}{\underset{1}{15}\,min} = 200\,mL/hr$$

Infusion pump rate calculation: 200 mL/hr

9. 1 g = 1000 mg (use conversion table as needed) of Maxipime

a. *Drug calculation:*

$$\frac{D}{H} \times V = \frac{\overset{3}{750}\,mg}{\underset{4}{1000}\,mg} \times 10\,mL = \frac{30}{4} = 7.5\,mL \text{ drug solution}$$

Amount of solution: 7.5 mL + 100 mL = 107.5 mL

b. *Infusion pump rate calculation:*

$$107.5 \text{ mL} \div \frac{30 \text{ min to administer}}{60 \text{ min/hr}} = 107.5 \text{ mL} \times \frac{\overset{2}{\cancel{60}}}{\underset{1}{\cancel{30}}} = 215 \text{ mL/hr pump rate}$$

10. *Amount of solution:* 10 mL + 500 mL = 510 mL

   a. *Infusion pump rate calculation:* $510 \text{ mL} \div \dfrac{180 \text{ min}}{60 \text{ min/hr}} = 510 \text{ mL} \times \dfrac{\overset{1}{\cancel{60}}}{\underset{3}{\cancel{180}}} = \dfrac{510}{3} = 170 \text{ mL/hr}$

11. **a.** See page 225 for mixing ADD-Vantage drugs. Mix 2 g of cefoxitin (Mefoxin) using ADD-Vantage vial with ADD-Vantage 100 mL diluent bag.

    b. *Infusion pump rate calculation (mL/hr):*

$$100 \text{ mL} \div \frac{30 \text{ min to administer}}{60 \text{ min/hr}} =$$

$$100 \text{ mL} \times \frac{\overset{2}{\cancel{60}}}{\underset{1}{\cancel{30}}} = 200 \text{ mL/hr}$$

12. **a.** BSA: 1.74 m²; see Figure 7-1, page 100.

    b. *Drug calculation:*
    1.5 mg × 1.74 m² = 2.61 or 2.6 mg/m²/day

$$\text{BF: } \frac{D}{H} \times V = \frac{2.6 \text{ mg}}{\underset{2}{\cancel{4}} \text{ mg}} \times \overset{3}{\cancel{6}} \text{ mL} = \frac{7.8}{2} = 3.9 \text{ mL or 4 mL}$$

   Amount of solution: 4 mL + 100 mL = 104 mL

    c. *Infusion pump rate calculation (mL/hr):*

$$104 \text{ mL} \div \frac{30 \text{ min to administer}}{60 \text{ min/hr}} = 104 \times \frac{\overset{2}{\cancel{60}}}{\underset{1}{\cancel{30}}} = 208 \text{ mL/hr}$$

13. **a.** 2.05 m² (BSA)

    b. *Drug calculation:*
    3.7 mg × 2.05 m² = 7.58 or 7.6 mg/m²
    Velban 10 mg diluted in 10 mL
    Each mg = 1 mL; 7.6 mg = 7.6 mL
    Amount of solution: 7.6 mL + 250 mL = 257.6 mL

    c. *Infusion pump rate calculation (mL/hr):*

$$257.6 \text{ mL} \div \frac{60}{60} = 257.6 \times \frac{\overset{1}{\cancel{60}}}{\underset{1}{\cancel{60}}} = 257.6 \text{ or 258 mL/hr}$$

14. **a.** *Drug calculation:*

$$\text{BF: } \frac{D}{H} \times V = \frac{20 \text{ mEq}}{40 \text{ mEq}} \times 20 \text{ mL} = \frac{400}{40} = 10 \text{ mL KCl}$$

   or
$$\text{FE: } \frac{H}{V} = \frac{D}{X} = \frac{40 \text{ mEq}}{20 \text{ mL}} = \frac{20 \text{ mEq}}{X \text{ mL}}$$

   (Cross multiply) 40 X = 400
                          X = 10 mL

   Amount of solution: 150 mL + 10 mL = 160 mL

   or
   RP: H : V ::   D :X
        40 mEq : 20 mL :: 20 mEq : X
               40 X = 400
                  X = 10 mL KCl

   or
$$\text{DA: mL} = \frac{20 \text{ mL} \times \overset{1}{\cancel{20}} \text{ mEq}}{\underset{2}{\cancel{40}} \text{ mEq} \times 1} = \frac{20}{2} = 10 \text{ mL}$$

b. *Infusion pump rate calculation:*

$$160 \text{ mL} \div \frac{120 \text{ min to administer}}{60 \text{ min/hr}} = 160 \times \frac{1}{2} = 80 \text{ mL/hr}$$

Set pump rate at 80 mL/hr to deliver KCl 20 mEq in 2 hours.

15. *Drug calculation:*

a. 1 mL = 500 mg and 2 mL = 1 g

b. BF: $\dfrac{D}{H} \times V = \dfrac{5 \text{ g}}{1 \text{ g}} \times 2 = 10 \text{ mL}$

or

RP: H : V :: D : X

1 : 2 :: 5 : X

X = 10

X = 10 mL KCl magnesium sulfate

or

FE: $\dfrac{H}{V} = \dfrac{D}{X} = \dfrac{1 \text{ g}}{2 \text{ mL}} = \dfrac{5 \text{ g}}{X \text{ mL}}$

(Cross multiply) X = 10 mL of magnesium sulfate

or

DA: mL $= \dfrac{1 \text{ mL} \times \overset{2}{\cancel{1000}} \text{ mg} \times 5 \cancel{\text{g}}}{\underset{1}{\cancel{500}} \text{ mg} \times 1 \cancel{\text{g}} \times 1} = 10 \text{ mL}$

Amount of solution: 10 mL + 100 mL = 110 mL

c. *Infusion pump rate calculation:*

$$110 \text{ mL} \div \frac{\overset{3}{\cancel{180}} \text{ min to administer}}{\underset{1}{\cancel{60}} \text{ min/hr}} = 110 \times \frac{1}{3} = 36.6 \text{ or } 37 \text{ mL/hr}$$

Set pump rate at 37 mL/hr to deliver magnesium sulfate 5 g in 3 hours.

16. a. *Drug calculation:*

BF: $\dfrac{D}{H} \times V = \dfrac{16 \text{ mEq}}{4.65 \text{ mEq}} \times 10 \text{ mL} = 34.4 \text{ mL}$

or

RP: H : V :: D : X

4.65 mEq : 10 mL :: 16 mEq : X mL

4.65 X = 160

X = 34.4 mL

or

FE: $\dfrac{H}{V} = \dfrac{D}{X} = \dfrac{4.65}{10} = \dfrac{16}{X}$

4.65 X = 160

X = 34.4 mL

or

DA: mL $= \dfrac{10 \text{ mL} \times 16 \cancel{\text{mEq}}}{4.65 \cancel{\text{mEq}} \times 1} = 34.4 \text{ mL}$

Amount of solution: 34.4 mL + 100 mL = 134.4 mL

b. *Infusion pump rate calculation:*

$$134.4 \text{ mL} \div \frac{\overset{1}{\cancel{30}} \text{ min to administer}}{\underset{2}{\cancel{60}} \text{ min/hr}} = 134.4 \times \frac{2}{1} = 268.8 \text{ or } 269 \text{ mL/hr}$$

evolve   Additional practice problems are available in the Intravenous Calculations and Advanced Calculations sections of Drug Calculations Companion, version 5, on Evolve.

PART IV

CALCULATIONS FOR SPECIALTY AREAS

CHAPTER 12

Pediatrics

FACTORS INFLUENCING PEDIATRIC DRUG ADMINISTRATION

Drug dosages for children differ greatly from those for adults because of the physiological differences between the two groups. Neonates and infants have immature kidney and liver function, which delays metabolism and elimination of many drugs. Drug absorption in neonates is different as a result of slow gastric emptying. Decreased gastric acid secretion in children younger than 3 years contributes to altered drug absorption. Neonates and infants have a lower concentration of plasma proteins, which can cause toxic effects with drugs that are highly bound to proteins. They have less total body fat and more total body water. Therefore lipid-soluble drugs require smaller doses because less than normal fat is present, and water-soluble drugs can require larger doses because of a greater percentage of body water. As children grow, changes in fat, muscle, body water, and organ maturity can alter the pharmacokinetic effects of drugs. Most drugs are dosed according to weight, and doses are specifically calculated for each child. For example, a dose of cefazolin for a 34-kg, 12-year-old child is larger than a dose for a 7-kg, 8-month-old infant. It is the nurse's responsibility to ensure that a safe drug dosage is given and to closely monitor signs and symptoms of adverse reactions to drugs. The purpose of learning how to calculate pediatric drug doses is to ensure that each child receives the correct dose within the therapeutic range.

Oral

Oral pediatric drug delivery often requires the use of a metric dosing device because most drugs for small children are provided in liquid form. The metric measuring device can be a small plastic cup, an oral dropper, a measuring spoon, an oral syringe, or a specially designed pediatric medication dispenser such as the medibottle (Figure 12-1). The medibottle is a specially designed pediatric medication dispenser that provides optimum drug delivery by allowing small volumes of medication to be swallowed with oral fluids. Some liquid medications come with their own calibrated droppers. The type of measuring device chosen depends on the developmental level of the child. For infants and toddlers, the oral syringe, dropper, and medibottle provide better drug delivery than is provided by a small cup. A young child who is cooperative is able to use a small cup or measuring spoon. All liquid medications can be drawn up with an oral syringe to ensure accuracy and then are transferred to a small cup or measuring spoon. It may be necessary to refill the cup or spoon with water or juice and to have the child drink that as well to ensure that all prescribed medication has been administered. Medicine should not be mixed in the infant's or toddler's bottle because the full dose will not be administered if the child doesn't finish the bottle. Any medication with a strong taste should not be mixed in formula because the infant could begin to refuse formula. Avoid giving oral medications to a crying child or infant, who could easily aspirate the medication. Some chewable medications are available for administration to the older child. Because many drugs are enteric-coated or are provided in timed-release form, the child must be told which medications are to be swallowed and not chewed.

Intramuscular

Intramuscular sites are chosen on the basis of the age and muscle development of the child (Table 12-1). All injections should be given in a manner that minimizes physical and psychosocial trauma. The child must be adequately restrained, if necessary, and provided with a momentary distraction. The procedure must be performed quickly, with comfort measures immediately following.

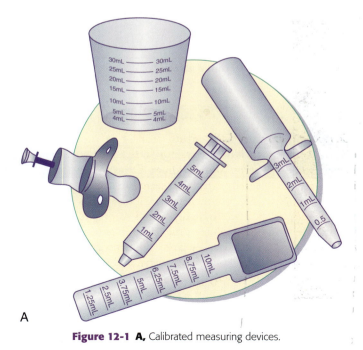

A

Figure 12-1 A, Calibrated measuring devices.

Continued

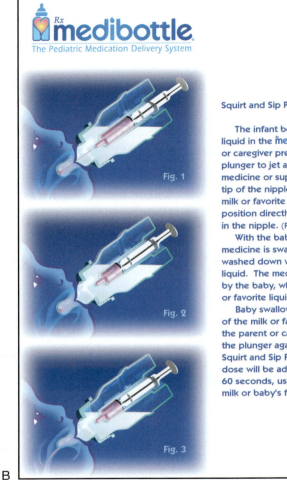

Squirt and Sip Process:

The infant begins to drink the liquid in the medibottle. The parent or caregiver presses the dispenser's plunger to jet a small squirt of medicine or supplements to the tip of the nipple. (Fig. 1) The baby's milk or favorite liquid will then be in position directly behind the medicine in the nipple. (Fig. 2)

With the baby's next sip, this medicine is swallowed and immediately washed down with the milk or favorite liquid. The medicine is undetected by the baby, who tastes only the milk or favorite liquid. (Fig. 3)

Baby swallows several more sips of the milk or favorite liquid before the parent or caregiver presses the plunger again to repeat the Squirt and Sip Process. The entire dose will be administered in 60 seconds, using one ounce of milk or baby's favorite liquid.

Figure 12-1, cont'd B, Medibottle. (**B,** from The Medicine Bottle Company, Inc.)

TABLE 12-1 Pediatric Guidelines for Intramuscular Injections According to Muscle Group*

	AMOUNT BY MUSCLE GROUP (mL)				
	Vastus Lateralis	Rectus Femoris	Ventro-gluteal	Dorsal Gluteal	Deltoid
Neonates	0.5 mL	Not safe	Not safe	Not safe	Not safe
Infants 1-12 months	0.5-1 mL	Not safe	Not safe	Not safe	Not safe
Toddlers 1-2 years	0.5-2 mL	0.5-1 mL	Not safe	Not safe	0.5-1 mL
Preschool 3-5 years	0.5-2 mL	0.5-1 mL	0.5-1 mL	Not safe	0.5-1 mL
School age 6-12 years	2 mL	2 mL	0.5-3 mL	0.5-2 mL	0.5-1 mL
Adolescent 12-18 years	2 mL	2 mL	2-3 mL	2-3 mL	1-1.5 mL

*The safe use of all sites is based on normal muscle development and size of the child. Follow institutional policies and procedures.

TABLE 12-2 Pediatric Guidelines for 24-Hour Intravenous Fluid Therapy

100 mL/kg for first 10 kg body weight
50 mL/kg for the next 10 kg body weight
20 mL/kg after 20 kg body weight

Example: Child's weight 25 kg

100 mL/kg × 10 kg = 1000 mL
50 mL/kg × 10 kg = 500 mL
20 mL/kg × 5 kg = 100 mL
1600 mL for 24 hours, or 66.6 mL/hr, or 67 mL

NOTE

The usual needle length and gauge for pediatric clients are ⅝ of an inch to 1 inch long and 22 to 27 gauge. Another method of estimating needle length is to grasp the muscle for injection between the thumb and the forefinger; half the distance would be the needle length.

Intravenous

For children, the maximum amount of intravenous (IV) fluid varies with body weight. Their 24-hour fluid status must be monitored closely to prevent overhydration. The amount of fluid given with IV medication must be considered in the planning of their 24-hour intake (Table 12-2). After the correct dosage of drug is obtained, it may need further dilution and to be given over a specified time, as mentioned in Chapter 11. Usually, the drug is diluted with 5 to 60 mL of IV fluid, depending on the drug or dosage, placed in a calibrated cylinder or syringe pump, and infused over 20 to 60 minutes, depending on the type of drug. After the drug has been infused, the cylinder is flushed with 3 to 20 mL of IV fluid to ensure that the child has received all of the medication and to prevent admixture. All fluid volume is considered intake. Refer to Chapter 11 for methods of calculating IV infusion rates.

The safety factors that must be considered when medications are administered to children are similar to those for adults. See Appendix A for more detailed information on safe nursing practice for drug administration.

PEDIATRIC DRUG CALCULATIONS

The two main methods of determining drug dosages for pediatric drug administration are body weight and body surface area (BSA). For both, a current weight is essential. The first method uses a specific number of milligrams, micrograms, or units for each kilogram of body weight (mg/kg, mcg/kg, unit/kg). Usually, drug data for pediatric dosage (mg/kg) are supplied by manufacturers in a drug information insert. BSA, measured in square meters (m^2), is considered a more accurate method than body weight. BSA takes into consideration the relation between basal metabolic rate and surface area, which correlates with blood volume, cardiac output, and organ growth and development. Although BSA has been used primarily to calculate the dosage of antineoplastic agents, BSA is used when there is a narrow margin between therapeutic and toxic doses. Pharmaceutical manufacturers are including BSA parameters (mg/m^2, mcg/m^2, $units/m^2$) in the drug information.

If the manufacturer does not supply data for pediatric dosing, the child's dosage can be determined from the adult dose. The BSA formula is used to calculate the pediatric dose. The BSA formula is considered more accurate than previously used formulas, such as Clark's, Young's, and Fried's rules. Drug calculations performed according to the BSA formula are safer than those done with formulas that rely solely on the child's age or weight. The West nomogram for infants and children (Figure 12-2) can also be used to determine BSA or to verify BSA results. It is important to follow institutional policies regarding the calculation of BSA (see Chapter 7). Although the BSA formula has improved the accuracy of drug dosing in infants and children, calculation of drug doses for neonates and preterm infants are weight based because BSA does not guarantee complete accuracy.

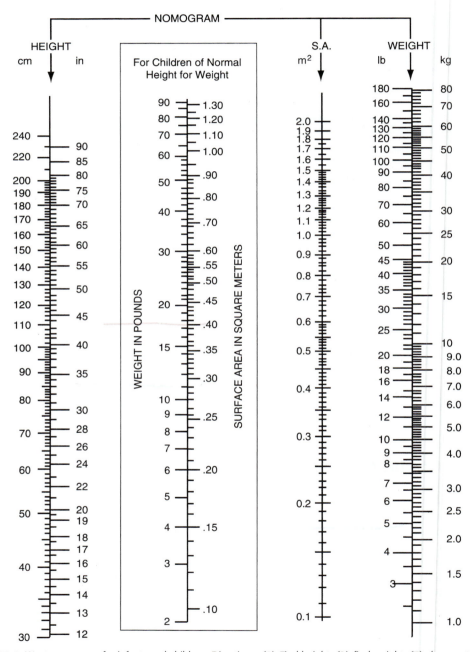

Figure 12-2 West nomogram for infants and children. *Directions: (1) Find height; (2) find weight; (3) draw a straight line connecting the height and weight. Where the line intersects on the S.A. (surface area) column is the body surface area in square meters (m²).* (Modified from data by E. Boyd & C. D. West. In Kliegman, R. M., Stanton, B. F., St. Geme, J. W., et al [2011]: *Nelson textbook of pediatrics,* ed. 19, Philadelphia: Saunders.)

Dosage per Kilogram Body Weight

The following information is needed to calculate the dosage:

a. Physician's order with the name of the drug, the dosage, and the frequency of administration.

b. The child's age and weight in kilograms:

$$1 \text{ kg} = 2.2 \text{ lb}$$

c. The pediatric dosage as listed by the manufacturer or hospital formulary.

d. Information on how the drug is supplied.

EXAMPLES   **PROBLEM 1**

a. Order: amoxicillin (Amoxil) 60 mg, po, tid.

Child's age and weight: 4 months, 12.5 lb.

b. Change pounds to kilograms.

$$\frac{12.5 \text{ lb/kg}}{2.2 \text{ kg}} = 5.7 \text{ kg}$$

c. Pediatric dosage for children older than 3 months old: 20-40 mg/kg/day in three equal doses.

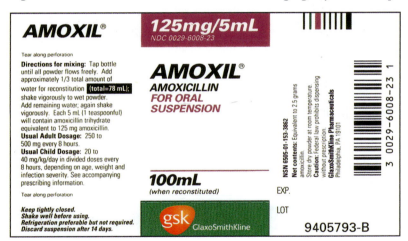

Step 1: Check dosing parameters by multiplying the child's weight by the minimum and maximum daily dose of the drug.

$$20 \text{ mg/kg/day} \times 5.7 \text{ kg} = 114 \text{ mg/day}$$
$$40 \text{ mg/kg/day} \times 5.7 \text{ kg} = 228 \text{ mg/day}$$

Step 2: Multiply the dosage by the frequency to determine the daily dose.

The order for amoxicillin 60 mg, po, tid means that three doses will be given per day.

$$60 \text{ mg} \times 3 = 180 \text{ mg}$$

Because the daily dose of amoxicillin 180 mg falls within the recommended range, it is considered a safe dose.

d. Drug preparation:

Use the basic formula (BF), ratio and proportion (RP), fractional equation (FE) method, or dimensional analysis (DA).

Basic Formula

$$\text{BF: } \frac{D}{H} \times V = \frac{60 \text{ mg}}{125 \text{ mg}} \times 5 \text{ mL} = 2.4 \text{ mL}$$

or

RP: *Ratio and Proportion*

125 mg : 5 mL :: 60 mg : X mL

$$125 \text{ X} = 300$$
$$\text{X} = 2.4 \text{ mL}$$

or

$$\text{DA: mL} = \frac{5 \text{ mL} \times 60 \text{ mg}}{125 \text{ mg} \times 1} = \frac{300}{125} = 2.4 \text{ mL}$$

or

FE: *Fractional Equation*

$$\frac{H}{V} = \frac{D}{X} = \frac{125 \text{ mg}}{5 \text{ mL}} = \frac{60 \text{ mg}}{X}$$

(Cross multiply) 125 X = 300

$$\text{X} = 2.4 \text{ mL}$$

Answer: amoxicillin 60 mg, po = 2.4 mL

PROBLEM 2

a. Order: ampicillin 350 mg, IV, q6h.

Child's weight and age: 61.5 lb and 9 years old.

Dilution instructions: Mix with 20 mL of $D_5/1/4$ NS; infuse over 20 minutes.

Flush with 15 mL at same infusion rate.

b. Change pounds to kilograms.

$$\frac{61.5}{2.2} = 27.95 \text{ or } 28 \text{ kg}$$

c. Pediatric dose is 25 to 50 mg/kg/day in divided doses.

Step 1: Multiply weight by minimum and maximum daily dose:

$$25 \text{ mg} \times 28 \text{ kg} = 700 \text{ mg/day}$$
$$50 \text{ mg} \times 28 \text{ kg} = 1400 \text{ mg/day}$$

Step 2: Multiply the dose by the frequency:

$$350 \text{ mg} \times 4 = 1400 \text{ mg/day}$$

The dose is considered safe because it does not exceed the therapeutic range.

d. Drug available: When diluted, 500 mg = 2 mL. Use your selected formula to calculate the dosage.

NDC 0015-7403-20
NSN 6505-00-946-4700
EQUIVALENT TO
500 mg AMPICILLIN
STERILE AMPICILLIN SODIUM, USP
For IM or IV Use
CAUTION: Federal law prohibits dispensing without prescription.

For IM use, add 1.8 mL diluent (read accompanying circular). Resulting solution contains 250 mg ampicillin per mL. Use solution within 1 hour. This vial contains ampicillin sodium equivalent to 500 mg ampicillin. Usual Dosage: Adults—250 to 500 mg IM q. 6h. READ ACCOMPANYING CIRCULAR for detailed indications, IM or IV dosage and precautions. APOTHECON® A Bristol-Myers Squibb Company Princeton, NJ 08540 USA 740320DRL-2

Cont:
Exp. Date:

$$\text{BF: } \frac{D}{H} \times V = \frac{350 \text{ mg}}{500 \text{ mg}} \times 2 \text{ mL} = 1.4 \text{ mL}$$

or
RP: 500 mg : 2 mL :: 350 mg : X mL
$$500 \, X = 700$$
$$X = 1.4 \text{ mL}$$

or

or
FE: $\dfrac{H}{V} = \dfrac{D}{X} = \dfrac{500 \text{ mg}}{2 \text{ mL}} = \dfrac{350 \text{ mg}}{X}$
$$500 \, X = 700$$
$$X = 1.4 \text{ mL}$$

DA: no conversion factor

$$mL = \dfrac{2 \text{ mL} \times \overset{7}{\cancel{350 \text{ mg}}}}{\underset{10}{\cancel{500 \text{ mg}}} \times 1} = \dfrac{14}{10} = 1.4 \text{ mL}$$

Answer: Each dose is 1.4 mL.

e. Amount of fluid to infuse medication:

$$1.4 \text{ mL} + 20 \text{ mL (dilution)} = 21.4 \text{ mL}$$

f. Flow rate calculation (60 gtt/mL set):

$$\dfrac{\text{Amount of solution} \times \text{gtt/mL (set)}}{\text{Minutes to administer}} = \text{gtt/min}$$

$$\dfrac{21.4 \text{ mL} \times \overset{3}{\cancel{60}} \text{ gtt/mL}}{\underset{1}{\cancel{20}} \text{ min}} = 64.2 \text{ gtt/min or 64 gtt/min}$$

g. Infusion pump setting

$$\text{Amount of solution} \div \dfrac{\text{Minutes to administer}}{60 \text{ min/hr}} = 21.4 \text{ mL} \div \dfrac{20 \text{ min}}{60 \text{ min}} =$$

$$21.4 \times \dfrac{60}{20} = 64.2 \text{ mL/hr or 64 mL (round off to whole number).}$$

YOU MUST REMEMBER

- The IV flush (3-20 mL) is part of the total IV fluids necessary for medication administration and must be included in patient intake. The flush is started after IV medication infusion is completed, and it is infused at the same rate.
- For a 60-gtt/mL set, the drop per minute rate is the same as the milliliter per minute rate.

Dosage per Body Surface Area

The following information is needed to calculate the dosage:
a. Physician's order with name of drug, dosage, and time frame or frequency.
b. Child's height, weight in kilograms, and age.
c. Information on how the drug is supplied.
d. Pediatric dosage (in m^2) as listed by manufacturer or hospital formulary.
e. BSA with square root.
f. BSA nomogram for children (Figure 12-2).

EXAMPLES **PROBLEM 1**

a. Order: methotrexate 50 mg, IV, × 1.
b. Child's height, weight, age: 134 cm, 32.5 kg, 9 years.
c. Pediatric dose: 25-75 mg/m² per week.
d. Drug preparation: 25 mg/mL.
e. BSA with square root (see BSA metric formula on p. 99)

$$\sqrt{\frac{134 \times 32.5}{3600}} = 1.09 \text{ m}^2$$

$$25 \text{ mg/m}^2 \times 1.09 \text{ m}^2 = 27.25 \text{ or } 27 \text{ mg}$$
$$75 \text{ mg/m}^2 \times 1.09 \text{ m}^2 = 81.75 \text{ or } 82 \text{ mg}$$

Compare answer with nomogram.

f. BSA nomogram for children: The child's height (134 cm) and weight (32.5 kg) intersect at 1.11 m² BSA.
Multiply the BSA, 1.11 m², by the minimum and maximum dose. (Substitute BSA for weight.)

$$25 \text{ mg/m}^2 \times 1.11 \text{ m}^2 = 28.0 \text{ mg}$$
$$75 \text{ mg/m}^2 \times 1.11 \text{ m}^2 = 83.0 \text{ mg}$$

This dose is considered safe because it is within the therapeutic range for the child's BSA.

g. Calculate drug dose: For determination of the amount of drug to be administered, either formula can be used:

$$\text{BF: } \frac{D}{H} \times V = \frac{50 \text{ mg}}{25 \text{ mg}} \times 1 \text{ mL} = 2 \text{ mL}$$

or
$$\text{FE: } \frac{H}{V} = \frac{D}{X} = \frac{25 \text{ mg}}{1 \text{ mL}} = \frac{50 \text{ mg}}{X \text{ mL}}$$

(Cross multiply) $25 X = 50$
$$X = 2 \text{ mL}$$

or
RP: 25 mg : 1 mL :: 50 mg : X mL
$$25 X = 50$$
$$X = 2 \text{ mL}$$

or
$$\text{DA: mL} = \frac{1 \text{ mL} \times \overset{2}{\cancel{50 \text{ mg}}}}{\underset{1}{\cancel{25 \text{ mg}}} \times 1} = 2 \text{ mL}$$

Answer: methotrexate 50 mg = 2 mL

SUMMARY PRACTICE PROBLEMS

Answers can be found on pages 269 to 277.

In the following dosage problems for oral, IM, and IV administration, determine whether the ordered drug is a safe pediatric dose, and calculate the dose.

I Oral

1. Child with a streptococcal soft tissue infection.
   Order: clindamycin 90 mg, po, qid.
   Child's weight and age: 68 lb, 6 years.
   Pediatric dose: 4-6 mg/lb/day in 3 doses.

Drug available: clindamycin 75 mg/5 mL.

$$\frac{Desired}{Have} \times volume$$

$$\frac{90\,mg}{75\,mg} \times 5\,mL$$

$$= 6\,mL$$

$90\,mg \times 4 = 360\,mg$ day total

Drug is safe & therapeutic

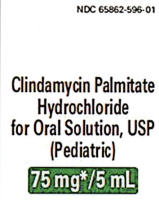

Clindamycin Palmitate Hydrochloride for Oral Solution, USP (Pediatric)

NDC 65862-596-01

75 mg*/5 mL when reconstituted

Rx only 100 mL (when mixed)

AUROBINDO

2. Child with seizures.
   Order: phenobarbital 25 mg, po, bid.
   Child's weight and age: 7.2 kg, 9 months.
   Pediatric dose: 5-7 mg/kg/day.
   Drug available: phenobarbital 20 mg/5 mL.

$25\,bid$
$\times 2$
$\boxed{\frac{50\,mg}{day}}$
safe +

$7.2\,kg \times 5\,mg = \boxed{36\,mg} $ day
$7.2\,kg \times 7\,mg = \boxed{50.4\,mg}$ day

$$\frac{25\,mg}{20\,mg} \times 5 = \boxed{6.25\,mL}$$

3. Child with lower respiratory tract infection.
   Order: cefprozil (Cefzil) 100 mg, po, q12h.
   Child's weight and age: 17 lb, 6 months.
   Pediatric dose greater than 6 months: 15 mg/kg/q12h.
   Drug available:

$17\,lbs \div 2.2 = 7.73\,kg$
$\times 15\,mg$
$115.9\,mg$ q 12 hrs

NDC 0087-7718-40 50 mL
Cefzil® (CEFPROZIL) for Oral Suspension
EQUIVALENT TO
125 mg/5 mL anhydrous cefprozil when constituted according to directions.
U.S. Patent No. 4,520,022
CAUTION: Federal law prohibits dispensing without prescription.
Bristol-Myers Squibb Company Princeton, New Jersey 08543 U.S.A.

$$\frac{100\,mg}{125\,mg} \times 5\,mL = \boxed{4\,mL}$$

4. Child with pain.
   Order: codeine 7.5 mg, po, q4h, prn × 6 doses/day.
   Child's height, weight, and age: 43 inches, 50 lb; 5 years.
   Pediatric dose: 100 mg/m²/day (see Figure 12-2), or solve by square root.
   Drug available: codeine 15-mg tablets.

5. Child with seizures.
   Order: Zarontin 125 mg, po, bid.
   Child's weight and age: 13 kg, 36 months.
   Pediatric dose: 15-40 mg/kg/day.
   Drug available:

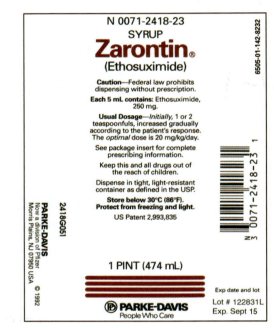

6. Child with seizures.
   Order: Dilantin 40 mg, po, bid.
   Child's weight and age: 6.7 kg, 3 months.
   Pediatric dose: 5-7 mg/kg/day.
   Drug available: Dilantin 125 mg/5 mL.

7. Child with acute urinary tract infection.
   Order: Bactrim 600 mg/120 mg, po, bid.
   Child's weight and age: 66 lb, 9 years.
   Pediatric dose: Bactrim 40 mg/kg/day sulfamethoxazole and 6-10 mg/kg/day trimethoprim.
   Drug available: Bactrim 400 mg/80 mg. For this drug, calculate the trimethoprim only.

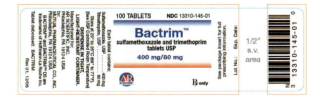

8. Infant with upper respiratory tract infection.
   Order: Augmentin oral suspension 75 mg, po, q8h.
   Child's weight and age: 8 kg, 7 months.
   Pediatric dose: 20-40 mg/kg/day.
   Drug available:

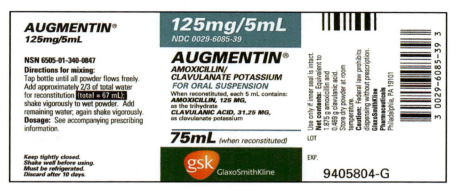

9. Child with poison ivy.
   Order: Benadryl 25 mg, po, q6h.
   Child's weight and age: 25 kg, 7 years.
   Pediatric dose: 5 mg/kg/day.
   Drug available: Benadryl 12.5 mg/5 mL.

10. Child with cystic fibrosis exposed to influenza A.
    Order: oseltamivir (Tamiflu) 45 mg, po, bid × 5 days.
    Child's weight and age: 16 kg, 4 years.
    Pediatric dose: 90 mg/day for 16-23 kg.
    Drug available: oseltamivir 12 mg/mL.

11. Order: cefaclor (Ceclor) 50 mg, qid.
    Child's weight and age: 15 lb, age 4 months.
    Pediatric dose: 20-40 mg/kg/day in three or four divided doses.
    Drug available:

12. Child with nausea and vomiting from chemotherapy.
    Order: ondansetron (Zofran) 2 mg, po 30 minutes before administration, q8h, prn.
    Child's weight and age: 80 lb, 10 years.
    Pediatric dose: 0.04-0.87 mg/kg/day.
    Drug available:

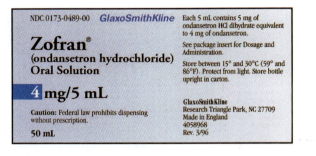

13. Child, 7 years old, with pinworms.
    Order: Pyrantel pamoate suspension 250 mg.
    Child's weight: 50 lbs.
    Pediatric dose: 11 mg/kg.
    Drug available: Pyrantel pamoate 50 mg/mL.

II Intramuscular

Determine whether dose is safe and calculate dose.

14. Child with pain after surgery.
    Order: morphine 4.5 mg, IM × 1.
    Child's weight and age: 45 kg, 14 years.
    Pediatric dose: 0.1 mg/kg.
    Drug available: morphine 10 mg/mL.

15. Child has strep throat (streptococcal pharyngitis).
    Order: Bicillin C-R, 1,000,000 units, IM × 1.
    Child's weight: 44 lb.
    Pediatric dose: 30-60 lb: 900,000-1,200,000 units daily.
    Drug available: Bicillin C-R, 1,200,000 units/2 mL.

16. Child receiving preoperative medication (may solve by nomogram or square root).
    Order: hydroxyzine (Vistaril) 25 mg, IM.
    Child's height and weight: 47 inches, 45 lb.
    Pediatric dose: 30 mg/m².
    Drug available:

17. Child receiving preoperative medication.
    Order: atropine 0.2 mg, IM.
    Child's weight and age: 12 kg, 7 months.
    Pediatric dose: 0.01-0.02 mg/kg/dose, not to exceed 0.4 mg/dose.
    Drug available:

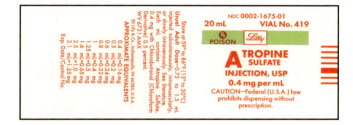

18. Child with cancer.
    Order: methotrexate 40 mg, IM, weekly (may solve by nomogram or square root).
    Child's height and weight: 56 inches, 100 lb.
    Pediatric dose: 7.5-30 mg/m²/wk.
    Drug available: methotrexate 2.5 mg/mL; 25 mg/mL; 100 mg/mL.

19. Order: A newborn is to receive AquaMEPHYTON (vitamin K) 0.5 mg IM immediately after delivery.
    Pediatric dose: 0.5-1 mg.
    Drug available:

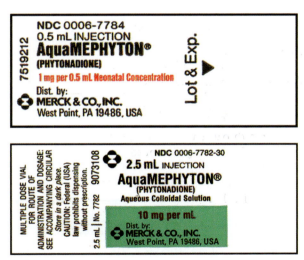

    a. Which AquaMEPHYTON container would you select? _____

    b. How many milliliters (mL) should the newborn receive? _____

    c. Is drug dose within the safe range? _____

20. Child with severe croup.
    Order: Dexamethasone 6 mg, IM × 1.
    Child's height, weight, and age: 42 inches, 44 lb, 4 years.
    Pediatric dose: 0.6 mg/m² to 9 mg/m²
    Drug available:
    a. Determine if dosage is safe.
    b. Calculate dose.

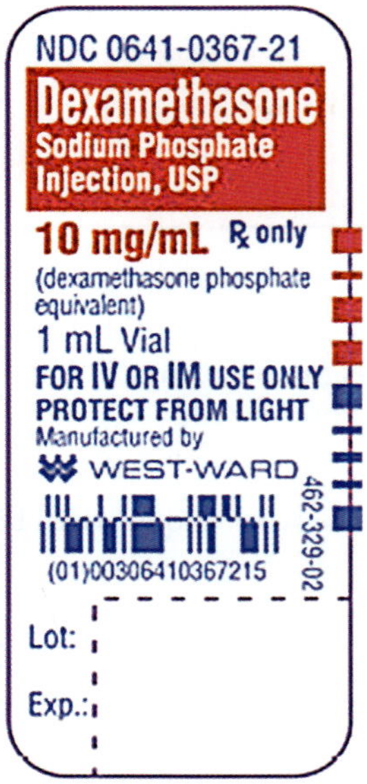

NDC 0641-0367-21

Dexamethasone
Sodium Phosphate
Injection, USP

10 mg/mL R only
(dexamethasone phosphate
equivalent)
1 mL Vial
FOR IV OR IM USE ONLY
PROTECT FROM LIGHT
Manufactured by
WEST-WARD

462-329-02

(01)00306410367215

Lot:

Exp.:

III Intravenous

21. Adolescent with progressive hip pain secondary to rheumatoid arthritis.
    Order: morphine sulfate 2.5 mg, IV piggyback, in 10 mL NS over 5 minutes. Flush with 5 mL.
    Child's weight and age: 50 kg, 16 years.
    Pediatric dose: 50-100 mcg/kg/dose for IV.
    Drug available:

$$\frac{D}{H} \times V = \frac{2.5\,mg}{5\,mg} \times 1mL = 0.5\,mL$$

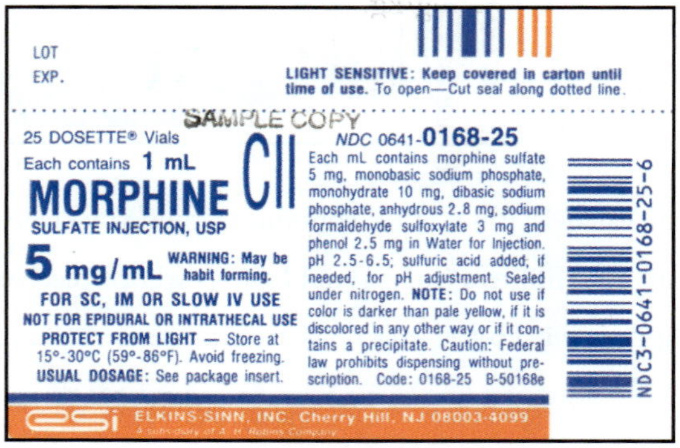

Handwritten notes (left margin):
50 → .05 mg
100 → 0.1 mg
× 50 kg
[2.5 - 5 mg]
Range

LOT
EXP.

LIGHT SENSITIVE: Keep covered in carton until
time of use. To open—Cut seal along dotted line.

SAMPLE COPY
25 DOSETTE® Vials
Each contains 1 mL
MORPHINE CII
SULFATE INJECTION, USP
5 mg/mL WARNING: May be
habit forming.
FOR SC, IM OR SLOW IV USE
NOT FOR EPIDURAL OR INTRATHECAL USE
PROTECT FROM LIGHT — Store at
15°-30°C (59°-86°F). Avoid freezing.
USUAL DOSAGE: See package insert.

NDC 0641-0168-25
Each mL contains morphine sulfate
5 mg, monobasic sodium phosphate,
monohydrate 10 mg, dibasic sodium
phosphate, anhydrous 2.8 mg, sodium
formaldehyde sulfoxylate 3 mg and
phenol 2.5 mg in Water for Injection.
pH 2.5-6.5; sulfuric acid added; if
needed, for pH adjustment. Sealed
under nitrogen. NOTE: Do not use if
color is darker than pale yellow, if it is
discolored in any other way or if it contains a precipitate. Caution: Federal
law prohibits dispensing without prescription. Code: 0168-25 B-50168e

NDC3-0641-0168-25-6

ESi ELKINS-SINN, INC. Cherry Hill, NJ 08003-4099

Handwritten notes (right margin):
$$\frac{10.5\,mL \times 60\,gtt/mL}{5\,min} = 126\,gtt/min$$

a. Determine if dosage is safe. **Yes**
b. Calculate dose. **0.5 mL**
c. How many mL should infuse?
d. How many gtt/min should infuse? **126 gtt/min**
e. What is the total amount of fluid given?

Handwritten notes (bottom):
0.5 mL + 10 mL = 10.5 mL   + Flush 5 mL = 15.5 mL total fluid

22. Treatment to reverse postoperative narcotic depression.
Order: Narcan (naloxone) 1.8 mg IV push.
Child's weight and age: 18 kg, 3 years.
Pediatric dose: 0.1 mg/kg
Drug available:

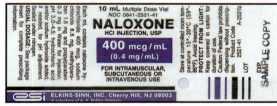

    a. Determine if dosage is safe.   **b.** Calculate dose.

23. Infant with sepsis.
Order: Amikin 40 mg, IV, q12h, in D$_5$W 5 mL, over 20 minutes. Flush with 3 mL.
Child's weight and age: 5.3 kg, 1 year.
Pediatric dose: 15 mg/kg/day.
Drug available:

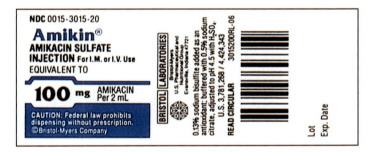

    a. Determine if dosage is safe.   **d.** How many gtt/min should infuse?
    b. Calculate dose.   **e.** What is the total amount of fluid given?
    c. How many mL should infuse?

24. Treatment for child with cerebral palsy having spasticity after spinal fusion.
Order: lorazepam 3 mg IV q6h.
Child's weight and age: 47 kg, 17 years.
Pediatric dose: 0.05-0.1 mg/kg.
Drug available: lorazepam 4 mg/mL.
    a. Determine if dosage is safe.
    b. Calculate dose.

25. Child with pneumonia.
    Order: cefazolin (Ancef) 500 mg, IV, q6h, in D_5W 20 mL, over 30 minutes.
    Flush with 10 mL.
    Child's weight and age: 5.6 kg, 2 months.
    Pediatric dose: 25-100 mg/kg/day in four divided doses.
    Drug available:

EXP.	**equivalent to** **1 gram** cefazolin NDC 0007-3130-16 **ANCEF®** **CEFAZOLIN FOR INJECTION (LYOPHILIZED)** Formerly sterile cefazolin sodium (lyophilized)	NSN 6505-01-262-9508 Before reconstitution protect from light and store between 15° and 30°C (59° and 86°F). **Usual Adult Dosage:** 250 mg to 1 gram every 6 to 8 hours. See accompanying prescribing information. For I.M. administration add 2.5 mL of Sterile Water for Injection. SHAKE WELL. Withdraw entire contents. Provides an approximate volume of 3.0 mL (330 mg/mL). For I.V. administration see accompanying prescribing information. Reconstituted Ancef is stable for 24 hours at room temperature or for 10 days if refrigerated (5°C or 41°F). **GlaxoSmithKline Pharmaceuticals** Philadelphia, PA 19101 694115-P
LOT	**25 Vials for Intramuscular or Intravenous Use**	**K3130-16**

    a. Determine if dosage is safe.
    b. Calculate dose.
    c. How many mL should infuse?
    d. How many gtt/min should infuse?
    e. What is the total amount of fluid given?

26. Child with sepsis.
    Order: gentamicin 10 mg, IV, q8h, in D_5W, 4 mL, over 30 minutes. Flush with 3 mL.
    Child's height, weight, and age: 21 inches, 4 kg, 1 month.
    Pediatric dose: more than 7 days old: 5-7.5 mg/kg/day in three divided doses.
    Drug available: gentamicin 10 mg/mL.
    a. Determine if dosage is safe.
    b. Calculate dose.
    c. How many mL should infuse?
    d. How many gtt/min should infuse?
    e. What is the total amount of fluid given?

27. Child with postoperative wound infection.
    Order: cefazolin 185 mg, IV, q6h, in D_5W 20 mL, over 20 minutes. Flush with 15 mL.
    Child's weight: 15 kg.
    Pediatric dose: 25-50 mg/kg/day.
    Drug available:

    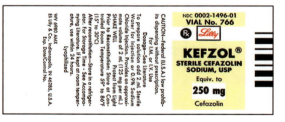

    a. Determine if dosage is safe.
    b. Calculate dose.
    c. How many mL should infuse?
    d. How many gtt/min should infuse?
    e. What is the total amount of fluid given?

28. Child with staphylococcus scalded skin syndrome.
   Order: clindamycin 50 mg IV q8h.
   Dilution instructions: mix in 10 mL NS over 15 min via syringe pump.
   Child's weight and age: 7.5 kg, 5 months.
   Pediatric dose: 16-20 mg/kg/day.
   Drug available: clindamycin 150 mg/mL.
   a. Determine if dosage is safe.
   b. Calculate dose.

29. Child with congestive heart failure.
   Order: digoxin 40 mcg, IV, bid, in NS 2 mL, over 1 minute.
   Child's weight and age: 6 lb, 1 month.
   Pediatric dose: 2 weeks to 2 years: 25-50 mcg/kg.
   Drug available: digoxin 0.1 mg/mL.
   a. Determine if dosage is safe.
   b. Calculate dose.

30. Child with lymphoma.
   Order: Cytoxan 125 mg, IV, in $D_5\frac{1}{2}$ NS, 300 mL, over 3 hours, no flush to follow.
   Child's weight and height: 16 kg, 75 cm (may solve by nomogram or square root).
   Pediatric dose: 60-250 mg/m²/day.
   Drug available:

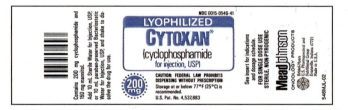

   a. Determine if dosage is safe.
   b. Calculate dose.

31. Child with pertussis.
   Order: azithromycin (Zithromax) 300 mg/day.
   Child's weight and age: 55 lb, 8 years.
   Pediatric dose: 10 mg/kg/day × 5 days.
   Drug available: azithromycin 200 mg/5 mL.

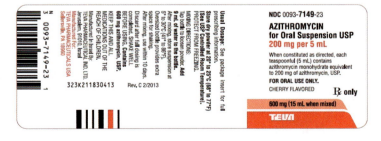

   a. Determine if dosage is safe.
   b. Calculate dose.

32. Child with severe systemic infection.
    Order: tobramycin (Nebcin) 15 mg, IV, q6h.
    Child's weight and age: 10 kg, 18 months.
    Pediatric dose parameters: 6-7.5 mg/kg/day in four divided doses.
    Drug available:

    ```
    NDC 0002-0501-01
    2 mL      VIAL No. 782

    Rx  Lilly

    NEBCIN®
    PEDIATRIC
    TOBRAMYCIN
    SULFATE
    INJECTION
    USP
    Equiv. to Tobramycin

    20  mg
        per
        2 mL

    Multiple Dose
    For I.M. or I.V. Use
    Must dilute for I.V. use.
    YE 1170 AMX
    Eli Lilly & Company
    Indpls., IN 46285, U.S.A.
    Exp. Date/Control No.
    ```

    a. Determine if dosage is safe.
    b. Calculate dose.

33. Child with acute lymphocytic leukemia.
    Order: daunorubicin HCl 40 mg, IV, daily.
    Pediatric dose parameters: more than 2 yr: 25-45 mg/m^2/day.
    Child's age, weight, and height: 10 years, 72 lb, 60 inches.
    Drug available: daunorubicin 20 mg/4 mL.
    Instructions: Mix in 100 mL D$_5$W; infuse in 45 minutes via pump.

    a. The BSA is _____

    b. How many milliliters should be mixed in the D$_5$W? _____

    c. Is the drug dose within the safe range? _____

    d. How many milliliters per hour should infuse? _____

34. Child with a serious fungal infection.
    Order: fluconazole (Diflucan) 200 mg, IV, per day for 10 days.
    Child's weight and age: 55 lb, 7 years.
    Pediatric dose: 6-12 mg/kg/day.
    Drug available: fluconazole 400 mg/200 mL.

    a. How many kilograms does the child weigh? _____

    b. Is the dose safe? _____

    c. How many milliliters should the child receive per dose? _____

IV Neonates

35. Neonate with bradycardia, heart rate less than 60 beats/min.
    Order: epinephrine 0.25 mg IV now.
    Pediatric dose: 0.1 mg/kg.

Neonate weight: 2.5 kg.
Drug available:

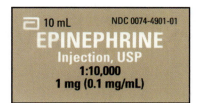

a. Determine if dosage is safe.
b. Calculate dose.

36. Neonate with respiratory depression after delivery; mother received Stadol during labor.
Neonate weight: 8 lb 12 oz.
Order: naxolone 0.04 mg IM now.
Pediatric dose: 0.01 mg/kg.
Drug available: naxolone 0.4 mg/mL.

a. Determine if dosage is safe.
b. Calculate dose.

37. Neonate with bacterial meningitis.
Neonate weight: 2.5 kg.
Order: ampicillin 125 mg IV push over 2 minutes.
Pediatric dose parameters: 50-75 mg/kg/dose.
Drug available:

APOTHECON®
Mfg. by Bristol-Myers Squibb Company
Princeton, NJ 08543 USA
Dist. by Geneva Pharmaceuticals, Inc. 740499FF-5
Dayton, NJ 08810 USA   1132495

740499

Exp.:

Lot:

NOV2018

1M38605

3-0015-7404-99-8

NDC 0015-7404-99

EQUIVALENT TO
1 gram AMPICILLIN
**Ampicillin
for Injection, USP**
For IM or IV Use
Rx only

NDC 0015	Label Claim	Recommended Amount of Diluent	Withdrawable Volume	Concentration (in mg/mL)
7401-20	125 mg	1.2 mL	1.0 mL	125 mg
7402-20	250 mg	1.0 mL	1.0 mL	250 mg
7403-20	500 mg	1.8 mL	2.0 mL	250 mg
7404-20	1 gram	3.5 mL	4.0 mL	250 mg
7405-20	2 gram	6.8 mL	8.0 mL	250 mg

a. Determine if dosage is safe.
b. Calculate dose.

38. Neonate with IV fluids for sepsis.
Neonate weight: 2.5 kg.
Order: D$_5$W 80 mL/kg for 24 hours.
a. How much D$_5$W should be given in 24 hours?
b. How many milliliters per hour should be infused?

39. Neonate with sepsis.
Neonate weight: 2.5 kg.
Order: gentamicin 10 mg q24h.
Pediatric dosage parameters: 4-5 mg/kg.
Drug available: gentamicin 40 mg/mL.
a. Determine if dosage is safe.
b. Calculate dose.

PEDIATRIC DOSAGE FROM ADULT DOSAGE

Body Surface Area Formula

The following information is needed to calculate the pediatric dosage with the BSA formula:
a. Physician's order with the name of the drug, the dosage, and the time frame or frequency.
b. The child's height and weight.
c. A BSA nomogram for children (p. 252).
d. The adult drug dosage.
e. The BSA formula:

$$\frac{\text{BSA (m}^2)}{1.73 \text{ m}^2} \times \text{Adult dose} = \text{Child dose}$$

EXAMPLE PROBLEM

a. Erythromycin 80 mg, po, qid.
b. Child's height is 34 inches and weight is 28.5 lb.
   Note: *Height and weight do not have to be converted to the metric system.*
c. Height (34 inches) and weight (28.5 lb) intersect the nomogram at 0.57 m². See BSA nomogram, Figure 12-2.
d. The adult drug dosage is 1000 mg/24 hr.
e. BSA formula:

$$\frac{\text{BSA (m}^2)}{1.73 \text{ m}^2} \times \text{Adult dose} = \frac{0.57 \text{ m}^2}{1.73 \text{ m}^2} \times 1000 \text{ mg}$$

$$= 0.33 \times 1000 \text{ mg}$$

$$= 330 \text{ mg/24 hr}$$

Dose frequency: $330 \text{ mg} \div 4 \text{ doses} = 82.5 \text{ or } 80 \text{ mg/dose}$

$80 \text{ mg} \times 4 \text{ times per day} = 320 \text{ mg/day}$

Dosage is safe.

Age Rules

Fried's rule and Young's rule are two methods for determining pediatric drug doses based on the child's age. Fried's rule is used primarily for children younger than 1 year of age, whereas Young's rule is used for children between 2 and 12 years of age. In current practice, these rules are infrequently used. Because the maturational development of infants and children is variable, age cannot be an accurate basis for drug dosing.

Fried's Rule:

$$\frac{\text{Age in months}}{150} \times \text{Adult dose} = \text{Infant dose}$$

Young's Rule:

$$\frac{\text{Child's age in years}}{\text{Age in years} + 12} \times \text{Adult dose} = \text{Child dose}$$

> **NOTE**
>
> The age rules should not be used if a pediatric dose is provided by the manufacturer.

ANSWERS   Summary Practice Problems

I Oral

1. Dosage parameters: 4 mg $\times$ 68 lb = 272 mg
   6 mg $\times$ 68 lb = 408 mg
Dosage frequency: 90 mg $\times$ 4 = 360 mg/day
Dosage is safe.

BF: $\dfrac{D}{H} \times V = \dfrac{90 \text{ mg}}{75 \text{ mg}} \times 5 \text{ mL} = 6 \text{ mL}$

or
DA: $\text{mL} = \dfrac{V \times D}{H \times X} = \dfrac{5 \text{ mL} \times 90 \text{ mL}}{75 \text{ mg} \times 1} = \dfrac{450}{75} = 6 \text{ mL}$

or
RP: H : V :: D :X
   75 mg:5 mL::90 mg:X
      75 X = 450
         X = 6 mL

or
FE: $\dfrac{H}{V} = \dfrac{D}{X} = \dfrac{75 \text{ mg}}{5 \text{ mL}} = \dfrac{90 \text{ mg}}{X}$

(Cross multiply) 75 X = 450
            X = 6 mL

2. Dosage parameters: 5 mg/kg/day $\times$ 7.2 kg = 36 mg/day
   7 mg/kg/day $\times$ 7.2 kg = 50.4 mg/day
Dose frequency: 25 mg $\times$ 2 = 50 mg
Dosage is safe.

BF: $\dfrac{D}{H} \times V = \dfrac{25 \text{ mg}}{20 \text{ mg}} \times 5 \text{ mL} = 6.25 \text{ mL/dose}$

or
DA: $\text{mL} = \dfrac{5 \text{ mL} \times \overset{5}{25 \text{ mg}}}{\underset{4}{20 \text{ mg}} \times 1} = \dfrac{25}{4} = 6.25 \text{ mL}$

3. Dosage parameters: 15 mg/kg, q12h $\times$ 8 kg = 120 mg, q12h
Dosage frequency: 100 mg, q12h
Dosage is safe.

BF: $\dfrac{D}{H} \times V = \dfrac{100 \text{ mg}}{125 \text{ mg}} \times 5 \text{ mL} = 4 \text{ mL/dose}$

or
FE: $\dfrac{H}{V} = \dfrac{D}{X} = \dfrac{125 \text{ mg}}{5 \text{ mL}} = \dfrac{100 \text{ mg}}{X}$

(Cross multiply) 125 X = 500
            X = 4 mL

4. Height and weight intersect at 0.84 m² with nomogram.
Dosage parameters: 100 mg/0.84 m²/day = 84 mg/day
Dose frequency: 84 mg/day $\div$ 6 = 14 mg/dose
Dosage is safe.
BSA with the Square Root: BSA Pounds and Inches Formula, see p. 99.

$$\sqrt{\dfrac{43 \times 50}{3131}} = \sqrt{0.686} = 0.828 \text{ or } 0.83 \text{ m}^2$$

Dosage parameters: 100 mg/0.83 m² = 83 mg/day (compare with nomogram)
Dosage frequency: 83 mg/day/6 = 13.8 or 14 mg/dose
Dosage is safe.

BF: $\dfrac{D}{H} \times V = \dfrac{7.5 \text{ mg}}{15 \text{ mg}} \times 1 = 0.50 \text{ or } \frac{1}{2} \text{ tablet}$

or
RP: H : V :: D :X
   15 mg : 1 tab :: 7.5 mg:X
      15 X = 7.5
         X = ½ tablet

5. Dosage parameters: 15 mg/kg/day $\times$ 13 kg = 195 mg/day
   40 mg/day $\times$ 13 kg = 520 mg/day
   Dose frequency: 125 mg $\times$ 2 = 250 mg/day
   Dosage is safe.

   BF: $\dfrac{D}{H} \times V = \dfrac{125 \text{ mg}}{250 \text{ mg}} \times 5 \text{ mL} = 2.5 \text{ mL}$

6. Dosage parameters: 5 mg/kg/day $\times$ 6.7 kg = 33.5 mg/day
   7 mg/kg/day $\times$ 6.7 kg = 46.9 mg/day
   Dose frequency: 40 mg $\times$ 2 = 80 mg/day
   Dosage exceeds the therapeutic range. Dosage is *not safe.*

7. Pounds to kilograms

   $\dfrac{66 \text{ lb}}{2.2 \text{ lb/kg}} = 30 \text{ kg}$

   Dosage parameters: 6 mg/kg/day $\times$ 30 kg = 180 mg/day
   10 mg/kg/day $\times$ 30 kg = 300 mg/day
   Dosage frequency: 2 times a day $\times$ 120 mg = 240 mg/day
   Dosage is safe.

   BF: $\dfrac{D}{H} \times \dfrac{120 \text{ mg}}{80 \text{ mg}} \times 1 = 1.5$ tablets

   or

   RP: H :V::   D :X
   80 mg : 1 :: 120 mg : X
   80 X = 120
   X = 1.5 tablets

   or
   DA: tab $= \dfrac{1 \text{ tab} \times 120 \text{ mg}}{80 \text{ mg} \times 1} = \dfrac{120}{80} = 1.5$ tablets

   or
   FE: $\dfrac{H}{V} = \dfrac{D}{X} = \dfrac{80 \text{ mg}}{1 \text{ tab}} = \dfrac{120 \text{ mg}}{X}$
   80 X = 120
   X = 1.5 tablets

8. Dosage parameters: 20 mg/kg/day $\times$ 8 kg = 160 mg/day
   40 mg/kg/day $\times$ 8 kg = 320 mg/day
   Dose frequency: 75 mg $\times$ 3 = 225 mg
   Dosage is safe.

   BF: $\dfrac{D}{H} \times V = \dfrac{75 \text{ mg}}{125 \text{ mg}} \times 5 \text{ mL} = 3 \text{ mL}$

   or
   RP: H : V :: D :X
   125 mg : 5 mL :: 75 mg : X
   125 X = 375
   X = 3 mL

   or
   FE: $\dfrac{H}{V} = \dfrac{D}{X} = \dfrac{125 \text{ mg}}{5 \text{ mL}} = \dfrac{75 \text{ mg}}{X} =$
   125 X = 375
   X = 3 mL

9. Dosage parameters: 5 mg/kg/day $\times$ 25 kg = 125 mg/day
   Dose frequency: 25 mg $\times$ 4 = 100 mg/day
   Dosage is safe.

   BF: $\dfrac{D}{H} \times V = \dfrac{25 \text{ mg}}{12.5 \text{ mg}} \times 5 \text{ mL} = 10 \text{ mL}$

   or
   DA: mL $= \dfrac{5 \text{ mL} \times \overset{2}{\cancel{25}} \text{ mg}}{\underset{1}{\cancel{12.5}} \text{ mg} \times 1} = 10 \text{ mL}$

   or
   FE: $\dfrac{H}{V} = \dfrac{D}{X} = \dfrac{12.5 \text{ mg}}{5 \text{ mL}} = \dfrac{25 \text{ mg}}{X \text{ mL}}$
   12.5 X = 125
   X = 10 mL

10. Dosing parameters: 90 mg/day
Dosing frequency: 45 mg $\times$ 2 = 90 mg
Dosage is safe.

$$\text{BF: } \frac{D}{H} \times V = \frac{45 \text{ mg}}{12 \text{ mg}} \times 1 \text{ mL} = 3.75 \text{ mL}$$

or
$$\text{DA: mL} = \frac{1 \text{ mL} \times 45 \text{ mg}}{12 \text{ mg} \times 1} = 3.75 \text{ mL}$$

11. 15 lb $\div$ 2.2 = 6.8 kg
Dosage parameters: 20 mg $\times$ 6.8 kg = 136 mg/day
                                40 mg $\times$ 6.8 kg = 272 mg/day
Dose frequency: 50 mg $\times$ 4 = 200 mg/day
Dosage is safe.

$$\text{BF: } \frac{D}{H} \times V = \frac{50}{125} \times 5 = \frac{250}{125} = 2 \text{ mL}$$

or
RP: H : V :: D : X
    125 mg:5 mL::50 mg:X mL
          125 X = 250
                X = 2 mL

or
$$\text{FE: } \frac{H}{V} = \frac{D}{X} = \frac{125 \text{ mg}}{5 \text{ mL}} = \frac{50 \text{ mg}}{X}$$

(Cross multiply) 125 X = 250
                        X = 2 mL

or
$$\text{DA: mL} = \frac{5 \text{ mL} \times \overset{2}{\cancel{50}} \text{ mg}}{\underset{5}{\cancel{125}} \text{ mg} \times 1} = \frac{10}{5} = 2 \text{ mL}$$

12. Pounds to kilograms

$$\frac{80 \text{ lb}}{2.2 \text{ lb/kg}} = 36.4 \text{ kg}$$

Dosing parameters:
    0.04 mg $\times$ 36.4 kg/day = 1.46 mg/kg/day
    0.87 mg $\times$ 36.4 kg/day = 31.7 mg/kg/day
Dosage frequency: 3 times a day $\times$ 2 mg = 6 mg
Dosage is safe.

$$\text{BF: } \frac{D}{H} \times V = \frac{2 \text{ mg}}{4 \text{ mg}} \times 5 \text{ mL} = 2.5 \text{ mL}$$

or
$$\text{DA: mL} = \frac{5 \text{ mL} \times \overset{1}{\cancel{2}} \text{ mg}}{\underset{2}{\cancel{4}} \text{ mg} \times 1} = \frac{5}{2} = 2.5 \text{ mL}$$

13. a. Pounds to kilograms

$$\frac{50 \text{ lbs}}{2.2 \text{ lbs/kg}} = 22.7 \text{ kg}$$

b. 22.7 kg $\times$ 11 mg/kg = 249.9 or 250 mg
Dosage is safe.

c. BF: $\frac{D}{H} \times V$

$$\frac{250 \text{ mg}}{50 \text{ mg}} \times 1 \text{ mL} = 5 \text{ mL}$$

or
$$\text{DA: mL} = \frac{1 \text{ mL} \times \overset{5}{\cancel{250}} \text{ mg}}{\underset{1}{\cancel{50}} \text{ mg} \times 1} = \frac{\overset{5}{\cancel{250}}}{\underset{1}{\cancel{50}}} = 5 \text{ mL}$$

or
$$\text{FE: } \frac{50 \text{ mg}}{1} = \frac{250 \text{ mg}}{X} =$$

                50 X = 250
                    X = 5 mL

or
RP: H : V :: D   :X
    50 mg:1 mL::250 mg:X
          50 X = 250 mg
                X = 5 mL

II Intramuscular

14. Dosing parameters: 0.1 mg/kg $\times$ 45 kg = 4.5 mg
Dosing frequency: one time.
Dosage is safe.

$$\text{BF:} \frac{D}{H} \times V = \frac{4.5 \text{ mg}}{10 \text{ mg}} \times 1 = 0.45 \text{ mL} \qquad\qquad \textit{or} \quad \text{DA: mL} = \frac{1 \text{ mL} \times 4.5 \text{ mg}}{10 \text{ mg}} = \frac{4.5}{10} = 0.45 \text{ mL}$$

15. Dosage parameters: Child's weight is 44 lb, which falls in the 30- to 60-lb pediatric dosage range.
Dose frequency: The one-time dose of 1,000,000 units falls within the pediatric dosage range.
Dosage is safe.

$$\text{BF:} \frac{D}{H} \times V = \frac{1,000,000 \text{ Units}}{1,200,000 \text{ Units}} \times 2 \text{ mL} = 1.666 \text{ or } 1.7 \text{ mL (round off to tenths)}$$

16. Height and weight intersect at 0.82 m^2 with the nomogram.
BSA with Square Root (Pounds and Inches Formula)

$$\sqrt{\frac{47 \text{ inches} \times 45 \text{ pounds}}{3131}} = \sqrt{0.675} = 0.82 \text{ m}^2 \text{ (same as the nomogram)}$$

Dosage parameters: 30 mg/m^2 $\times$ 0.82 m^2 = 24.6 mg or 25 mg
Dose frequency: 25 mg IM/dose
Dosage is safe.

$$\text{BF:} \frac{D}{H} \times V = \frac{25 \text{ mg}}{25 \text{ mg}} \times 1 = 1.0 \text{ mL} \qquad\qquad \textit{or} \quad \text{DA: mL} = \frac{1 \text{ mL} \times \overset{1}{25} \text{ mg}}{\underset{1}{25} \text{ mg} \times 1} = 1 \text{ mL}$$

17. Dosing parameters: 0.01 mg/kg/dose $\times$ 12 kg = 0.12 mg/dose
0.02 mg/kg/dose $\times$ 12 kg = 0.24 mg/dose
Dosage is safe.

$$\text{BF:} \frac{D}{H} \times V = \frac{0.2}{0.4} \times 1 = 0.5 \text{ mL}$$

18. Height and weight intersect at 1.38 m^2 with the nomogram.
Dosing parameters for nomogram: 7.5 mg $\times$ 1.38 m^2 = 10.35 mg/wk
30 mg $\times$ 1.38 m^2 = 41.4 mg/wk
BSA with Square Root (Pounds and Inches Formula)

$$\sqrt{\frac{56 \text{ inches} \times 100 \text{ pounds}}{3131}} = \sqrt{1.788} = 1.34 \text{ m}^2$$

Dosing parameter for BSA formula: 7.5 mg $\times$ 1.34 m^2 = 10.05 mg/wk
30 mg $\times$ 1.34 m^2 = 40.2 mg/wk
Dose frequency: 40 mg/wk IM
Dosage is safe.

$$\text{BF:} \frac{D}{H} \times V = \frac{40 \text{ mg}}{100 \text{ mg}} \times 1 \text{ mL} = 0.4 \text{ mL} \qquad\qquad \textit{or} \quad \text{DA: mL} = \frac{1 \text{ mL} \times 40 \text{ mg}}{100 \text{ mg} \times 1} = \frac{40}{100} = 0.4 \text{ mL}$$

19. a. Preferred selection is AquaMEPHYTON 1 mg = 0.5 mL
b. *AquaMEPHYTON 1 mg = 0.5 mL:*

$$\text{BF:} \frac{D}{H} \times V = \frac{0.5 \text{ mg}}{1.0 \text{ mg}} \times 0.5 \text{ mL} = \frac{0.25}{1.0} = 0.25 \text{ mL}$$

or

RP: H :   V   ::   D   :X
    1 mg:0.5 mL::0.5 mg:X
          X = 0.25 mL

AquaMEPHYTON 10 mg = 1 mL:

BF: $\dfrac{D}{H} \times V = \dfrac{0.5 \text{ mg}}{10 \text{ mg}} \times 1.0 \text{ mL} = \dfrac{0.5}{10} = 0.05 \text{ mL}$

or

FE: $\dfrac{H}{V} = \dfrac{D}{X} = \dfrac{10 \text{ mg}}{1 \text{ mL}} = \dfrac{0.5 \text{ mg}}{X \text{ mL}}$

$10\,X = 0.5$
$X = 0.05 \text{ mL}$

For AquaMEPHYTON 1 mg = 0.5 mL, give 0.25 mL (use a tuberculin syringe).
For AquaMEPHYTON 10 mg = 1 mL, give 0.05 mL (use a tuberculin syringe; however, it would be diffi-
    cult to give this small amount).
c. Drug dose is within the safe range.

20. Height and weight intersect at 0.78 m² with the nomogram.
Dosage parameters: 0.6 mg/m² × 0.78 m² = 0.46 mg
          9 mg/m² × 0.78 m² = 7.02 mg
a. Dosage is safe.

b. BF: $\dfrac{D}{H} \times V = \dfrac{6 \text{ mg}}{10 \text{ mg}} \times 1 \text{ mL} = 0.6 \text{ mL}$

or

DA: $\text{mL} = \dfrac{1 \text{ mL}}{10 \text{ mg}} \times \dfrac{6 \text{ mg}}{1} = 0.6 \text{ mL}$

or

RP: H :   V   ::   D   :X
    10 mg:1 mL::6 mg:X
          10 X = 6
          X = 0.6 mL

or

FE: $\dfrac{H}{V} = \dfrac{D}{H} = \dfrac{10 \text{ mg}}{1 \text{ mL}} = \dfrac{6 \text{ mg}}{X}$

(Cross multiply) 10 X = 6
          X = 0.6 mL

III Intravenous

21. Dosage parameters: 50 mcg/kg/dose × 50 kg = 2500 mcg/dose or 2.5 mg/dose
          100 mcg/kg/dose × 50 kg = 5000 mcg/dose or 5 mg/dose
a. Dosage is safe.

b. BF: $\dfrac{D}{H} \times V = \dfrac{2.5}{5} \times 1 = 0.5 \text{ mL}$

or

DA: $\text{mL} = \dfrac{1 \text{ mL} \times \overset{1}{2.5 \text{ mg}}}{\underset{2}{5 \text{ mg}} \times 1} = \dfrac{1}{2} \text{ or } 0.5 \text{ mL}$

c. Amount of fluid to be infused: 0.5 mL + 10 mL = 10.5 mL

d. $\dfrac{10.5 \text{ mL} \times \overset{12}{60} \text{ gtt/mL}}{\underset{1}{5} \text{ minutes}} = 126 \text{ gtt/min}$

e. Total fluid for medication infusion plus flush: 10.5 mL + 5 mL = 15.5 mL.

22. Dosing parameter: 0.1 mg/kg × 18 kg = 1.8 mg.
a. Dosage is safe.

b. BF: $\dfrac{D}{H} \times V = \dfrac{1.8 \text{ mg}}{0.4 \text{ mg}} \times 1 \text{ mL} = 4.5 \text{ mL}$ by IV push

23. Dosage parameters: 15 mg/kg/day $\times$ 5.3 = 79.5 mg/day.
    Dose frequency: 40 mg IV $\times$ 2 = 80 mg. 79.5 mg is rounded off to 80 mg.
    a. Dosage is safe.

    b. BF: $\dfrac{D}{H} \times V = \dfrac{40 \text{ mg}}{100 \text{ mg}} \times 2 = 0.8$ mL

    or
    RP: H : V :: D :X
    100 mg : 2 mL :: 40 mg : X
    100 X = 80
    X = 0.8 mL

    or
    FE: $\dfrac{H}{V} = \dfrac{D}{X} = \dfrac{100 \text{ mg}}{2 \text{ mL}} = \dfrac{40 \text{ mg}}{X}$

    (Cross multiply) 100 X = 80
    X = 0.8 mL

    c. Amount of fluid to be infused: 0.8 mL + 5 mL = 5.8 mL

    d. $\dfrac{5.8 \text{ mL} \times \overset{3}{\cancel{60}} \text{ gtt/mL}}{\underset{1}{\cancel{20}} \text{ minutes}} = 17.4$ gtt/min or 17 gtt/min

    e. Total fluid for medication infusion plus flush: 5.8 mL + 3 mL = 8.8 mL.

24. Dosing parameters: 0.05 mg/kg $\times$ 47 kg = 2.35 mg
    0.1 mg/kg $\times$ 47 kg = 4.7 mg
    a. Dosage is safe.

    b. BF: $\dfrac{D}{H} \times V = \dfrac{3 \text{ mg}}{4 \text{ mg}} \times 1$ mL = 0.75 mL

    or
    RP: H : V :: D :X
    4 mg : 1 mL :: 3 mg : X
    4 X = 3
    X = 0.75 mL

    or
    FE: $\dfrac{H}{V} = \dfrac{D}{X} = \dfrac{4 \text{ mg}}{1 \text{ mL}} = \dfrac{3 \text{ mg}}{X} =$

    (Cross multiply) 4 X = 3
    X = 0.75 mL

25. Dosage parameters: 25-100 mg/kg/day in four divided doses.
    25 mg $\times$ 5.6 kg = 140 mg/day
    100 mg $\times$ 5.6 kg = 560 mg/day
    560 mg $\div$ 4 = 140 mg/dose
    Dose frequency: 500 mg $\times$ 4 = 2000 mg/day
    Dose exceeds therapeutic range of 560 mg/day. Dosage is *not safe*.

26. Dosage parameters: 5 mg/kg/day $\times$ 4 kg = 20 mg/day
    7.5 mg/kg/day $\times$ 4 kg = 30 mg/day
    Dose frequency: 10 mg $\times$ 3 times/day = 30 mg
    a. Dosage is safe.

    b. BF: $\dfrac{D}{H} \times V = \dfrac{10 \text{ mg}}{10 \text{ mg}} \times 1$ mL = 1 mL

    or
    RP: H : V :: D : X
    10 mg : 1 mL :: 10 mg : X mL
    10 X = 10
    X = 1 mL

    or
    DA: mL = $\dfrac{1 \text{ mL} \times \overset{1}{\cancel{10 \text{ mg}}}}{\underset{1}{\cancel{10 \text{ mg}}} \times 1} = 1$ mL

    or
    FE: $\dfrac{H}{V} = \dfrac{D}{X} = \dfrac{10 \text{ mg}}{1 \text{ mL}} = \dfrac{10 \text{ mg}}{X \text{ mL}}$

    c. Amount of fluid to be infused: 1 mL + 4 mL = 5 mL

    (Cross multiply) 10 X = 10
    X = 1 mL

    d. $\dfrac{5 \text{ mL} \times \overset{2}{\cancel{60}} \text{ gtt/mL}}{\underset{1}{\cancel{30}} \text{ minutes}} = 10$ gtt/min

    e. Total fluid for medication infusion plus flush: 5 mL + 3 mL = 8 mL

27. Dosage parameters: 25 mg/kg/day $\times$ 15 kg = 375 mg/day
                     50 mg/kg/day $\times$ 15 kg = 750 mg/day
Dose frequency: 185 mg $\times$ 4 = 740 mg/day
  a. Dosage is safe.

  b. BF: $\dfrac{D}{H} \times V = \dfrac{185 \text{ mg}}{125 \text{ mg}} \times 1 \text{ mL} = 1.48$ or 1.5 mL

       Reconstitution information: 125 mg = 1 mL

or

RP: H : V :: D :X
           125 mg : 1 mL :: 185 mg : X
               125 X = 185
                  X = 1.5 mL

  c. Amount of fluid to be infused: 1.5 mL + 20 mL = 21.5 mL

  d. $\dfrac{21.5 \text{ mL} \times \overset{3}{\cancel{60}} \text{ gtt/mL}}{\underset{1}{\cancel{20}} \text{ minutes}} = 64.5$ gtt/min

  e. Total fluid for medication infusion plus flush: 21.5 mL + 15 mL = 36.5 mL

28. Dosing parameter: 16 mg/kg/day $\times$ 7.5 kg = 120 mg/day
               20 mg/kg/day $\times$ 7.5 kg = 150 mg/day
Dosing frequency: 50 mg $\times$ 3 = 150 mg
  a. Dosage is safe.

  b. BF: $\dfrac{D}{H} \times V = \dfrac{50 \text{ mg}}{150 \text{ mg}} \times 1 \text{ mL} = 0.33$ mL or 0.3 mL

or

RP: H : V :: D :X
           150 mg : 1 mL :: 50 mg : X mL
               150 X = 50
                 $X = \dfrac{50}{150} = 0.3$ mL

or
DA: mL = $\dfrac{1 \text{ mL} \times \overset{1}{\cancel{50 \text{ mg}}}}{\underset{3}{\cancel{150 \text{ mg}}} \times 1} = 0.33$ mL or 0.3 mL

or
FE: $\dfrac{H}{V} = \dfrac{D}{X} = \dfrac{150 \text{ mg}}{1 \text{ mL}} = \dfrac{50 \text{ mg}}{X \text{ mL}} =$

(Cross multiply) 150 X = 50
              $X = \dfrac{50}{150}$
              X = 0.3 mL

29. Dosage parameters: 25 mcg/kg/day $\times$ 2.72 kg = 68 mcg
               50 mcg/kg/day $\times$ 2.72 kg = 136 mcg
Dose frequency: 40 mcg $\times$ 2 = 80 mcg
  a. Dosage is safe.

  b. BF: $\dfrac{D}{H} \times V = \dfrac{40 \text{ mcg}}{100 \text{ mcg}} \times 1 = 0.4$ mL

0.1 mg = 100 mcg

30. Height and weight intersect at 0.6 m² according to the nomogram.
Dosing parameters for nomogram: 60 mg/m²/day $\times$ 0.6 m² = 36 mg/day.
                             250 mg/m²/day $\times$ 0.6 m² = 150 mg/day.

BSA with the square root (metric formula)

$\dfrac{\sqrt{16 \text{ kg} \times 75 \text{ cm}}}{3600} = \sqrt{0.333} = 0.58 \text{ m}^2$

Dosage parameters for BSA formula: 60 mg/m²/day $\times$ 0.58 m² = 34.8 mg/day
                               250 mg/m²/day $\times$ 0.58 m² = 145 mg/day

  a. Dosage is safe.

  b. BF: $\dfrac{D}{H} \times V = \dfrac{125 \text{ mg}}{200 \text{ mg}} \times 10 \text{ mL} = 6.25$ mL

or
DA: mL = $\dfrac{10 \text{ mL} \times \overset{5}{\cancel{125 \text{ mg}}}}{\underset{8}{\cancel{200 \text{ mg}}} \times 1} = \dfrac{50}{8} = 6.25$ mL

31. Dosage parameters: 55 lb ÷ 2.2 = 25 kg
$$25 \text{ kg} \times 10 \text{ mg/kg} = 250 \text{ mg}$$
$$25 \text{ kg} \times 12 \text{ mg/kg} = 300 \text{ mg}$$

   a. Dosage is safe.

   b. BF: $\dfrac{D}{H} \times V = \dfrac{300 \text{ mg}}{200 \text{ mg}} \times \dfrac{5 \text{ mL}}{1} = 7.5 \text{ mL}$

   or

   RP: H : V :: D : X
   $$200 \text{ mg} : 5 \text{ mL} :: 300 \text{ mg} : X \text{ mL}$$
   $$200 \text{ X} = 1500$$
   $$X = 7.5 \text{ mL}$$

   or

   DA: $\text{mL} = \dfrac{300 \text{ mg} \times 5 \text{ mL}}{200 \text{ mg} \times 1} = 7.5 \text{ mL}$

   FE: $\dfrac{H}{V} = \dfrac{D}{X} = \dfrac{200 \text{ mg}}{5 \text{ mL}} = \dfrac{300 \text{ mg}}{X}$

   (Cross multiply) 200 X = 1500
   $$X = 7.5 \text{ mL}$$

32. Pediatric dosage parameters: 6 mg × 10 kg/day = 60 mg/day
$$7.5 \text{ mg} \times 10 \text{ kg/day} = 75 \text{ mg/day}$$
$$15 \text{ mg} \times 4 \text{ (q6h)} = 60 \text{ mg/day}$$

   a. Drug dosage per day is within the safe range.

   b. BF: $\dfrac{15}{\underset{10}{\cancel{20}}} \times \overset{1}{\cancel{2}} \text{ mL} = \dfrac{15}{10} = 1.5 \text{ mL of Nebcin}$

   or

   RP: 20 mg : 2 mL :: 15 mg : X
   $$20 \text{ X} = 30$$
   $$X = 1.5 \text{ of Nebcin}$$

33. **a.** The BSA using inches and pound formula is 1.17.
   b. 8 mL of daunorubicin HCl mixed in 100 mL D_5W.
   c. Dosage parameters: 25 mg × 1.17 m² = 29.3 mg/day
$$45 \text{ mg} \times 1.17 \text{ m}^2 = 52.7 \text{ mg/day or 53 mg/day}$$
   Child is to receive 40 mg of daunorubicin HCl per day.
   Drug dose is within the safe range.

   d. $108 \text{ mL} \div \dfrac{45 \text{ min}}{60 \text{ min}} = 108 \times \dfrac{\overset{4}{\cancel{60}}}{\underset{3}{\cancel{45}}} = 144 \text{ mL}$

   Pump setting: 144 mL/hr

34. **a.** 55 lb ÷ 2.2 lb/kg = 25 kg
   b. Yes. 6 mg/kg × 25 kg = 150 mg
   12 mg/kg × 25 kg = 300 mg
   Drug dosage is safe.

   c. BF: $\dfrac{D}{H} \times V = \dfrac{200 \text{ mg}}{400 \text{ mg}} \times 200 \text{ mL} = 100 \text{ mL of Diflucan per dose}$

IV Neonates

35. **a.** 0.1 mg/kg × 2.5 kg = 0.25 mg
   Drug dosage is safe.

   b. BF: $\dfrac{0.25 \text{ mg}}{0.1 \text{ mg}} \times 1 \text{ mL} = 2.5 \text{ mL}$

   or

   DA: $\text{mL} = \dfrac{1 \text{ mL} \times 0.25 \text{ mg}}{0.1 \text{ mg} \times 1} = \dfrac{0.25}{0.1} = 2.5 \text{ mL}$

   or

   FE: $\dfrac{H}{V} = \dfrac{D}{X} = \dfrac{0.1 \text{ mg}}{1 \text{ mL}} = \dfrac{0.25 \text{ mg}}{X} =$

   (Cross multiply) 0.1 X = 0.25
   $$X = 2.5 \text{ mL}$$

36. a. $\dfrac{8.75}{2.2} = 3.97$ kg or 4 kg

0.01 mg/kg $\times$ 4 kg $= 0.04$ mg dose
Drug dosage is safe.

b. BF: $\dfrac{D}{H} \times V = \dfrac{0.04 \text{ mg}}{0.4 \text{ mg}} \times 1 \text{ mL} = 0.1 \text{ mL}$

or
RP: H : V ::   D   : X
       0.4 mg : 1 mL :: 0.04 mg : X mL
             $0.4\,X = 0.04$
                $X = 0.1$ mL

37. Dosage parameters: 50 mg/kg $\times$ 2.5 kg $= 125$ mg
              75 mg/kg $\times$ 2.5 kg $= 187.5$ mg
a. Drug dosage is within safe range.

b. BF: $\dfrac{125 \text{ mg}}{500 \text{ mg}} \times 2 \text{ mL} = 0.5 \text{ mL}$

or
DA: mL $= \dfrac{2 \text{ mL} \times \overset{1}{\cancel{125}} \text{ mg}}{\underset{4}{\cancel{500}} \text{ mg} \times 1} = \dfrac{2}{4} = 0.5$ mL

or
FE: $\dfrac{H}{V} = \dfrac{D}{X} = \dfrac{500 \text{ mg}}{2 \text{ mL}} = \dfrac{125 \text{ mg}}{X} =$

(Cross multiply) $500\,X = 250$
                 $X = 0.5$ mL

38. a. 80 mL/kg $\times$ 2.5 kg $= 200$ mL D_5W in 24 hours

b. $\dfrac{200 \text{ mL}}{24 \text{ hr}} = 8.3 \text{ mL/hr}$

39. Dosage parameters: 4 mg/kg $\times$ 2.5 kg $= 10$ mg
              5 mg/kg $\times$ 2.5 kg $= 12.5$ mg
a. Drug dosage is safe.

b. BF: $\dfrac{D}{H} \times V = \dfrac{10 \text{ mg}}{40 \text{ mg}} \times 1 \text{ mL} = 0.25 \text{ mL}$

or
RP: H : V ::   D : X
       40 mg : 1 mL :: 10 mg : X mL
             $40\,X = 10$
                $X = 0.25$ mL

---

evolve   Additional practice problems are available in the Pediatric Calculations section of Drug Calculations Companion, version 5, on Evolve.

CHAPTER 13

Critical Care

Objectives
- Calculate the prescribed concentration of a drug in solution.
- Identify the units of measure designated for the amount of drug in solution.
- Describe the four determinants of infusion rates.
- Calculate the concentration of drug per unit of time for a specific body weight.
- Recognize the variables needed for the basic fractional formula.
- Describe how the titration factor is used when infusion rates are changed.
- Recognize the methods of determining the total amount of drug infused over time.

In critical care areas, medication is primarily given intravenously and therefore has an immediate systemic effect on the patient. Drug dosages can be highly individualized, which necessitates close patient monitoring for improvement or stabilization in parameters such as vital signs, urine output, cardiac index, level of consciousness, or whatever is appropriate for the medication. Because intravenous (IV) medication can have immediate effects and have a narrow therapeutic range, the patient can be at great risk if these medications are administered incorrectly. Therefore it is essential that the nurse understand the drug's mechanism of action and the calculations necessary for safe drug administration.

Administration of potent drugs—drugs that cause major physiological changes—may be delivered in milligrams, micrograms, or units per body weight or unit time. The physician determines the drug dosage and rate of infusion either per body weight or unit time, per hour or per minute. Depending on the medication, the physician may give the type of IV solution for the dilution. Most institutions have their own pharmacy guidelines or protocols for preparation of drugs for continuous IV infusion in critical care areas. Premixed, ready-to-use IV drugs in solution are also available from drug manufacturers with standardized dosages. The nurse is the last step in the administration process and must make sure that the dosage is accurate and the infusion rate is correct.

National research has shown a high incidence of IV drug errors committed by pharmacists, physicians, and nurses. Complete examination of medication processes is under way across the country in an effort to eliminate adverse drug errors. One step in the process has been to identify drugs with the highest potential to do harm when used in error. Now these drugs are referred to as "high-alert" drugs and identified in some facilities with special labeling (Table 13-1). Another effort under way is the increasing use of programmable infusion pump technology or "smart pumps." These pumps have drug menus called "libraries" entered into their software with safe dosing limits called guardrails. The pump will alarm if the limits are breached and prevent infusion of an unsafe dose. The smart pump's technology allows a facility to program the pump for specific areas, i.e., adult, pediatric, oncology, and anesthesia.

When the nurse uses the smart pump, she or he first selects the drug from the drug library. The library list of drugs is distinguished by capitalized letters that emphasize spelling differences for drugs with similar names. The nurse selects the amount of the drug and the amount of the prescribed soluton for infusion, and the pump calculates the *concentration of solution*. If the drug is dosed based on patient weight, the most current weight in kilograms is entered, allowing the smart pump to calculate the drug's dosage per kilogram of body weight per minute. Depending on the drug that is selected from the library, the smart pump will use volume per hour or volume per minute to calculate the dosage.

TABLE 13-1 High-Alert Drug Examples

Drug Class	Examples
Adrenergic agonists	Epinephrine, norepinephrine, dopamine, dobutamine
Adrenergic antagonists	Esmolol
Anesthetics	Propofol
Antiarrhythmics	Amiodarone, lidocaine
Anticoagulants	Heparin, bivalirudin, argatroban, lepirudin
Antineoplastics	
Dextrose, hypertonic, 20% or greater	
Electrolyte solutions	Potassium chloride, potassium phosphate, magnesium sulfate
Fibrinolytics	Streptokinase, anistreplase, alteplase
Glycoprotein IIb/IIIa inhibitors	Eptifibatide
Inotropics	Milrinone
Insulin	
Liposomal forms of drugs	Liposomal amphotericin
Moderate sedatives	Midazolam, lorazepam, diazepam
Neuromuscular blockers	Atracurium, vecuronium, cisatracurium
Opiates	
Total parenteral nutrition solutions	
Vasodilators	Nitroglycerin, nitroprusside, nesiritide

Adapted from Dennison, Robin D. High-alert drugs: Strategies for some IV infusions. *American Nurse Today,* November, 2006. Retrieved from http://www.americannursetoday.com/high-alert-drugs-strategies-for-safe-i-v-infusions/.

The smart pump is an effective tool for drug administration, but the nurse must know all the drug calculation formulas used in the critical care setting and how they are applied to verify that the dose is correct before it is given to the patient. Nurses working in these areas need to be able to calculate for:

1. Concentration of the solution.
2. Concentration per hour or per minute.
3. Volume per hour or minute.
4. Dosage per kilogram body weight per minute.

For high-alert drugs it is recommended that two nurses independently do the drug calculations and verify the results. If any questions arise regarding dosing or infusion rates, the pharmacist and the physician should be consulted before the drug is administered to the patient.

CALCULATING AMOUNT OF DRUG OR CONCENTRATION OF A SOLUTION

The first step in administering a medication is to determine the concentration of the solution, which is the amount of drug in each milliliter (mL) of solution. This is written as units per milliliter, milligrams per milliliter, or micrograms per milliliter and must be calculated for individualized patient dosage. For all problems, remember to convert to like units before solving.

Calculating Units per Milliliter

EXAMPLE Infuse heparin 5000 units in D_5W 250 mL at 30 mL/hr. What will be the concentration of heparin in each milliliter of D_5W?
Method: units/mL

Set up a ratio and proportion. Solve for X.	$5000 \text{ units} : 250 \text{ mL} :: X \text{ units} : \text{mL}$ $250 X = 5000$ $X = 20 \text{ units}$

Answer: The D_5W with heparin will have a concentration of 20 units/mL of solution.

Calculating Milligrams per Milliliter

EXAMPLE Infuse lidocaine 2 g in 500 mL D_5W at 2 mg/min. What will be the concentration of lidocaine in each milliliter of D_5W?
Method: mg/mL

Convert grams to milligrams. Set up a ratio and proportion and solve for X.	$2 \text{ g} = 2000 \text{ mg}$ $2000 \text{ mg} : 500 \text{ mL} :: X \text{ mg} : \text{mL}$ $500 X = 2000$ $X = 4 \text{ mg}$

Answer: The D_5W with lidocaine has a concentration of 4 mg/mL of solution.

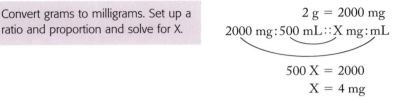

NOTE

At the beginning of his or her shift, the nurse must check the infusion pump to verify the medication and concentration that are programmed in the device match the order on the MAR/eMAR.

Calculating Micrograms per Milliliter

EXAMPLE Infuse dobutamine 250 mg in 500 mL D_5W at 650 mcg/min. What is the concentration of dobutamine in each milliliter of D_5W?
Method: mcg/mL

Convert milligrams to micrograms. Set up a ratio and proportion and solve for X.

$$250 \text{ mg} = 250,000 \text{ mcg}$$
$$250,000 \text{ mcg} : 500 \text{ mL} :: X \text{ mcg} : \text{mL}$$

$$500 \text{ X} = 250,000$$
$$X = 500 \text{ mcg/mL}$$

Answer: The D_5W with dobutamine will have a concentration of 500 mcg/mL of solution.

PRACTICE PROBLEMS: ▶ I CALCULATING CONCENTRATION OF A SOLUTION

Answers can be found on pages 294 to 295.

1. **Order:** heparin 10,000 units in 250 mL D_5W at 30 mL/hr.
2. **Order:** propofol 1000 mg in 100 mL at 30 mL/hr.
3. **Order:** regular insulin 100 units in 500 mL NS at 30 mL/hr.
4. **Order:** lidocaine 1 g in 1000 mL D_5W at 30 mL/hr.
5. **Order:** norepinephrine 4 mg in 500 mL D_5W at 15 mL/hr.
6. **Order:** dopamine 500 mg in 250 mL D_5W at 10 mL/hr.
7. **Order:** dobutamine 400 mg in 250 mL D_5W at 20 mL/hr.
8. **Order:** Isuprel 2 mg in 250 mL D_5W at 10 mL/hr.
9. **Order:** streptokinase 750,000 units in 50 mL D_5W over 30 minutes.
10. **Order:** nitroprusside 50 mg in 500 mL D_5W at 50 mcg/min.
11. **Order:** aminophylline 1 g in 250 mL D_5W at 20 mL/hr.
12. **Order:** Pronestyl 2 g in 250 mL D_5W at 16 mL/hr.
13. **Order:** heparin 25,000 units in 250 mL D_5W at 5 mL/hr.
14. **Order:** aminophylline 1 g in 500 mL D_5W at 40 mL/hr.
15. **Order:** nitroglycerin 50 mg in 250 mL D_5W at 50 mcg/min.
16. **Order:** alteplase 100 mg in NS 100 mL over 2 hours.
17. **Order:** theophylline 800 mg in D_5W 500 mL at 0.5 mg/kg.
18. **Order:** milrinone 20 mg in D_5W 100 mL at 0.50 mcg/kg/min.
19. **Order:** streptokinase 1.5 million units in D_5W 100 mL over 60 minutes.
20. **Order:** amiodarone 150 mg in D_5W 100 mL over 10 minutes.

CALCULATING INFUSION RATE FOR CONCENTRATION AND VOLUME PER UNIT TIME

The second step for administering medication is to calculate the *infusion rate* of the drug per *unit time*. Infusion rates can mean two things: the rate of volume (mL) given or the rate of concentration (units, mg, mcg) administered. *Unit time* means per hour or per minute. For drugs administered by continuous infusion, the four most important determinants are the concentration per hour and minute and the volume per hour and minute. Infusion rates are part of the physician's continuous infusion order, and they may be stated in concentration or volume per unit time.

Today's technology has produced smart pumps that are easily programmable, have built-in safety features, and can calculate and deliver appropriate drug dosages. The smart pump's conrol panel allows the user to select or enter (1) the name of the drug, (2) the concentration of the drug, (3) the volume of the solution, (4) the patient's weight in kilograms, and (5) the drug's dosage parameter per unit time (e.g., mg/min, units/hr, mcg/min) (Figure 13-1).

Not all facilities have infusion pumps with advanced technology; therefore the nurse must be able to calculate the infusion rates. For general-purpose infusion pumps that deliver mL/hr, the volume per hour of the drug must be known. *Remember:* If an infusion device is unavailable, a microdrip IV administration set is the appropriate set to use because the drops per minute rate (gtt/min) corresponds to the volume per hour rate (mL/hr).

Complete infusion rates for the volume and concentration are given in the examples and practice problems. In clinical practice, not all of the data is needed or pertinent for each drug to infuse. For example, when administering a heparin infusion, the concentration per minute is not as vital as the concentration per hour. However, vasoactive drugs such as dobutamine focus heavily on the concentration per minute and not the concentration per hour. Both of these drugs can use the same methods of calculation in order to obtain the same information. The nurse must have knowledge of pharmacology and clinical practice to determine the data that will be the most beneficial.

Concentration and Volume per Hour and Minute With a Drug in Units

EXAMPLES Infuse heparin 5000 units in D_5W 250 mL at 30 mL/hr. Concentration of solution is 20 units/mL. (Also note that volume/hour is given.) How many milliliters will be infused per minute?

Find volume per minute:
Method: mL/min

Set up a ratio and proportion. Use volume/hour, 30 mL/hr, or 30 mL/60 min as the known variable.	$30 \text{ mL} : 60 \text{ min} :: X \text{ mL} : \text{min}$ $60 X = 30$ $X = 0.5 \text{ mL}$

Answer: The infusion rate for volume per minute is 0.5 mL/min and the hourly rate is 30 mL/hr.

What is the concentration per minute and hour?
Find concentration per minute:
Method: units/min

Multiply the concentration of solution by the volume per minute.	$20 \text{ units/mL} \times 0.5 \text{ mL/min} = 10 \text{ units/min}$

Find concentration per hour:
Method: units/hr

Multiply the volume per minute by 60 min/hr.	$10 \text{ units/min} \times 60 \text{ min/hr} = 600 \text{ units/hr}$

Answer: The concentration per minute of heparin is 10 units/min and the concentration per hour is 600 units/hr.

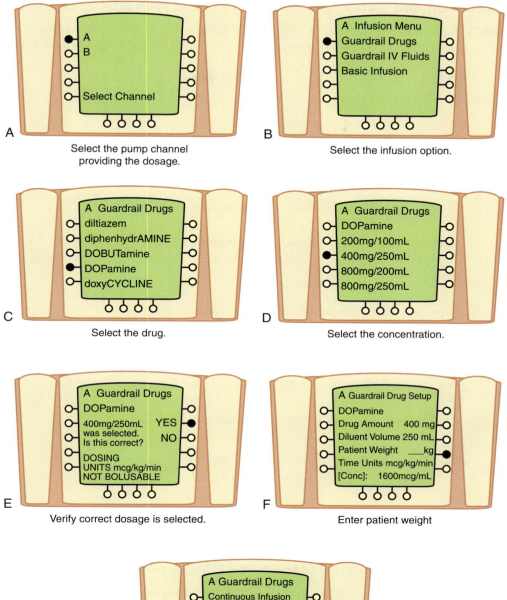

A. Select the pump channel providing the dosage.

B. Select the infusion option.

C. Select the drug.

D. Select the concentration.

E. Verify correct dosage is selected.

F. Enter patient weight

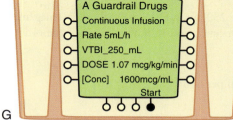

G. Verify information is correct and start infusion.

Figure 13-1 Examples of display screens of a dose rate calculator on an advanced infusion pump. (Modified from the Alaris System with Guardrail, Suite MX software. CareFusion 2011, San Diego, Calif.)

Concentration and Volume per Hour and Minute With a Drug in Milligrams

EXAMPLES Infuse lidocaine 2 g in D_5W 500 mL at 2 mg/min. Concentration of solution is 4 mg/mL. (Also note that concentration/minute is given.) How many milligrams will be infused per hour?

Find concentration per hour:
Method: mg/hr

Find the concentration/minute. Multiply concentration/minute × 60 min/hr.	lidocaine 2 mg/min 2 mg/min × 60 min = 120 mg/hr

Answer: The amount of lidocaine infused per hour is 120 mg/hr.

How many milliliters of lidocaine will be infused in 1 hour?
Find volume per hour:
Method: mL/hr

Calculate concentration of solution. Divide the concentration/hour by the concentration of solution.	lidocaine 4 mg/mL $\dfrac{120 \text{ mg/hr}}{4 \text{ mg/mL}} = 30 \text{ mL/hr}$

Answer: The infusion rate in milliliters for lidocaine 2 mg/min is 30 mL/hr.

How many milliliters of lidocaine will be infused in 1 minute?

Divide the concentration/minute by the concentration of the solution.	$\dfrac{2 \text{ mg/min}}{4 \text{ mg/mL}} = 0.5 \text{ mL/min}$

Answer: The infusion rate for lidocaine 2 mg/min is 0.5 mL/min.

Concentration and Volume per Hour and Minute With a Drug in Micrograms

EXAMPLES Infuse dobutamine 250 mg in D_5W 500 mL at 650 mcg/min. Concentration of solution is 500 mcg/mL. (Also note that concentration/minute is given in the order.) How many micrograms will be infused in 1 hour?

Find concentration per hour:
Method: mcg/hr

Find the concentration/minute. Multiply concentration/minute by 60 min/hr.	dobutamine 650 mcg/min 650 mcg/min × 60 min/hr = 39,000 mcg/hr

Answer: The concentration of dobutamine infused per hour is 39,000 mcg/hr.

How many milliliters of dobutamine will be infused in 1 hour?
Find volume per hour:
Method: mL/hr

| Calculate concentration of solution. Divide the concentration/hour by the concentration of solution. | dobutamine 500 mcg/mL $$\frac{39{,}000 \text{ mcg/hr}}{500 \text{ mcg/mL}} = 78 \text{ mL/hr}$$ |

Answer: The infusion rate for dobutamine 650 mcg/min is 78 mL/hr.

How many milliliters of dobutamine should be infused in 1 minute?
Find volume per minute:
Method: mL/min

| Divide concentration/minute by concentration of solution. | $$\frac{650 \text{ mcg/min}}{500 \text{ mcg/mL}} = 1.3 \text{ mL/min}$$ |

Answer: The infusion rate for dobutamine is 1.3 mL/min.

PRACTICE PROBLEMS: ▶ II CALCULATING INFUSION RATE

Answers can be found on pages 296 to 301.

Use the examples to find the following information:
• Concentration of the solution
• Infusion rates per unit time:
  a. Volume per minute
  b. Volume per hour
  c. Concentration per minute
  d. Concentration per hour

1. **Order:** heparin 1000 units in D_5W 500 mL at 50 mL/hr.
2. **Order:** nitroprusside 100 mg in D_5W 500 mL at 60 mL/hr.
3. **Order:** nitroprusside 25 mg in D_5W 250 mL at 50 mcg/min.
4. **Order:** dopamine 800 mg in D_5W 500 mL at 400 mcg/min.
5. **Order:** norepinephrine 2 mg in D_5W 250 mL at 45 mL/hr.
6. **Order:** dobutamine 1000 mg in D_5W 500 mL at 12 mL/hr.
7. **Order:** dobutamine 250 mg in D_5W 250 mL at 10 mL/hr.
8. **Order:** lidocaine 2 g in D_5W 500 mL at 4 mg/min.
9. **Order:** dopamine 400 mg in D_5W 250 mL at 60 mL/hr.
10. **Order:** isoproterenol 4 mg in D_5W 500 mL at 65 mL/hr.
11. **Order:** morphine sulfate 50 mg in 150 mL NS at 3 mg/hr.
12. **Order:** regular Humulin insulin 50 units in 250 mL NS at 4 units/hr.
13. **Order:** aminophylline 2 g in 250 mL D_5W at 20 mL/hr.
14. **Order:** nitroglycerin 50 mg in 250 mL D_5W at 24 mL/hr.
15. **Order:** heparin 25,000 units in 500 mL D_5W at 10 mL/hr.
16. **Order:** amiodarone 900 mg in D_5W 500 mL at 33.3 mL/hr.
17. **Order:** procainamide 1 g in D_5W 250 mL at 4 mg/min.
18. **Order:** diltiazem 100 mg in 100 mL NS at 10 mg/hr.
19. **Order:** streptokinase 750,000 units in 250 mL NS at 100,000 units/hr.
20. **Order:** bretylium 1 g in 250 mL D_5W at 1 mg/min.

CALCULATING INFUSION RATES OF A DRUG FOR SPECIFIC BODY WEIGHT PER UNIT TIME

The last method is calculating infusion rates for the amount of drug per unit time for a specific body weight. The weight parameter is an accurate means of dosing for a therapeutic effect. The metric system is used for all drug dosing, so pounds must be changed to kilograms. The physician orders the *desired dose per kilogram of body weight* and the *concentration of the solution*. From this information, infusion rates can be calculated for administering an individualized dose. Accurate daily weights are essential for the correct dosage.

The previous methods for calculating *concentration of solution* and *infusion rates* for concentration and volume are used, with one addition. The *concentration per minute* is obtained by multiplying the *body weight* by the *desired dose per kilogram per minute*, which must be done before the other infusion rates can be calculated. For many vasoactive drugs given as examples in this chapter, the most useful information clinically is the concentration per minute for the specific body weight, volume per minute, and volume per hour, because these parameters determine the infusion pump settings (see Figure 13-1).

New volumetric infusion pumps can now deliver fractional portions of a milliliter from tenths to hundredths in addition to calculating dosages for infusion rates. If the infusion pumps available do not have this feature and the volume per hour is a fractional amount, it must be rounded off to a whole number (1.8 mL/hr = 2 mL/hr). When calculating concentration per minute and hour and volume per minute, carry out the problem to three decimal places, if necessary, before rounding off. The volume per hour, if fractional, can then be rounded off, making the volume per hour as accurate as possible. There are two important factors to consider when rounding off fractional infusion rates:

1. If the patient's condition is labile, the difference between 1 or 2 mL could be important.
2. The ordering physician should be consulted if rounding off would significantly change the drug dosage.

Micrograms per Kilogram Body Weight

EXAMPLES Infuse dobutamine 250 mg in 500 mL D$_5$W at 10 mcg/kg/min. Patient weighs 143 lb. Concentration of solution is 500 mcg/mL. How many micrograms of dobutamine would be infused per minute? Per hour?

Convert pounds to kilograms:

Divide pounds by 2.2.	$\dfrac{143 \text{ lb}}{2.2 \text{ lb/kg}} = 65 \text{ kg}$

Find concentration per minute:
Method: mcg/min

Multiply patient's weight by the desired dose of mcg/kg/min.	$65 \text{ kg} \times 10 \text{ mcg/kg/min} = 650 \text{ mcg/min}$

Find concentration per hour:
Method: mcg/hr

Multiply concentration/min by 60 min/hr.	$650 \text{ mcg/min} \times 60 \text{ min/hr} = 39,000 \text{ mcg/hr}$

Answer: The concentration of dobutamine infused per minute and per hour is 650 mcg/min and 39,000 mcg/hr for the patient's body weight.

How many milliliters of dobutamine will be infused per minute? Per hour? Find volume per minute:
Method: mL/min

Divide the concentration/minute by the concentration of the solution.	$\dfrac{650 \text{ mcg/min}}{500 \text{ mcg/mL}} = 1.3 \text{ mL/min}$

Find volume per hour:
Method: mL/hr

Multiply volume/minute by 60 min/hr.	$1.3 \text{ mL/min} \times 60 \text{ min/hr} = 78 \text{ mL/hr}$

Answer: The volume of dobutamine infused per minute is 1.3 mL/min, and the infusion rate is 78 mL/hr.

BASIC FRACTIONAL FORMULA

A fractional equation can create a basic formula that can be used as another quick method to determine any one of the following quantities: concentration of solution, volume per hour, and desired concentration per minute ($\times$ kilogram of body weight, if required). The equation has one constant, the drop rate of the IV set, 60 gtt/mL. The unknown quantity can be represented by X. (See Chapter 6 for fractional equations.) The basic formula is not accurate to the nearest hundredth, as are the other methods in this section:

$$\frac{\text{Concentration of solution (units, mg, mcg/mL)}}{\text{Drop rate of set (60 gtt/mL)}} = \frac{\text{Desired concentration} \times \text{kg body weight}}{\text{Volume/hr (mL/hr or gtt/min)}}$$

Using Basic Formula to Find Volume per Hour or Drops per Minute

EXAMPLE Infuse heparin 5000 units in 250 mL D_5W at 0.15 units/kg/min.

Patient weighs 70 kg. The concentration of solution is 20 units/mL.

Desired concentration/minute: 0.15 units/kg/min $\times$ 70 kg = 10.5 units/min

$$\frac{20 \text{ units/mL}}{60 \text{ gtt/mL}} = \frac{10.5 \text{ units/min}}{X \text{ (mL/hr or gtt/min)}}$$

$$20\,X = 630$$
$$X = 31 \text{ mL/hr or 31 gtt/min}$$

Using Basic Formula to Find Desired Concentration per Minute

EXAMPLE Infuse lidocaine 2 g in 500 mL D_5W at 30 mL/hr. The concentration of the solution is 4 mg/mL.

$$\frac{4 \text{ mg/mL}}{60 \text{ gtt/mL}} = \frac{X}{30 \text{ mL/hr}}$$

$$60\,X = 120$$
$$X = 2 \text{ mg/min}$$

Using Basic Formula to Find Concentration of Solution

EXAMPLE Infuse dobutamine 250 mg in D_5W 500 mL at 10 mcg/kg/min with rate of 78 mL/hr. Patient weighs 65 kg.

$$\text{Desired concentration per minute} = 10 \text{ mcg/kg/min} \times 65 \text{ kg}$$
$$= 650 \text{ mcg/min}$$

$$\frac{X}{60 \text{ gtt/mL}} = \frac{650 \text{ mcg/min}}{78 \text{ mL/hr}}$$

$$78\,X = 39{,}000$$
$$X = 500 \text{ mcg/mL}$$

PRACTICE PROBLEMS: ▶ III CALCULATING INFUSION RATE FOR SPECIFIC BODY WEIGHT

Answers can be found on pages 301 to 304.

Determine the infusion rates for specific body weight by calculating the following:
- Concentration of the solution
- Weight in kilograms
- Infusion rates:
  a. Concentration per minute
  b. Concentration per hour (not always measured)
  c. Volume per minute
  d. Volume per hour

You can use the basic fractional formula and compare answers.

1. Infuse dobutamine 500 mg in 250 mL D_5W at 5 mcg/kg/min. Patient weighs 182 lb.
2. Infuse amrinone 250 mg in 250 mL NS at 5 mcg/kg/min. Patient weighs 165 lb.
3. Infuse vecuronium 20 mg in 100 mL NS at 0.8 mcg/kg/min. Patient weighs 202 lb.
4. Infuse nitroprusside 100 mg in 500 mL D_5W at 3 mcg/kg/min. Patient weighs 55 kg.
5. Infuse Precedex 200 mcg in 50 mL NS at 0.3 mcg/kg/hr. Patient weighs 158 lb. Hourly rate only.
6. Infuse propofol (Diprivan) 500 mg/50 mL infusion bottle at 10 mcg/kg/min. Patient weighs 187 lb.
7. Infuse alfentanil (Alfenta) 10,000 mcg in D_5W 250 mL at 0.5 mcg/kg/min. Patient weighs 175 lb.
8. Infuse milrinone (Primacor) 20 mg in D_5W 100 mL at 0.375 mcg/kg/min. Patient weighs 160 lb.
9. Infuse theophylline 400 mg in D_5W 500 mL at 0.55 mg/kg/hr. Patient weighs 70 kg. Hourly rate only.
10. Infuse esmolol 2.5 g in NS 250 mL at 150 mcg/kg/min. Patient weighs 148 lb.

TITRATION OF INFUSION RATE

High-alert drugs are given to improve a physiological function that is causing a life-threatening condition for the patient. Every high-alert drug produces a physiological response that should be closely monitored and evaluated for effectiveness. For example, a patient receiving aminophylline should be monitored for improved respiratory rate and breath sounds. Another example is nitroprusside, where a patient's decrease in blood pressure is the goal of therapy. Monitoring parameters should be a part of the physician's order and followed closely by the nurse.

The purpose of titration in medication administration is to give the least amount of drug in the therapeutic range to elicit the appropriate targeted physiological response. With the smart pump, the therapeutic ranges are calculated. If a general-purpose infusion pump is used, the nurse should calculate the upper and lower limits of the therapeutic range.

Titration of drugs administered by infusion is based on (1) *concentration of solution,* (2) *infusion rates,* (3) *specific concentration per kilogram of body weight,* and (4) *titration factor.* The *titration factor* is the concentration of drug per drop in units (units/gtt), milligrams (mg/gtt), or micrograms (mcg/gtt). For the programmable volumetric infusion pump, the titration factor is the increment of increase or decrease in units, micrograms, or milligrams. If the only IV equipment available has the mL/hr feature, the titration factor of concentration per drop can be used. Smart pumps can infuse medication volume in increments of 0.01 mL/hr. Other pump features include a drug-specific dose calculator that allows the nurse to select a drug name and input the dosage, the concentration of the drug, and the weight of the patient (see Figure 13-1). These infusion pumps make drug delivery and titration easier for the nurse and safer for the patient. Any dose changes can be easily reprogrammed by the pump's drug-specific dose calculator. The smart pump's safety features help to decrease medication errors. Many drug manufacturers are recommending smart pumps for the delivery of all vasoactive medications used in the critical care setting.

Calculating the titration factor is necessary when the technology of the advanced infusion pump is unavailable. The titration factor can be added to or subtracted from the baseline infusion rate to determine the exact concentration of an infusion. Because the titration method of drug administration is primarily used when a patient's condition is labile, calculating the titration factor gives the nurse the means of determining the exact amount of drug to be infused.

Medication protocols of the institution or drug infusion charts (developed by the drug manufacturer or the hospital's pharmacy) can be used to adjust infusion rates at the appropriate increments when titrating medications via the physician's order. It is imperative that critical care nurses are knowledgeable on the expected effects of a given medication, its titration factor, and its minimum and maximum dosage when titrating. Often, the amount of drug being infused falls between calibrations on the charts. When this occurs, the titration factor can be used to determine the exact concentration of drug being administered. The titration factor can also be used to verify the correct selection from the chart.

EXAMPLE Infuse isuprel 2 mg in 250 mL D$_5$W. Titrate 1 to 3 mcg/min to maintain heart rate greater than 50 beats/min and less than 130 beats/min and blood pressure greater than 90 mm Hg systolic.

a. Find concentration of solution:

Convert mg to mcg. Set up ratio and proportion.	$2 \text{ mg} = 2000 \text{ mcg}$
	$2000 \text{ mcg} : 250 \text{ mL} :: X \text{ mcg} : \text{mL}$
	$250 \, X = 2000$
	$X = 8 \text{ mcg}$
	8 mcg/mL

b. Infusion rate by volume per unit time:
Desired infusion rate by concentration is stated in the problem.
Note that the upper dosage and lower dosage must be determined.

Find volume rate per minute: mL/min:

Divide concentration/minute by concentration of solution.	*Lower*	*Upper*
	$\dfrac{1 \text{ mcg/min}}{8 \text{ mcg/mL}}$	$\dfrac{3 \text{ mcg/min}}{8 \text{ mcg/mL}}$
	$= 0.125 \text{ mL/min}$	$= 0.375 \text{ mL/min}$

Find volume rate per hour: mL/hr (equivalent to gtt/min):

Multiply volume rate/minute by 60 min.	*Lower* $0.125 \text{ mL/min} \times 60 \text{ min/hr}$ $= 7.5 \text{ mL/hr}$ *Upper* $0.375 \text{ mL/hr} \times 60 \text{ min/hr}$ $= 22.5 \text{ mL/hr}$

Dosage range is 7.5 mL/hr at 1 mcg/min, the lowest dose ordered, to 22.5 mL/hr at 3 mcg/min, the highest dose ordered.

Determine Titration Factor Using Infusion Pump

When the amount of fluid being titrated is 1 mL or greater (0.1 mL/hr lowest increment of infusion), the concentration of the solution multiplied by the volume per hour will give the total concentration to be given in 1 hour. The total volume in 1 hour divided by 60 min/hr will yield the concentration per minute.

EXAMPLE Increase isuprel from 7.5 mL/hr to 9 mL/hr.

Multiply concentration of solution by volume/hr. Then divide by 60 min/hr.	$9 \text{ mL/hr} \times 8 \text{ mcg/mL} = 72 \text{ mcg/hr}$ $\dfrac{72 \text{ mcg/hr}}{60 \text{ min/hr}} = 1.2 \text{ mcg/min}$

When increments of less than 1 mL are being titrated, multiply the concentration by the lowest increment of infusion.

Multiply concentration of solution by 0.1 mL/hr to get the concentration/hr.	$8 \text{ mcg/mL} \times 0.1 \text{ mL/hr} = 0.8 \text{ mcg/hr}$

Find rate in mcg/min by dividing concentration/hr by 60 min/hr.	$\dfrac{0.8 \text{ mcg/hr}}{60 \text{ min/hr}} = 0.013 \text{ mcg/min}$

Titration factor is 0.8 mcg/hr or 0.013 mcg/min for the solution of isuprel 2 mg in 250 mL D_5W with 0.1 mL/hr as the lowest increment of infusion. If the baseline rate is 7.5 mL/hr and 1 mcg/min, increasing the rate by 0.1 mL/hr to 7.6 mL/hr will increase the per minute dose to 1.013 mcg/min. Since isuprel is ordered in mcg/min, using the titration factor in mcg/min would give a very accurate dose if increases or decreases are needed.

Increasing or Decreasing Infusion Rates Using Infusion Pump

When increasing infusion rate (0.1 mL/hr lowest increment of infusion) from baseline, multiply the titration factor by the number of increases and add to beginning rate.

EXAMPLE   **Baseline Data**

Order	isuprel 2 mg in 250 mL
Concentration of solution	8 mcg/mL
Beginning rate	1 mcg/min
Volume per hour	7.5 mL/hr
Lowest increment of infusion	0.1 mL/hr (lowest pump setting)
Titration factors	0.8 mcg/hr or 0.013 mcg/min

Since the order is given in mcg/min, the titration factor of mcg/min should be used. To increase infusion rate from 7.5 mL/hr to 7.7 mL/hr, a 0.2-mL increase on the infusion pump, multiply titration factor by 2. Multiply 2×0.013 mcg/min = 0.026 mcg/min, then add to baseline of 1 mcg/min and now the concentration per minute is 1.026 mcg/min. Incremental increases can be easily calculated by multiplying the titration factor by the number of increases, then adding to baseline.

EXAMPLE

Hourly Rate (mL/hr)	Titration Factor	Concentration/min (ADD)
7.5 mL/hr	0.013 mcg/min	1 mcg/min
7.6 mL/hr	0.013 mcg/min $\times$ 1 = 0.013	1.013 mcg/min
7.7 mL/hr	0.013 mcg/min $\times$ 2 = 0.026	1.026 mcg/min
7.8 mL/hr	0.013 mcg/min $\times$ 3 = 0.039	1.039 mcg/min

To titrate downward, multiply titration factor by the number of decreases and subtract each decrease from current infusion rate.

EXAMPLE

Hourly Rate (mL/hr)	Titration Factor	Concentration/min (SUBTRACT)
10 mL/hr	0.013 mcg/min	1.33 mcg/min
9.8 mL/hr	0.013 mcg/min $\times$ 2 = 0.026	1.299 mcg/min
9.4 mL/hr	0.013 mcg/min $\times$ 6 = 0.078	1.247 mcg/min

Determine Titration Factor Using a Microdrip IV Set

A microdrip IV set has a drop factor of 60 gtt/mL, so the number of drops per minute is the same as the hourly rate. In a situation where infusion pumps are not available, a microdrip IV set should be the only option to deliver small amounts of IV medication. Using the isuprel data, the mL/hr rate will be 7.5 gtt counted per minute from the drip chamber. The titration factor is the amount of isuprel in each drop.

Determine the titration factor:

Find rate in gtt/min. Divide concentration/minute by gtt/min.	7.5 gtt/min $$\frac{1 \text{ mcg/\cancel{min}}}{7.5 \text{ gtt/\cancel{min}}} = 0.133 \text{ mcg/gtt}$$

The *titration factor* is 0.133 mcg/gt in a solution of isuprel 2 mg in 250 mL D$_5$W. In other words, changing drops per minute results in a corresponding change in milliliters per hour. If the baseline infusion rates are **1 mcg/min** for concentration and **7.5 mL/hr** for volume, increasing the infusion rate by **1 gt/min** changes the concentration/minute by **0.133 mcg** and increases the hourly volume by **1 mL** to give a rate of **8.5 mL/hr.**

Increasing or Decreasing Infusion Rates Using a Microdrip IV Set

To increase the infusion rate by 5 gtt/min from a baseline rate of 1 mcg/min, set up a ratio and proportion or multiply the titration factor (mcg/gt) by 5 to obtain the increment of increase.

EXAMPLES

Set up a ratio and proportion with rate in gtt/min as the known variable.

7.5 gtt : 1 mcg :: 5 gtt : X mcg

7.5 X = 5

X = 0.666 mcg

5 gtt/0.66 mcg

or

Multiply titration factor in mcg/gt by 5.

0.133 mcg/gt × 5 gtt = 0.665 mcg

Adding 5 gtt/min increases the volume infusion rate by 5 mL/hr, from 7.5 to 12.5 mL/hr. The concentration of drug delivered is increased by 0.665 mcg/min to 1.665 mcg/min. For example,

$$
\begin{array}{ll}
1.000 \text{ mcg/min} & \text{baseline rate} \\
+\,0.665 \text{ mcg/min} & \text{increment of rate increased} \\
\hline
1.665 \text{ mcg/min} & \text{adjusted infusion rate}
\end{array}
$$

Suppose the infusion rate was 3 mcg/min and a decrease was needed. To decrease the infusion rate by 10 gtt, set up another ratio and proportion or multiply the titration factor (mcg/gt) by 10.

EXAMPLES

Set up a ratio and proportion with rate in gtt/mcg as the known variable.

7.5 gtt : 1 mcg :: 10 gtt : X mcg

7.5 X = 10

X = 1.33 mcg

1.33 mcg/10 gtt

or

Multiply titration factor in mcg/gt by 10.

0.133 mcg/gt × 10 gtt = 1.33 mcg

Subtracting 10 gtt/min decreases the infusion rate by 10 mL/hr, from 22.5 to 12.5 mL/hr. The amount of drug delivered is decreased by 1.33 mcg/min to 1.67 mcg/min. For example,

$$
\begin{array}{ll}
3.00 \text{ mcg/min} & \text{baseline infusion rate} \\
-1.33 \text{ mcg/min} & \text{increment of rate decreased} \\
\hline
1.67 \text{ mcg/min} & \text{adjusted infusion rate}
\end{array}
$$

PRACTICE PROBLEMS: ▶ IV TITRATION OF INFUSION RATE

Answers can be found on pages 304 to 305.

1. What are the units of measure for the following terms?
   a. Concentration of solution per minute for specific body weight
   b. Concentration of solution
   c. Volume per hour
   d. Concentration per minute
   e. Volume per minute
   f. Concentration per minute
   g. Titration factor

2. Order: nitroprusside 50 mg in 250 mL D_5W. Titrate 0.5 to 1.5 mcg/kg/min to maintain mean systolic blood pressure at 100 mm Hg. Patient weighs 70 kg.

   Find the following:
   a. Concentration of solution
   b. Concentration per minute
   c. Volume per minute and hour
   d. Titration factor for infusion pump; for microdrop set
   e. Increase infusion rate of 10.5 mL/hr by 0.5 mL to 11 mL/hr with infusion pump. What is the concentration per minute?
   f. Increase infusion rate from 11 mL/hr to 20 mL/hr. What is the concentration per minute?
   g. Increase the infusion rate of 11 gtt/min by 5 gtt. What is the concentration per minute? What is the volume per hour?
   h. Increase the infusion rate of 16 gtt/mL by 13 gtt. What is the concentration per minute? What is the volume per hour?

3. Order: dopamine 400 mg in 250 mL D_5W. Titrate beginning at 4 mcg/kg/min to maintain a mean systolic blood pressure of 100 to 120 mm Hg. Patient weighs 75 kg.

   Find the following:
   a. Concentration of solution
   b. Concentration per minute
   c. Volume per minute and hour
   d. Titration factor for infusion pump; for microdrip set
   e. With the infusion pump, increase infusion rate from 11.4 mL/hr to 12 mL/hr. What is the concentration per minute?
   f. With the infusion pump, increase the infusion rate to 12.5 mL/hr. What is the concentration per minute?
   g. Using a microdrip set, increase the infusion rate of 13 gtt/min by 7 gtt. What is the concentration per minute? What is the volume per hour?
   h. Using a microdrip set, decrease the infusion rate of 20 mL/hr (20 gtt/min) by 5 gtt. What is the concentration per minute? What is the volume per hour?

TOTAL AMOUNT OF DRUG INFUSED OVER TIME

Determining the total amount of drug infused over time is useful when changes in drug therapy occur. If adverse effects, toxic levels, therapeutic failure, or discontinuance of a drug occurs, knowing the amount that was administered can be important for charting and for determining future therapies.

For this calculation, the concentration of the drug in its solution must be known, as well as the time that the drug therapy began to the nearest minute. Again, with 60-gtt sets, the hourly rate is the same as the drip rate per minute.

EXAMPLES Heparin 10,000 units in 250 mL D_5W at 30 mL/hr has been infusing for 3 hours. The drug is discontinued.

How much heparin did the patient receive?
Find concentration of solution:

Set up a ratio and proportion. Solve for X.	10,000 units : 250 mL :: X units : mL 250 X = 10,000 X = 40 units 40 units/mL

Find concentration per hour:

Multiply concentration of solution by volume/hour.	40 units/mL × 30 mL/hr = 1200 units/hr

Calculate total amount of drug infused:

Multiply concentration/hour by length of administration.	1200 units/hr × 3 hr = 3600 units/hr

Answer: The total amount of heparin infused over 3 hours was 3600 units.

PRACTICE PROBLEMS: ▶ V TOTAL AMOUNT OF DRUG INFUSED OVER TIME

Answers can be found on page 306.

Solve for the amount of drug infused over time.
1. In 1 hour, a patient received two boluses of lidocaine 100 mg and an IV infusion of 4 mg/mL at 40 mL/hr for 30 minutes. How many milligrams have been infused?

   Note: Do not exceed 300 mg/hr of lidocaine.

2. Heparin 20,000 units in 500 mL D_5W at 50 mL/hr has been infused for 5½ hours. The drug is discontinued. How much heparin has been given?

ANSWERS

I Calculating Concentration of a Solution

1. 10,000 units : 250 mL :: X units : mL
   250 X = 10,000
   X = 40 units
   The concentration of solution is 40 units/mL.

2. 1000 mg : 100 mL :: X mg : mL
   100 X = 1000 mg
   X = 10 mg
   The concentration of solution is 10 mg/mL.

3. 100 units : 500 mL :: X units : mL
$$500\,X = 100$$
$$X = 0.2 \text{ units}$$
The concentration of solution is 0.2 units/mL.

4.
$$1\,g = 1000\,mg$$
1000 mg : 1000 mL :: X mg : mL
$$1000\,X = 1000$$
$$X = 1\,mg$$
The concentration of solution is 1 mg/mL.

5.
$$4\,mg = 4000\,mcg$$
4000 mcg : 500 mL :: X mcg : mL
$$500\,X = 4000$$
$$X = 8\,mcg$$
The concentration of solution is 8 mcg/mL.

6. 500 mg : 250 mL :: X mcg : mL
$$250\,X = 500$$
$$X = 2\,mg$$
The concentration of solution is 2 mg/mL.

7. 400 mg : 250 mL :: X mg : mL
$$250\,X = 400$$
$$X = 1.6\,mg$$
The concentration of solution is 1.6 mg/mL.

8.
$$2\,mg = 2000\,mcg$$
2000 mcg : 250 mL :: X mcg : mL
$$250\,X = 2000$$
$$X = 8\,mcg$$
The concentration of solution is 8 mcg/mL.

9. 750,000 units : 50 mL :: X units : mL
$$50\,X = 750{,}000$$
$$X = 15{,}000 \text{ units}$$
The concentration of solution is 15,000 units/mL.

10.
$$50\,mg = 50{,}000\,mcg$$
50,000 mcg : 500 mL :: X mcg : mL
$$500\,X = 50{,}000$$
$$X = 100\,mcg$$
The concentration of solution is 100 mcg/mL.

11.
$$1\,g = 1000\,mg$$
1000 mg : 250 mL :: X mg : mL
$$250\,X = 1000$$
$$X = 4\,mg$$
The concentration of solution is 4 mg/mL.

12.
$$2\,g = 2000\,mg$$
2000 mg : 250 mL :: X mg : mL
$$250\,X = 2000$$
$$X = 8\,mg$$
The concentration of solution is 8 mg/mL.

13. 25,000 units : 250 mL :: X mg : mL
$$250\,X = 25{,}000$$
$$X = 100 \text{ units}$$
The concentration of solution is 100 units/mL.

14.
$$1\,g = 1000\,mg$$
1000 mg : 500 mL :: X mg : mL
$$500\,X = 1000$$
$$X = 2\,mg$$
The concentration of solution is 2 mg/mL.

15.
$$50\,mg = 50{,}000\,mcg$$
50,000 mcg : 250 mL :: X mcg : mL
$$250\,X = 50{,}000$$
$$X = 200\,mcg$$
The concentration of solution is 200 mcg/mL.

16. 100 mg : 100 mL :: X mg : mL
$$100\,X = 100$$
$$X = 1\,mg/mL$$
The concentration of solution is 1 mg/mL.

17. 800 mg : 500 mL :: X mg : mL
$$500\,X = 800$$
$$X = 1.6\,mg/mL$$
The concentration of solution is 1.6 mg/mL.

18. 20 mg : 100 mL :: X mg : mL
$$100\,X = 20$$
$$X = 0.2\,mg/mL$$
The concentration of solution is 0.2 mg/mL.

19. 1,500,000 units : 100 mL :: X mg : mL
$$100\,X = 1{,}500{,}000$$
$$X = 15{,}000 \text{ units/mL}$$
The concentration of solution is 15,000 units/mL.

20. 150 mg : 100 mL :: X mg : mL
$$100\,X = 150$$
$$X = 1.5\,mg/mL$$
The concentration of solution is 1.5 mg/mL.

II Calculating Infusion Rate

1. *Concentration of solution:*
   1000 units : 500 mL = X units : mL
   $$500\,X = 1000$$
   $$X = 2 \text{ units}$$
   The concentration of solution is 2 units/mL.
   Infusion rates:
   a. Volume/min:
   50 mL : 60 min :: X mL : min
   $$60\,X = 50$$
   $$X = 0.833 \text{ mL or } 0.83 \text{ mL or } 0.8 \text{ mL}$$
   $$0.8 \text{ mL/min}$$
   b. Volume/hr:
   50 mL/hr

   c. Concentration/min:
   2 units/mL × 0.8 mL/min = 1.60 units/min

   d. Concentration/hr:
   1.60 units/min × 60 min/hr = 96 units/hr

2. *Concentration of solution.*
   100 mg : 500 mL :: X mg : mL
   $$500\,X = 100$$
   $$X = 0.2 \text{ mg}$$
   The concentration of solution is 0.2 mg/mL.
   Infusion rates:
   a. Volume/min:
   60 mL : 60 min :: X mL : min
   $$60\,X = 60$$
   $$X = 1 \text{ mL}$$
   $$1 \text{ mL/min}$$
   b. Volume/hr:
   60 mL/hr

   c. Concentration/min:
   0.2 mg/mL × 1 mL/min = 0.2 mg/min

   d. Concentration/hr:
   0.2 mg/min × 60 min/hr = 12 mg/hr

3. *Concentration of solution:*
   25 mg = 25,000 mcg
   25,000 mcg : 250 mL :: X mcg : mL
   $$250\,X = 25,000$$
   $$X = 100 \text{ mcg}$$
   The concentration of solution is 100 mcg/mL.
   Infusion rates:
   a. Volume/min:
   $$\frac{50 \text{ mcg/min}}{100 \text{ mcg/mL}} = 0.5 \text{ mL/min}$$
   b. Volume/hr:
   0.5 mL/min × 60 min/hr = 30 mL/hr

   c. Concentration/min:
   50 mcg/min

   d. Concentration/hr:
   50 mcg/min × 60 min/hr = 3000 mcg/hr

4. *Concentration of solution:*
$$800 \text{ mg} = 800,000 \text{ mcg}$$
$$800,000 \text{ mcg}:500 \text{ mL}::X \text{ mcg}:mL$$
$$500 \text{ X} = 800,000$$
$$X = 1600 \text{ mcg}$$
The concentration of solution is 1600 mcg/mL.
Infusion rates:
a. Volume/min:
$$\frac{400 \text{ mcg/min}}{1600 \text{ mcg/mL}} = 0.25 \text{ mL/min}$$
b. Volume/hr:
0.25 mL/min × 60 min/hr = 15 mL/hr

c. Concentration/min:
400 mcg/min

d. Concentration/hr:
400 mcg/min × 60 min/hr = 24,000 mcg/hr

5. *Concentration of solution:*
$$2 \text{ mg} = 2000 \text{ mcg}$$
$$2000 \text{ mcg}:250 \text{ mL}::X \text{ mcg}:mL$$
$$250 \text{ X} = 2000$$
$$X = 8 \text{ mcg}$$
The concentration of solution is 8 mcg/mL.
Infusion rates:
a. Volume/min:
$$45 \text{ mL}:60 \text{ min}::X \text{ mL}:min$$
$$60 \text{ X} = 45$$
$$X = 0.75 \text{ mL/min}$$
b. Volume/hr:
45 mL/hr

c. Concentration/min:
8 mcg/mL × 0.75 mL/min = 6 mcg/min

d. Concentration/hr:
6 mcg/min × 60 min/hr = 360 mcg/hr

6. *Concentration of solution:*
$$1000 \text{ mg} = 1,000,000 \text{ mcg}$$
$$1,000,000 \text{ mcg}:500 \text{ mL}::X \text{ mcg}:mL$$
$$500 \text{ X} = 1,000,000$$
$$X = 2000 \text{ mcg}$$
The concentration of solution is 2000 mcg/mL.
Infusion rates:
a. Volume/min:
$$12 \text{ mL}:60 \text{ min}::X \text{ mL}:min$$
$$60 \text{ X} = 12$$
$$X = 0.2 \text{ mL}$$
0.2 mL/min
b. Volume/hr:
12 mL/hr

c. Concentration/min:
2000 mcg/mL × 0.2 mL/min = 400 mcg/min

d. Concentration/hr:
400 mcg/min × 60 min/hr = 24,000 mcg/hr

7. *Concentration of solution:*
$$250 \text{ mg} = 250,000 \text{ mcg}$$
$$250,000 \text{ mcg}:250 \text{ mL}::X \text{ mcg}:mL$$
$$250 \text{ X} = 250,000$$
$$X = 1000 \text{ mcg}$$
The concentration of solution is 1000 mcg/mL.
Infusion rates:
a. Volume/min:
$$10 \text{ mL}:60 \text{ min}::X \text{ mL}:1 \text{ min}$$
$$60 \text{ X} = 10 \text{ mL}$$
$$X = 0.1666 \text{ mL or } 0.17 \text{ mL}$$
0.17 mL/min
b. Volume/hr:
10 mL/hr

c. Concentration/min:
1000 mcg/mL × 0.17 mL/min = 170 mcg/min

d. Concentration/hr:
170 mcg/min × 60 min/hr = 10,200 mcg/hr

8. *Concentration of solution:*

$$2 \text{ g} = 2000 \text{ mg}$$
$$2000 \text{ mg}:500 \text{ mL}::X \text{ mg}:mL$$
$$500 \text{ X} = 2000$$
$$X = 4 \text{ mg}$$

The concentration of solution is 4 mg/mL.

Infusion rates:

a. Volume/min:
$$\frac{4 \text{ mg/min}}{4 \text{ mg/mL}} = 1 \text{ mL/min}$$

b. Volume/hr:
1 mL/min × 60 min/hr = 60 mL/hr

c. Concentration/min:
4 mg/min

d. Concentration/hr:
4 mg/min × 60 min/hr = 240 mg/hr

9. *Concentration of solution:*

$$400 \text{ mg}:250 \text{ mL}::X \text{ mg}:mL$$
$$250 \text{ X} = 400$$
$$X = 1.6 \text{ mg}$$

The concentration of solution is 1.6 mg/mL.

Infusion rates:

a. Volume/min:
$$60 \text{ mL}:60 \text{ min}::X \text{ mL}:min$$
$$60 \text{ X} = 60$$
$$X = 1 \text{ mL}$$
$$1 \text{ mL/min}$$

b. Volume/hr:
60 mL/hr

c. Concentration/min:
1.6 mg/mL × 1 mL/min = 1.6 mg/min

d. Concentration/hr:
1.6 mg/min × 60 min/hr = 96 mg/hr

10. *Concentration of solution:*

$$4 \text{ mg} = 4000 \text{ mcg}$$
$$4000 \text{ mcg}:500 \text{ mL}::X \text{ mcg}:mL$$
$$500 \text{ X} = 4000$$
$$X = 8 \text{ mcg}$$

The concentration of solution is 8 mcg/mL.

Infusion rates:

a. Volume/min:
$$65 \text{ mL}:60 \text{ min}::X \text{ mL}:min$$
$$60 \text{ X} = 65$$
$$X = 1.083 \text{ mL or}$$
$$1.08 \text{ mL/min}$$

b. Volume/hr:
65 mL/hr

c. Concentration/min:
8 mcg/mL × 1.08 mL/min = 8.64 mcg/min

d. Concentration/hr:
8.64 mcg/min × 60 min/hr = 518.4 mcg/hr or
518 mcg/hr

11. *Concentration of solution:*

$$50 \text{ mg}:150 \text{ mL}::X \text{ mg}:mL$$
$$150 \text{ X} = 50$$
$$X = 0.33 \text{ mg}$$

The concentration of solution is 0.33 mg/mL.

Infusion rates:

a. Volume/min:
$$\frac{0.05 \text{ mg/min}}{0.33 \text{ mg/mL}} = 0.15 \text{ mL/min}$$

b. Volume/hr:
$$\frac{3 \text{ mg/hr}}{0.33 \text{ mg/mL}} = 9.09 \text{ or } 9 \text{ mL/hr}$$

c. Concentration/min:
$$3 \text{ mg}:60 \text{ min}::X \text{ mg}:min$$
$$60 \text{ X} = 3$$
$$X = 0.05 \text{ mg/min}$$

12. *Concentration of solution:*
$$50 \text{ units} : 250 \text{ mL} :: X \text{ mg} : \text{mL}$$
$$250 X = 50$$
$$X = 0.2 \text{ units}$$
The concentration of solution is 0.2 units/mL.
Infusion rates:
   a. Concentration/min:
$$4 \text{ units} : 60 \text{ min} :: X \text{ units} : \text{min}$$
$$60 X = 4$$
$$X = 0.066 \text{ units/min or } 0.07 \text{ units/min}$$
   b. Concentration/hr:
   4 units/hr

   c. Volume/min:
$$\frac{0.066 \text{ units/min}}{0.2 \text{ units/mL}} = 0.33 \text{ mL/min}$$
   d. Volume/hr:
$$\frac{4 \text{ units/hr}}{0.2 \text{ units/mL}} = 20 \text{ mL/hr}$$

13. *Concentration of solution:*
$$2 \text{ g} = 2000 \text{ mg}$$
$$2000 \text{ mg} : 250 \text{ mL} :: X \text{ mg} : \text{mL}$$
$$250 X = 2000$$
$$X = 8 \text{ mg}$$
The concentration of solution is 8 mg/mL.
Infusion rates:
   a. Volume/hr = 20 mL/hr

   b. Volume/min:
$$20 \text{ mL} : 60 \text{ min} :: X \text{ mL} : \text{min}$$
$$60 X = 20$$
$$X = 0.3 \text{ mL/min}$$

   c. Concentration/min:
   8 mg/mL × 0.3 mL/min = 2.4 mg/min
   d. Concentration/hr:
   2.4 mg/min × 60 min/hr = 144 mg/hr

14. *Concentration of solution:*
$$50 \text{ mg} = 50,000 \text{ mcg}$$
$$50,000 \text{ mcg} : 250 \text{ mL} :: X \text{ mg} : \text{mL}$$
$$250 X = 50,000$$
$$X = 200 \text{ mcg}$$
The concentration of solution is 200 mcg/mL.
Infusion rates:
   a. Volume/hr = 24 mL/hr

   b. Volume/min:
$$24 \text{ mL/hr} : 60 \text{ min/hr} :: X \text{ mL} : \text{min}$$
$$60 X = 24$$
$$X = 0.4 \text{ mL/min}$$

   c. Concentration/min:
   200 mcg/mL × 0.4 mL/min = 80 mcg/min
   d. Concentration/hr:
   80 mcg/min × 60 min = 4800 mcg/hr

15. *Concentration of solution:*
$$25,000 \text{ units} : 500 \text{ mL} :: X \text{ units} : \text{mL}$$
$$500 X = 25,000$$
$$X = 50 \text{ units}$$
The concentration of solution is 50 units/mL.
Infusion rates:
   a. Volume/hr:
   10 mL/hr
   b. Volume/min:
$$10 \text{ mL} : 60 \text{ min/hr} :: X \text{ mL} : \text{min}$$
$$60 X = 10$$
$$X = 0.166 \text{ mL/min}$$

   c. Concentration/hr:
   50 units/mL × 10 mL/hr = 500 units/hr
   d. Concentration/min:
   50 units/mL × 0.166 mL/min = 8.3 units/min

16. *Concentration of solution:*
    900 mg : 500 mL :: X mg : mL
    500 X = 900
    X = 1.8 mg/mL
    The concentration of solution is 1.8 mg/mL.
    Infusion rates:
    a. Volume/hr:
    33.3 mL/hr
    b. Volume/min:
    33.3 mL : 60 min :: X mL : min
    60 X = 33.3
    X = 0.55 mL/min
    c. Concentration/hr:
    1.8 mg/mL × 33.3 mL/hr = 59.9 mg/hr
    d. Concentration/min:
    1.8 mg/mL × 0.55 mL/min = 0.99 mg/mL or
    1.0 mg/mL

17. *Concentration of solution:*
    1 g = 1000 mg
    1000 mg : 250 mL :: X mg : mL
    250 X = 1000
    X = 4 mg/mL
    The concentration of solution is 4 mg/mL.
    Infusion rates:
    a. Volume/min:
    $$\frac{4 \text{ mg/min}}{4 \text{ mg/mL}} = 1 \text{ mL/min}$$
    b. Volume/hr:
    1 mL/min × 60 min/hr = 60 mL/hr
    c. Concentration/hr:
    4 mg/min × 60 min/hr = 240 mg/hr
    d. Concentration/min:
    4 mg/min

18. *Concentration of solution:*
    100 mg : 100 mL :: X mg : mL
    100 X = 100
    X = 1 mg/mL
    The concentration of solution is 1 mg/mL.
    Infusion rates:
    a. Volume/hr:
    $$\frac{10 \text{ mg/hr}}{1 \text{ mg/mL}} = 10 \text{ mL/hr}$$
    b. Volume/min:
    $$\frac{10 \text{ mL/hr}}{60 \text{ min/hr}} = 0.166 \text{ mL/min}$$
    c. Concentration/hr:
    10 mg/hr
    d. Concentration/min:
    1 mg/mL × 0.166 mL/min = 0.166 mg/min or
    0.17 mg/min

19. *Concentration of solution:*
    750,000 units : 250 mL :: X units : mL
    250 X = 750,000
    X = 3000 units/mL
    The concentration of solution is 3000 units/mL.
    Infusion rates:
    a. Volume/hr:
    $$\frac{100,000 \text{ units/hr}}{3000 \text{ units/mL}} = 33.3 \text{ mL/hr}$$
    b. Volume/min:
    $$\frac{33.3 \text{ mL/hr}}{60 \text{ min/hr}} = 0.55 \text{ mL/min}$$
    c. Concentration/hr:
    100,000 units/hr
    d. Concentration/min:
    $$\frac{100,000 \text{ units/hr}}{60 \text{ min/hr}} = 1666.6 \text{ units/min or } 1667 \text{ units/min}$$

20. *Concentration of solution:*
$$1 \text{ g} = 1000 \text{ mg}$$
$$1000 \text{ mg} : 250 \text{ mL} :: X \text{ mg} : \text{mL}$$
$$250 \text{ X} = 1000$$
$$X = 4 \text{ mg/mL}$$
The concentration of solution is 4 mg/mL.
Infusion rates:
a. Volume/min:
$$\frac{1 \text{ mg/min}}{4 \text{ mg/mL}} = 0.25 \text{ mL/min}$$

b. Volume/hr:
0.25 mL/min × 60 min/hr = 15 mL/hr

c. Concentration/hr:
4 mg/mL × 15 mL/hr = 60 mg/hr

d. Concentration/min:
1 mg/min

III Calculating Infusion Rate for Specific Body Weight

1. *Concentration of solution:*
$$500 \text{ mg} = 500,000 \text{ mcg}$$
$$500,000 : 250 \text{ mL} :: X \text{ mcg} : \text{mL}$$
$$250 \text{ X} = 500,000$$
$$X = 2000 \text{ mcg}$$
The concentration of solution is 2000 mcg/mL.
Infusion rates:
a. Concentration/min:
Body weight × Desired dose/kg/min
82.7 kg × 5 mcg/kg/min
= 413.5 mcg/min

b. Concentration/hr:
413.5 mcg/min × 60 min/hr = 24,810 mcg/hr

2. *Concentration of solution:*
$$250 \text{ mg} = 250,000 \text{ mcg}$$
$$250,000 \text{ mcg} : 250 \text{ mL} :: X \text{ mcg} : \text{mL}$$
$$250 \text{ X} = 250,000$$
$$X = 1000 \text{ mcg}$$
The concentration of solution is 1000 mcg/mL.
Infusion rates:
a. Concentration/min:
Body weight × Desired dose/kg/min
75 kg × 5 mcg/kg/min = 375 mcg/min

b. Concentration/hr:
375 mcg/min × 60 min/hr = 22,500 mcg/hr

Patient weight:
lb to kg: $\dfrac{182}{2.2} = 82.7 \text{ kg}$

c. Volume/min:
$$\frac{413.5 \text{ mcg/min}}{2000 \text{ mcg/mL}} = 0.206 \text{ mL/min or } 0.2 \text{ mL/min}$$

d. Volume/hr:
0.2 mL/min × 60 min/hr = 12 mL/hr

Patient weight:
lb to kg: $\dfrac{165}{2.2} = 75 \text{ kg}$

c. Volume/min:
$$\frac{375 \text{ mcg/min}}{1000 \text{ mcg/mL}} = 0.375 \text{ mL/min}$$

d. Volume/hr:
0.375 mL/min × 60 min/hr = 22.5 mL/hr

3. *Concentration of solution:*
$$20 \text{ mg} = 20{,}000 \text{ mcg}$$
$$20{,}000 \text{ mcg}:100 \text{ mL}::X \text{ mcg}:\text{mL}$$
$$100 \text{ X} = 20{,}000$$
$$X = 200 \text{ mcg}$$
The concentration of the solution is 200 mcg/mL.
Infusion rates:
a. Concentration/min:
   Body weight × Desired dose/kg/min
$$92 \text{ kg} \times 0.8 \text{ mcg/kg/min}$$
$$= 73.6 \text{ mcg/min}$$
b. Concentration/hr:
   73.6 mcg/min × 60 min/hr = 4,416 mcg/hr
4. *Concentration of solution:*
$$100 \text{ mg} = 100{,}000 \text{ mcg}$$
$$100{,}000 \text{ mcg}:500 \text{ mL}::X \text{ mg}:\text{mL}$$
$$500 \text{ X} = 100{,}000$$
$$X = 200 \text{ mcg}$$
The concentration of solution is 200 mcg/mL.
Infusion rates:
a. Concentration/min:
   3 mcg/kg/min × 55 kg = 165 mcg/min

b. Concentration/hr:
   165 mcg/min × 60 min/hr = 9900 mcg/hr

5. *Concentration of solution:*
$$200 \text{ mcg}:50 \text{ mL}::X \text{ mcg}:\text{mL}$$
$$50 \text{ X} = 200$$
$$X = 4 \text{ mcg}$$
The concentration of solution is 4 mcg/mL.
Infusion rates (hourly only, so no answers for a *or* c*):*
b. Concentration/hr:
   Body weight × Desired dose/kg/hr
$$72 \text{ kg} \times 0.3 \text{ mcg/kg/hr}$$
$$= 21.6 \text{ mcg/hr}$$

Patient weight:
lb to kg: $\dfrac{202}{2.2} = 92 \text{ kg}$

c. Volume/min:
$$\frac{73.6 \text{ mcg/min}}{200 \text{ mcg/mL}} = 0.368 \text{ mL/min}$$

d. Volume/hr:
   0.368 mL/min × 60 min/hr = 22.08 or 22.1 mL/hr
Patient weight:
55 kg

c. Volume/min:
$$\frac{165 \text{ mcg/min}}{200 \text{ mcg/mL}} = 0.825 \text{ mL/min}$$
d. Volume/hr:
   0.825 mL/min × 60 min/hr = 49.5 mL/hr

Patient weight:
lb to kg: $\dfrac{158 \text{ lb}}{2.2} = 72 \text{ kg}$

d. Volume/hr:
$$\frac{21.6 \text{ mcg/hr}}{4 \text{ mcg/mL}} = 5.4 \text{ mL/hr}$$

6. *Concentration of solution:*
$$500 \text{ mg} : 50 \text{ mL} :: X \text{ mg} : mL$$
$$50 X = 500$$
$$X = 10 \text{ mg/mL}$$
The concentration of solution is 10 mg/mL or 10,000 mcg/mL.
Infusion rates:

a. Concentration/min:
Body weight × Desired dose/kg/min
85 kg × 10 mcg/kg/min
= 850 mcg/min

b. Concentration/hr:
850 mcg/min × 60 min/hr = 51,000 mcg/hr
or 51 mg/hr

Patient weight:
lb to kg: $\dfrac{187}{2.2} = 85 \text{ kg}$

c. Volume/min:
$\dfrac{850 \text{ mcg/min}}{10,000 \text{ mcg/mL}} = 0.085 \text{ mL/min}$

d. Volume/hr:
0.085 mL/min × 60 min/hr = 5.1 mL/hr

7. *Concentration of solution:*
$$10,000 \text{ mcg} : 250 \text{ mL} :: X \text{ mcg} : mL$$
$$250 X = 10,000$$
$$X = 40 \text{ mcg/mL}$$

Infusion rates:

a. Concentration/min:
Body weight × Desired dose/kg/min
79.5 kg × 0.5 mcg/kg/min
= 39.75 mcg/min

b. Concentration/hr:
39.75 mcg/min × 60 min/hr = 2385 mcg/hr
or 2.4 mg/hr

Patient weight:
lb to kg: $\dfrac{175}{2.2} = 79.5 \text{ kg}$

c. Volume/min:
$\dfrac{39.75 \text{ mcg/min}}{40 \text{ mcg/mL}} = 0.99 \text{ mL/min or 1 mL/min}$

d. Volume/hr:
0.99 mL/min × 60 min/hr = 59.4 mL/hr

8. *Concentration of solution:*
$$20 \text{ mg} : 100 \text{ mL} :: X \text{ mg} : mL$$
$$100 X = 20$$
$$X = 0.2 \text{ mg/mL}$$
$$\text{or } 200 \text{ mcg/mL}$$

Infusion rates:

a. Concentration/min:
Body weight × Desired dose/kg/min
72.7 kg × 0.375 mcg/kg/min
= 27.2 mcg/min

b. Concentration/hr:
27.2 mcg/min × 60 min/hr = 1632 mcg/hr or
1.6 mg/hr

Patient weight:
lb to kg: $\dfrac{160}{2.2} = 72.7 \text{ kg}$

c. Volume/min:
$\dfrac{27.2 \text{ mcg/min}}{200 \text{ mcg/mL}} = 0.136 \text{ mL/min}$

d. Volume/hr:
0.136 mL/min × 60 min/hr = 8.16 mL/hr or
8.2 mL/hr

Patient weight:
70 kg

9. *Concentration of solution:*
$$400 \text{ mg} : 500 \text{ mL} :: X \text{ mg} : mL$$
$$500 X = 400$$
$$X = 0.8 \text{ mg/mL}$$

Infusion rates:

a. Concentration/hr:
Body weight × Desired dose/kg/min
70 kg × 0.55 mg/kg/min
= 38.5 mg/hr

b. Volume/hr:
$\dfrac{38.5 \text{ mg/hr}}{0.8 \text{ mg/mL}} = 48.125 \text{ mL/hr or 48 mL/hr}$

10. *Concentration of solution:*
$$2500 \text{ mg}:250 \text{ mL}::X \text{ mg}:\text{mL}$$
$$250 \text{ X} = 2500$$
$$X = 10 \text{ mg/mL}$$

Infusion rates:

a. Concentration/min:
Body weight × Desired dose/kg/min
$$67.3 \times 150 \text{ mcg/kg/min}$$
$$= 10{,}095 \text{ mcg/min or } 10 \text{ mg/min}$$

b. Concentration/hr:
10 mg/min × 60 min/hr = 600 mg/hr

Weight:

lb to kg: $\dfrac{148}{2.2} = 67.27 \text{ or } 67.3 \text{ kg}$

c. Volume/min:
$$\dfrac{10 \text{ mg/min}}{10 \text{ mg/mL}} = 1 \text{ mL/min}$$

d. Volume/hr:
1 mL/min × 60 min/hr = 60 mL/hr

IV Titration of Infusion Rate

1. a. (units, mg, mcg)/kg/min
   b. (units, mg, mcg)/mL
   c. mL/hr
   d. (units, mg, mcg)/min

   e. mL/min
   f. (units, mg, mcg)/min
   g. (units, mg, mcg)/min with infusion pump
      (units, mg, mcg)/gtt with microdrip IV set

2. a. Concentration of solution:
$$50 \text{ mg} = 50{,}000 \text{ mcg}$$
$$50{,}000 \text{ mcg}:250 \text{ mL}::X \text{ mcg}:1 \text{ mL}$$
$$250 \text{ X} = 50{,}000$$
$$X = 200 \text{ mcg}$$
The concentration of solution is 200 mcg/mL.

b. Concentration/min:
Lower: 0.5 mcg/kg/min × 70 kg = 35 mcg/min
Upper: 1.5 mcg/kg/min × 70 kg = 105 mcg/min

c. Volume/min and volume/hr:
Lower
$$\dfrac{35 \text{ mcg/min}}{200 \text{ mcg/mL}} = 0.175 \text{ mL/min} \times 60 \text{ min/hr} = 10.5 \text{ or } 11 \text{ mL/hr}$$
Upper
$$\dfrac{105 \text{ mcg/min}}{200 \text{ mcg/mL}} = 0.525 \text{ mL/min} \times 60 \text{ min/hr} = 31.5 \text{ or } 32 \text{ mL/hr}$$

d. Titration factor for infusion pump:

200 mcg/mL × 0.1 mL/hr = 20 mcg/hr

$$\dfrac{20 \text{ mcg/hr}}{60 \text{ min/hr}} = 0.333 \text{ or } 0.3 \text{ mcg/min}$$

Titration factor for microdrip

11 mL/hr = 11 gtt/min

$$\dfrac{35 \text{ mcg}}{11 \text{ gtt/min}} = 3.18 \text{ or } 3 \text{ mcg/gt}$$

e. Base rate 10.5 mL/hr or 35 mcg/min.
5 × 0.33/min = 1.65 mcg/min or 1.7 mcg/min
Add to base rate $\quad$ 35 $\quad$ mcg/min
$$\underline{+\ \ 1.7 \text{ mcg/min}}$$
$$36.7 \text{ mcg/min}$$

f. 200 mcg/hr × 20 mL/hr = 4000 mcg/hr

$$\frac{4000 \text{ mcg/hr}}{60 \text{ min/hr}} = 66.6 \text{ mcg/min}$$

g. Concentration/min and volume/hr using a microdrip set:
  5 gtt × 3 mcg/gt = 15 mcg
  15 mcg + 35 mcg/min = 50 mcg/min
  5 gtt + 11 gtt/min = 16 gtt/min or 16 mL/hr

h. Concentration/min and volume/hr using a microdrip set:
  13 gtt × 3 mcg/gt = 39 mcg
  39 mcg + 50 mcg = 89 mcg/min
  13 gtt + 16 gtt = 29 gtt/mL or 29 mL/hr

3. a. Concentration of solution:
  400 mg = 400,000 mcg
  400,000 mcg : 250 mL :: X mcg : 1 mL
  250 X = 400,000 mcg
  X = 1600 mcg

The concentration of solution is 1600 mcg/mL.

b. Concentration/min:
  4 mcg/kg/min × 75 kg = 300 mcg/min

c. Volume/min and volume/hr:

$$\frac{300 \text{ mcg/min}}{1600 \text{ mcg/mL}} = 0.1875 \text{ mL/min} \times 60 \text{ min/hr} = 11.25 \text{ or } 11 \text{ mL/hr}$$

d. Titration factor for infusion pump:
  1600 mcg/mL × 0.1 mL/hr = 160 mcg/hr

$$\frac{160 \text{ mcg/hr}}{60 \text{ min/hr}} = 2.66 \text{ or } 2.7 \text{ mcg/min}$$

Titration factor for microdrip:

  11 mL/hr = 11 gtt/min

$$\frac{300 \text{ mcg/min}}{11 \text{ gtt/min}} = 27.2 \text{ or } 27 \text{ mcg/gtt}$$

e. Base rate 11 mL/hr or 300 mcg/min
  6 × 2.7 mcg/min = 16.2 mcg/min

  300   mcg/min
  +16.25 mcg/min
  ─────────────
  316.2 mcg/min

f. 12.5 mL/hr × 1600 mcg/mL = 333 mcg/min
  = 20,000 mcg/hr

$$\frac{20,000 \text{ mcg/hr}}{60 \text{ min/hr}} = 333 \text{ mcg/min}$$

g. Concentration/min and volume/hr using a microdrip set:
  20 gtt/min × 27 mcg/gt = 540 mcg/min
  7 gtt + 13 gtt/min = 20 gtt/min or 20 mL/hr

h. Concentration/min and volume/hr using a microdrip set:
  15 gtt/min × 27 mcg/gt = 405 mcg/min
  20 gtt/min − 5 gtt = 15 gtt/min or 15 mL/hr

V Total Amount of Drug Infused Over Time

1. Lidocaine bolus:

    $$\begin{array}{r} 100\ mg \\ +100\ mg \\ \hline 200\ mg \end{array}$$

    Lidocaine IV infusion:

    a. Concentration of solution: given as 4 mg/mL in problem.

    b. Concentration/hr:
       4 mg/mL × 40 mL/hr = 160 mg/hr

    c. Concentration over ½ hour:

       $$160\ mg/hr \times \frac{30\ min}{60\ min/hr} = 80\ mg\ over\ 30\ min$$

    d. Amount of IV drug infused:
       Lidocaine per two boluses: 200 mg
       Lidocaine per IV infusion: +80 mg

       280 mg total amount infused over 1 hr

    Note: The infusion rate is close to exceeding the maximum therapeutic range, which is 200 to 300 mg/hr.

2. Concentration of solution:
    20,000 units : 500 mL :: X units : 1 mL

    $$500\ X = 20,000$$
    $$X = 40\ units$$

    a. The concentration of solution is 40 units/mL.

    b. Concentration/hr:
       40 units/mL × 50 mL/hr = 2000 units/hr

    c. Amount of IV drug infused over 5½ hours:

       $$2000\ units \times \frac{\overset{1}{\cancel{30}}\ min}{\underset{2}{\cancel{60}}\ min/hr} = 1000\ units\ over\ \tfrac{1}{2}\ hr$$

       $$\begin{array}{r} 10,000\ units \\ +1,000\ units \\ \hline 11,000\ units\ over\ 5\tfrac{1}{2}\ hr \end{array}$$

       $$2000\ units \times 5\ hr = 10,000\ units/5\ hr$$

---

evolve   Additional practice problems are available in the Advanced Calculations section of Drug Calculations Companion, version 5, on Evolve.

CHAPTER 14

Pediatric Critical Care

Objectives
- Recognize factors that contribute to errors in drug and fluid administration.
- Identify the steps in calculating dilution parameters.
- Determine the accuracy of the dilution parameters in a drug order.

Outline
FACTORS INFLUENCING INTRAVENOUS ADMINISTRATION
CALCULATING ACCURACY OF DILUTION PARAMETERS

In delivery of emergency drugs with complex dilution calculations, it is important for the nurse to evaluate the accuracy of the physician's order and to ensure that a child does not receive excessive fluids. Many institutions are attempting to standardize the concentration of the solution for various pediatric intravenous (IV) dosages to decrease the occurrence of miscalculations. National efforts are under way to standardize IV emergency drugs for infusion to eliminate medication errors.

As noted in Chapter 13, the concepts of concentration of the solution, infusion rates for concentration and volume, and concentration of a drug for specific body weight per unit time that are used in adult critical care are also used to prepare pediatric doses.

FACTORS INFLUENCING INTRAVENOUS ADMINISTRATION

Excess fluid can be given when the fluid volume of the emergency drug is not considered in the 24-hour fluid intake. Long IV tubing can be another source of fluid excess and can cause errors in drug delivery. When the priming or filling volume of the IV tubing is not considered, the child may receive extra fluid, especially if medication is added to the primary IV set via a secondary IV set. IV medication may not reach the child if the IV infusion rate is low, such as 1 mL/hr, or if the IV tubing has not been primed or filled with the medication before infusion. Most pediatric departments are developing protocols for safe and consistent IV drug delivery.

CALCULATING ACCURACY OF DILUTION PARAMETERS

The nurse may find it necessary to calculate the dilution parameters of a drug order that specifies the concentration per kilogram per minute and the volume per hour infusion rate. The physician should determine all drug dose parameters, including concentration per kilogram per minute, volume per hour, and dilution parameters. The nurse should check the accuracy of the dilution parameters to ensure that the correct drug dosage is given. These methods are also used to prepare the pediatric dose. In many pediatric critical care areas, IV fluids for drug administration are limited to prevent fluid overload. If the physician changes the drug dosage, rather than increasing the volume (mL), the concentration of the solution will be changed. It is important that all health care providers follow the policies and procedures of their institution regarding medication administration.

EXAMPLES **PROBLEM 1:** A 5-year-old-child, weight 14 kg, with septic shock.
Order: dobutamine 10 mcg/kg/min at 2.1 mL/hr; titrate to keep SBP >90.
Dilute as follows: dobutamine 200 mg in D_5W to make a total volume of 50 mL for a syringe pump.
Pediatric dosage: 2-20 mcg/kg/min.
Drug available: dobutamine 250 mg/20 mL.

Here are the following checks that can determine whether the infusion rate and the dilution orders will result in the correct concentration delivered according to weight.

Step 1: Calculate infusion concentration rates per minute and hour.
    a. Concentration per minute.

$$\text{Child's weight} \times \text{concentration/kg/min} =$$
$$14 \text{ kg} \times 10 \text{ mcg/kg/min} = 140 \text{ mcg/min}$$

    b. Concentration per hour.

$$140 \text{ mcg/min} \times 60 \text{ min/hr} = 8400 \text{ mcg/hr}$$

Step 2: Calculate the concentration of the solution. Check order by dividing concentration per hour by the ordered mL per hour. Results should match.

$$200 \text{ mg} = 200,000 \text{ mcg}$$
$$200,000 \text{ mcg} : 50 \text{ mL} :: X \text{ mcg} : 1 \text{ mL} \quad \textbf{and} \quad \frac{8400 \text{ mcg/hr}}{2.1 \text{ mL/hr}} = 4000 \text{ mcg/mL}$$
$$50 X = 200,000$$
$$X = 4000 \text{ mcg/mL}$$

The concentration solution matches.

Step 3: Calculate the infusion rate, volume per hour. Divide concentration per hour by concentration of solution. Results should confirm the infusion rate in order.

$$\frac{8400 \text{ mcg/hr}}{4000 \text{ mcg/mL}} = 2.1 \text{ mL/hr}$$

Infusion rate is correct.

Step 4: Calculate drug order.
$$\text{H} \quad : \quad \text{V} \quad :: \quad \text{D} \quad : \quad \text{V}$$
$$250 \text{ mg} : 20 \text{ mL} :: 200 \text{ mg} : X \text{ mL} \quad \textbf{or} \quad \frac{D}{H} \times V = \frac{200}{250} \times \frac{20}{1} = \frac{4000}{250} = 16 \text{ mL}$$
$$250 X = 4000$$
$$X = 16 \text{ mL}$$

Dobutamine 200 mg is 16 mL. Find the amount of D_5W by subtracting 16 mL of dobutamine drug volume from 50 mL; 34 mL of D_5W is needed to fill the 50-mL syringe.

PROBLEM 2: A 3-week-old premature infant, weight 1.6 kg, in shock.
Order: dopamine 2.5 mcg/kg/min at 0.6 mL/hr.
Dilute as follows: dopamine 20 mg in D_5W to make a total of 50 mL for syringe pump.

Dosage range: 2 to 20 mg/kg/min.
Drug available: dopamine 200 mg/5 mL.

Check to determine whether the infusion rate and the dilution orders will result in the correct concentration delivered according to weight.

Step 1: Calculate the concentration per minute and per hour, based on weight.
   a. Concentration rate per minute

$$\text{Infant's weight } 1.6 \text{ kg} \times 2.5 \text{ mcg/kg/min} = 4 \text{ mcg/min}$$

   b. Concentration rate per hour

$$4 \text{ mcg/min} \times 60 \text{ min/hr} = 240 \text{ mcg/hr}$$

Step 2: Calculate the concentration of the solution. Check order by dividing concentration per hour by the ordered mL per hour. Results should match.

$$20 \text{ mg} = 20,000 \text{ mcg}$$
$$20,000 \text{ mcg} : 50 \text{ mL} :: X \text{ mcg} : \text{mL} \quad \textbf{and} \quad \frac{240 \text{ mcg/hr}}{0.6 \text{ mL/hr}} = 400 \text{ mcg/mL}$$
$$50 X = 20,000$$
$$X = 400 \text{ mcg/mL}$$

The concentration of solution matches.

Step 3: Calculate the infusion rate, volume per hour. Divide concentration per hour by concentration solution. Results should confirm the infusion rate in order.

$$\frac{240 \text{ mcg/hr}}{400 \text{ mcg/mL}} = 0.6 \text{ mL/hr}$$

Infusion rate is correct.

Step 4: Calculate dilution orders.

$$\frac{D}{H} \times V = \frac{20 \text{ mg}}{200 \text{ mg}} \times 5 \text{ mL} = 0.5 \text{ mL} \quad \textbf{or} \quad \begin{array}{c} H \ : \ V \ :: \ D \ : \ V \\ 200 \text{ mg} : 5 \text{ mL} :: 20 \text{ mg} : X \text{ mL} \\ 200 X = 100 \\ X = 0.5 \text{ mL} \end{array}$$

Dopamine 20 mg is 0.5 mL. Find the amount of D_5W needed by subtracting 0.5 mL of dopamine drug volume from 50 mL; 49.5 mL of D_5W is needed to fill the 50-mL syringe.

PROBLEM 3: For the same infant, the physician increases the dose of dopamine.
Order: dopamine 15 mcg/kg/min at 1.8 mL/hr.
Dilution: Same, dopamine 20 mg in 50 mL with a syringe pump.
Pediatric dosage range: 2-20 mcg/kg/min.
Drug available: dopamine 200 mg/5 mL.

Check to determine whether the infusion rate and the dilution orders will result in the correct concentration delivered according to weight.

Step 1: Calculate the concentration per minute and per hour based on weight.
   a. Concentration rate per minute

$$\text{Infant's weight } 1.6 \text{ kg} \times 15 \text{ mcg/kg/min} = 24 \text{ mcg/min}$$

   b. Concentration rate per hour

$$24 \text{ mcg/min} \times 60 \text{ min/hr} = 1440 \text{ mcg/hr}$$

Step 2: Calculate the concentration of the solution. Check order by dividing concentration per hour by the ordered mL per hour.

400 mcg/mL (same as previous problem) **and** $\dfrac{1440 \text{ mcg/hr}}{1.8 \text{ mL/hr}} = 800 \text{ mcg/mL}$

Concentrations do not match. Physician must be consulted.

Step 3: Calculate the correct infusion rate per hour. Divide concentration per hour by concentration of solution.

$$\frac{1440 \text{ mcg/hr}}{400 \text{ mcg/mL}} = 3.6 \text{ mL/hr}$$

SUMMARY PRACTICE PROBLEMS

Answers can be found on pages 311 to 314.

Determine whether dilution orders will yield the correct concentration of solution.

1. A 5-year-old child with acute status asthmaticus.
   Child weighs 21 kg.
   Order: terbutaline 0.1 mcg/kg/min. Dilute 25 mg terbutaline in 25 mL D₅W to make a total volume of 50 mL. Infuse at 0.25 mL/hr with syringe pump.
   Pediatric dosage range: 0.02-0.25 mcg/kg/min.
   Drug available: terbutaline 1 mg/mL.

2. A 9-year-old child who is intubated postoperatively.
   Child weighs 30 kg.
   Order: fentanyl 0.03 mcg/kg/min. Dilute 2.5 mg fentanyl in 30 mL 0.9% saline to make a total volume of 50 mL. Infuse at 1 mL/hr with syringe pump.
   Pediatric dosage range: 0.01-0.05 mcg/kg/min.
   Drug available: fentanyl 2.5 mg/20 mL.

3. A 1-year-old child with septic shock.
   Child weighs 9 kg.
   Order: dopamine 5 mcg/kg/min. Dilute 40 mg dopamine in 49.5 mL D₅W to make a total volume of 50 mL. Infuse at 3.4 mL/hr with syringe pump.
   Pediatric dosage range: 2-20 mcg/kg/min.
   Drug available: dopamine 400 mg/5 mL.

4. A 3-year-old child with hypertension related to a tumor.
   Child weighs 16 kg.
   Order: sodium nitroprusside 2 mcg/kg/min. Dilute 50 mg nitroprusside in 45 mL D₅W to make a total volume of 50 mL. Infuse at 3 mL/hr with syringe pump.
   Pediatric dosage range: 200-500 mcg/kg/hr.
   Drug available: sodium nitroprusside 50 mg/5 mL.

5. A 10-year-old child with diabetic ketoacidosis.
   Child weighs 32 kg.
   Order: regular insulin 0.1 units/kg/hr.
   Dilute: regular insulin 50 units in 49.5 mL 0.9% saline, total volume 50 mL at 6.4 mL/hr with syringe pump.
   Pediatric dosage: 0.1 units/kg/hr.
   Drug available: regular insulin 100 units/mL.

6. A 2-day-old child with patent ductus arteriosus.
   Child weighs 3.4 kg.
   Order: alprostadil 0.1 mcg/kg/min.
   Dilute 0.1 mg of alprostadil in 50 mL D₅W to run at 2 mL/hr with syringe pump.
   Pediatric dosage range: 0.05-0.1 mcg/kg/min.
   Drug available: alprostadil 500 mcg/mL.

7. A 7-year-old child with pulmonary embolism.
   Child weighs 20 kg.
   Order: heparin 25 units/kg/hr using a premixed bag with a standard concentration of 200 units/mL. Run at 2.5 mL/hr with IV pump.
   Pediatric dosage range: 15-25 units/kg/hr.
   Drug available: heparin 50,000 units/250 mL.

ANSWERS   SUMMARY PRACTICE PROBLEMS

1. *Step 1:* Calculate the concentration per minute and hour based on weight.
   a. Concentration per minute.

   $$21 \text{ kg} \times 0.1 \text{ mcg/kg/min} = 2.1 \text{ mcg/min}$$

   b. Concentration per hour.

   $$2.1 \text{ mcg/min} \times 60 \text{ min/hr} = 126 \text{ mcg/hr} = 0.126 \text{ mg/hr}$$

   Step 2: Calculate the concentration of solution. Check order by dividing concentration per hour by the order mL per hour.

   $$25 \text{ mg} : 50 \text{ mL} :: X \text{ mg} : 1 \text{ mL} \quad \textbf{and} \quad \frac{126 \text{ mcg/hr}}{0.25 \text{ mL/hr}} = 504 \text{ mcg/mL} = 0.5 \text{ mg/mL}$$
   $$50 \, X = 25$$
   $$X = 0.5 \text{ mg/1 mL}$$

   The concentration of solution matches.

   Step 3: Calculate the infusion rate, volume per hour. Divide concentration per hour by concentration of solution.

   $$\frac{0.126 \text{ mg/hr}}{0.5 \text{ mg/mL}} = 0.25 \text{ mL/hr}$$

   Step 4: Calculate the drug order.

   $$\text{BF:} \frac{D}{H} \times V = \frac{25 \text{ mg}}{1 \text{ mg}} \times 1 \text{ mL} = \frac{25}{1} = 25 \text{ mL} \quad \textbf{or} \quad \text{RP: 1 mg} : 1 \text{ mL} :: 25 \text{ mg} : X \text{ mL}$$
   $$X = 25 \text{ mL}$$

   Drug order is correct.

2. *Step 1:* Calculate the concentration per minute and hour based on weight.
   a. Concentration per minute.

   $$30 \text{ kg} \times 0.03 \text{ mcg/kg/min} = 0.9 \text{ mcg/min}$$

   b. Concentration per hour.

   $$0.9 \text{ mcg/min} \times 60 \text{ min/hr} = 54 \text{ mcg/hr} = 0.054 \text{ mg/hr}$$

Step 2: Calculate the concentration of solution. Check order by dividing concentration per hour by the order mL per hour.

$$2.5 \text{ mg}:50 \text{ mL}::X \text{ mg}:1 \text{ mL} \quad \textbf{and} \quad \frac{54 \text{ mcg/hr}}{1 \text{ mL/hr}} = 54 \text{ mcg/mL} = 0.05 \text{ mg/mL}$$

$$50 X = 2.5$$
$$X = 0.05 \text{ mg/mL}$$

The concentration of solution matches.

Step 3: Calculate the infusion rate, volume per hour. Divide concentration per hour by concentration of solution.

$$\frac{0.054 \text{ mg/hr}}{0.05 \text{ mg/mL}} = 1 \text{ mL/hr}$$

Step 4: Calculate the drug order.

$$\text{BF:} \frac{D}{H} \times V = \frac{2.5 \text{ mg}}{2.5 \text{ mg}} \times 20 \text{ mL} = \frac{1}{1} \times 20 \text{ mL} = 20 \text{ mL} \quad \textbf{or} \quad \text{RP: } 2.5 \text{ mg}:20 \text{ mL}::2.5 \text{ mg}:X \text{ mL}$$
$$2.5 X = 50$$
$$X = 20 \text{ mL}$$

Drug order is correct.

3. *Step 1:* Calculate the concentration per minute and hour based on weight.
   a. Concentration per minute.

   $$9 \text{ kg} \times 5 \text{ mcg/kg/min} = 45 \text{ mcg/min}$$

   b. Concentration per hour.

   $$45 \text{ mcg/min} \times 60 \text{ min/hr} = 2700 \text{ mcg/hr} = 2.7 \text{ mg/hr}$$

   Step 2: Calculate the concentration of solution. Check order by dividing concentration per hour by the order mL per hour.

   $$40 \text{ mg}:50 \text{ mL}::X \text{ mg}:1 \text{ mL} \quad \textbf{and} \quad \frac{2700 \text{ mcg/hr}}{3.4 \text{ mL/hr}} = 794 \text{ mcg/mL} \quad \textbf{or} \quad 0.8 \text{ mg/mL}$$
   $$50 X = 40$$
   $$X = 0.8 \text{ mg/mL or } 800 \text{ mcg/mL}$$

   The concentration of solution matches.

   Step 3: Calculate the infusion rate, volume per hour. Divide concentration per hour by concentration of solution.

   $$\frac{2.7 \text{ mg/hr}}{0.8 \text{ mg/mL}} = 3.4 \text{ mL/hr } (3.375 \text{ mL/hr before rounding})$$

   Step 4: Calculate the drug order.

   $$\text{BF:} \frac{D}{H} \times V = \frac{40 \text{ mg}}{400 \text{ mg}} \times 5 \text{ mL} = \frac{200}{400} = 0.5 \text{ mL} \quad \textbf{or} \quad \text{RP: } 400 \text{ mg}:5 \text{ mL}::40 \text{ mg}:X \text{ mL}$$
   $$400 X = 200 \text{ mL}$$
   $$X = 0.5 \text{ mL}$$

   Drug order is correct.

4. *Step 1:* Calculate the concentration per minute and hour based on weight.
   a. Concentration per minute.

   $$16 \text{ kg} \times 2 \text{ mcg/kg/min} = 32 \text{ mcg/min}$$

   b. Concentration per hour.

   $$32 \text{ mcg/min} \times 60 \text{ min/hr} = 1920 \text{ mcg/hr} = 1.92 \text{ mg/hr}$$

Step 2: Calculate the concentration of solution. Check order by dividing concentration per hour by the order mL per hour.

$$50 \text{ mg}:50 \text{ mL}::X \text{ mg}:1 \text{ mL} \quad \textbf{and} \quad \frac{1920 \text{ mcg/hr}}{3 \text{ mL/hr}} = 640 \text{ mcg/mL}$$

$$50 \text{ X} = 50$$

$$X = 1 \text{ mg/mL or } 1000 \text{ mcg/mL}$$

The concentration of solution does not match and the order is incorrect. The physician must be consulted.

Step 3: Calculate the correct infusion rate, volume per hour. Divide concentration per hour by concentration of solution.

$$\frac{1920 \text{ mcg/hr}}{1000 \text{ mcg/mL}} = 1.9 \text{ mL/hr}$$

The concentration of solution is incorrect, and infusion rate cannot be confirmed until concentration of solution is clarified.

Step 4: Calculate the drug order.

$$\text{BF: } \frac{D}{H} \times V = \frac{50 \text{ mg}}{50 \text{ mg}} \times 5 \text{ mL} = \frac{250}{50} = 5 \text{ mL} \quad \textbf{or} \quad \text{RP: } 50 \text{ mg}:5 \text{ mL}::50 \text{ mg}:X \text{ mL}$$

$$50 \text{ X} = 250$$

$$X = 5 \text{ mL}$$

Drug order is correct.

5. *Step 1:* Calculate the concentration per hour based on weight.

$$32 \text{ kg} \times 0.1 \text{ units/kg/hr} = 3.2 \text{ units/hr}$$

Step 2: Calculate the concentration of the solution. Check order by dividing the concentration per hour by the order per mL per hour.

$$50 \text{ units}:50 \text{ mL}::X \text{ units}:1 \text{ mL} \quad \textbf{and} \quad \frac{3.2 \text{ units/hr}}{6.4 \text{ mL/hr}} = 0.5 \text{ units/mL}$$

$$50 \text{ X} = 50$$

$$X = 1 \text{ unit/mL}$$

The concentration of solution does not match. The physician must be consulted.

Step 3: Calculate the correct infusion rate, volume per hour. Divide concentration per hour by concentration of solution.

$$\frac{3.2 \text{ units/hr}}{1 \text{ unit/mL}} = 3.2 \text{ mL/hr}$$

The concentration of solution is incorrect and infusion rate cannot be confirmed.

Step 4: Calculate the drug order.

$$\frac{D}{H} = \frac{50 \text{ units}}{100 \text{ units}} \times 1 \text{ mL} = 0.5 \text{ mL} \quad \textbf{or} \quad \text{RP: } 100 \text{ units}:1 \text{ mL}::50 \text{ units}:X \text{ mL}$$

$$100 \text{ X} = 50$$

$$X = 0.5 \text{ mL}$$

Drug order is correct.

6. *Step 1:* Calculate the concentration per minute and hour based on weight.

   a. Concentration per minute.

   $$3.4 \text{ kg} \times 0.1 \text{ mcg/kg/min} = 0.34 \text{ mcg/min}$$

   b. Concentration per hour.

   $$0.34 \text{ mcg/min} \times 60 \text{ min} = 20.4 \text{ mcg/hr}$$

Step 2: Calculate the concentration of solution. Check order by dividing concentration per hour by the order mL per hour.

$$0.1 \text{ mg} = 100 \text{ mcg}$$

$$100 \text{ mcg} : 50 \text{ mL} :: X \text{ mcg} : \text{mL} \quad \textbf{and} \quad \frac{20.4 \text{ mcg/hr}}{2 \text{ mL/hr}} = 10.2 \text{ mcg/mL}$$

$$50 \text{ X} = 100$$

$$X = 2 \text{ mcg/mL}$$

The concentration of solution does not match. The physician must be consulted.

Step 3: Calculate the correct infusion rate, volume per hour. Divide the concentration per hour by the concentration of solution.

$$\frac{20.4 \text{ mcg/hr}}{2 \text{ mcg/mL}} = 10.2 \text{ mL/hr}$$

The concentration of solution is incorrect and infusion rate cannot be confirmed.

Step 4: Calculate the drug order.

$$\text{BF:} \frac{D}{H} = \frac{0.1 \text{ mg}}{0.5 \text{ mg}} \times 1 \text{ mL} = 0.2 \text{ mL} \quad \textbf{or} \quad \text{RP:} \ 0.5 \text{ mg} : 1 \text{ mL} :: 0.1 \text{ mg} : X \text{ mL}$$

$$0.5 \text{ X} = 0.1$$

$$X = 0.2 \text{ mL}$$

Drug order is correct.

7. *Step 1:* Calculate the concentration per hour based on weight.

Concentration per hour.

$$20 \text{ kg} \times 25 \text{ units/kg/hr} = 500 \text{ units/hr}$$

Step 2: Calculate the concentration of solution. Check order by dividing concentration per hour by the order mL per hour.

$$50,000 \text{ units} : 250 \text{ mL} :: X \text{ units} : \text{mL} \quad \textbf{and} \quad \frac{500 \text{ units/hr}}{2.5 \text{ mL/hr}} = 200 \text{ units/mL}$$

$$250 \text{ X} = 50,000$$

$$X = 200 \text{ units/mL}$$

The concentration of solution matches.

Step 3: Calculate infusion rate, volume per hour. Divide concentration per hour by concentration of solution.

$$\frac{500 \text{ units/hr}}{200 \text{ units/mL}} = 2.5 \text{ mL/hr}$$

Step 4: Calculate the drug order.

Premixed bag of heparin 50,000 units/250 mL.

---

evolve   Additional practice problems are available in the Intravenous Calculations and Advanced Calculations sections of Drug Calculations Companion, version 5, on Evolve.

CHAPTER 15

Labor and Delivery

Objectives
- State the complication related to intravenous fluid administration in the high-risk mother.
- Recognize the different types of fluid administration used in cases of high-risk labor.
- Determine the infusion rates of a drug in solution when the drug is prescribed by concentration or volume.

Outline
FACTORS INFLUENCING INTRAVENOUS FLUID AND DRUG MANAGEMENT
TITRATION OF MEDICATIONS WITH MAINTENANCE INTRAVENOUS FLUIDS
Administration by Concentration
Administration by Volume
INTRAVENOUS LOADING DOSE
INTRAVENOUS FLUID BOLUS

Drug calculations for labor and delivery are the same as those used in critical care. Determinations of the concentration of the solution, infusion rates, and titration factors are the primary calculation skills used. Accurate calculations are essential, as is the monitoring of intravenous (IV) fluid intake for medications and anesthetic procedures. Impaired renal filtration in patients with preeclampsia and the antidiuretic effect of tocolytic drugs make the monitoring of fluid intake vital. Accurate measurement of IV fluid intake along with pulmonary assessment can decrease the risk of fluid overload and the sequelae of acute pulmonary edema in women at high risk for complications.

Physicians' orders and hospital protocols give specific guidelines for administering IV drugs. Careful labeling of all IV fluids, IV medications, and IV lines is essential in preventing drug errors. The nurse is responsible for managing the IV drug therapy, monitoring the patient's fluid balance, and assessing the patient's response to drug therapy.

FACTORS INFLUENCING INTRAVENOUS FLUID AND DRUG MANAGEMENT

The most important concept in labor and delivery is that the drugs given to the mother also affect the unborn baby. Therefore the responses of both the mother and the unborn baby must be closely monitored. Vital signs and laboratory results, such as platelet counts, liver function studies, renal function, magnesium levels, reflexes, and contraction patterns, are the main indicators of the mother's status. For the fetus, the fetal heart pattern is the primary guide.

TITRATION OF MEDICATIONS WITH MAINTENANCE INTRAVENOUS FLUIDS

Women in labor receive IV fluids to prevent dehydration when oral intake is contraindicated. IV drugs are given to stimulate labor, treat preeclampsia, or inhibit preterm labor. Normally, 500 to 1000 mL of IV fluids may be given to initially hydrate the mother, especially in preterm labor or before administration of regional anesthesia. Any IV medications that are given by titration are a part of the hourly IV rate. The patient has a primary IV line and a secondary IV line for medications. All IV medications should be delivered by a volumetric pump, which ensures that the specified volume and correct dosage are delivered.

Titration of drugs is frequently done for women with preeclampsia and women experiencing preterm labor. The most common use of titration is for the induction or augmentation of labor. In the following example, an oxytocic drug is given, and the primary IV rate is adjusted with the secondary IV drug line to achieve a therapeutic effect and maintain adequate maternal hydration. Note that the drug is ordered to be given by concentration and that the infusion rates for volume per minute and hour must be determined.

Administration by Concentration

EXAMPLES
1. Give IV fluids at 100 mL/hr with lactated Ringer's solution (LR).
2. Mix 10 units of oxytocin in 1000 mL normal saline solution (NS). Start at 1 milliunit/min, increase by 1 or 2 milliunits/min, every 15-30 min, until uterine contractions are 2 to 3 minutes apart. Do not exceed 40 milliunits/min.

Note: 1 unit = 1000 milliunits

Available: Secondary set:
         oxytocin 10 units/mL
         1000 mL NS
         IV set drop factor 20 gtt/mL
         infusion pump
      Primary set:
         1000 mL LR
         IV set drop factor 20 gtt/mL
         infusion pump

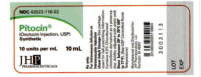

For the *secondary* IV set, the following calculations must be made:
1. Concentration of solution.
2. Infusion rates: volume per minute and volume per hour.
3. Titration factor in concentration per minute (milliunits/min).

For the *primary* IV set, the following calculations must be made:
1. Pump is used; set the rate at mL/hr.
2. Balance primary IV flow with secondary IV rate to achieve 100 mL/hr.

Secondary IV *(see Chapter 8 for formulas)*

1. Concentration of solution:

$$10\ \text{units} : 1000\ \text{mL} :: X : 1\ \text{mL}$$
$$1000\ X = 10$$
$$X = 0.01\ \text{unit or 10 milliunits}$$

The concentration of solution is 10 milliunits/mL.

2. Infusion rates for volume:

$$\frac{\text{Concentration/minute}}{\text{Concentration of solution}} = \text{Volume/min} \times 60 \text{ min} = \text{Volume/hr}$$

Volume per minute   **Volume per hour**

$$\frac{1 \text{ milliunit/min}}{10 \text{ milliunits/mL}} = 0.1 \text{ mL/min} \times 60 \text{ min} = 6 \text{ mL/hr}$$

$$\frac{2 \text{ milliunits/min}}{10 \text{ milliunits/mL}} = 0.2 \text{ mL/min} \times 60 \text{ min} = 12 \text{ mL/hr}$$

$$\frac{5 \text{ milliunits/min}}{10 \text{ milliunits/mL}} = 0.5 \text{ mL/min} \times 60 \text{ min} = 30 \text{ mL/hr}$$

3. Titration factor (see Chapter 12): To increase the concentration by increments of 1 milliunit/min, the hourly rate on the pump must be increased by 6 mL/hr. The titration factor for this problem is 6 mL/hr. To increase the concentration to a higher rate, multiply the rate of increase times 6 mL/hr. (Example: To increase infusion to 5 milliunits/min, multiply 5 by 6 mL = 30 mL/hr.)

For the secondary IV line, the concentration of the solution is 10 milliunits/mL of oxytocin, with the infusion rate of 6 mL/hr to be increased in increments of 1 to 2 milliunits every 15 to 30 minutes until contractions are 2 to 3 minutes apart.

Primary IV

The secondary IV rate will start at 6 mL/hr; therefore the primary rate will be 94 mL/hr. (A balance is needed to achieve 100 mL/hr.)

For every increase in rate from the secondary line, a corresponding decrease must be made with the primary IV line. If the rate of the secondary line exceeds the ordered hourly rate, the primary IV line may be shut off completely. The concentration of the solution may be changed by the physician if the mother is receiving too much fluid.

Administration by Volume

In the previous example, the oxytocin was ordered to be infused by concentration (milliunits/min), which is the recommended method for patient safety. Sometimes in clinical practice, the infusion rate may be ordered by volume (mL/hr).

EXAMPLES Mix 30 units of oxytocin in 500 mL NS. Start at 1 mL/hr and increase by 1 to 2 mL every 15-30 min until uterine contractions are 2 to 3 minutes apart. Notify physician before exceeding 40 milliunits/min.

To determine the concentration per hour of infusion, multiply concentration of the solution by volume/hr.

$$60 \text{ milliunits/mL} \times 1 \text{ mL/hr} = 60 \text{ milliunits/hr}$$

To determine the concentration of the infusion per minute, divide:

$$\frac{\text{Concentration/hr}}{60 \text{ min/hr}} = \text{Concentration/min}$$

$$\frac{60 \text{ milliunits/hr}}{60 \text{ min/hr}} = 1 \text{ milliunit/min}$$

Therefore an oxytocin solution with a concentration of 60 milliunits/mL infused at 1 mL/hr will administer 1 milliunit of the drug per minute.

INTRAVENOUS LOADING DOSE

Some situations require IV medications to be infused over a short period to obtain a serum level for a therapeutic effect. This type of IV drug administration is called a *loading dose*.

In the following example, a patient with preeclampsia receives a loading dose of magnesium sulfate, followed by a maintenance dose of magnesium sulfate via the secondary IV line. A primary IV line is also maintained after the loading dose is given. At the end of this example, the total IV intake is determined for an 8-hour period.

EXAMPLES
1. Mix magnesium sulfate 40 g in 1000 mL of sterile NS.
2. Infuse 4 g over 20 minutes, then maintain at 2 g/hr.
3. Start LR at 75 mL/hr after magnesium sulfate loading dose.

Available: Secondary set:
   magnesium sulfate 50% (5 g in 10-mL ampules)
   1000 mL IV fluid
   IV set 20 gtt/mL
   infusion pump
Primary set:
   1000 mL LR
   IV set drop factor 20 gtt/mL
   infusion pump

For the *secondary* IV line, the following calculations must be made:
1. Dose of magnesium sulfate in IV.
2. Concentration of solution.
3. Volume of loading dose and flow rate for infusion pump (see Chapter 10).
4. Infusion rate: volume per hour of magnesium sulfate infusion.

For the *primary* IV line, the following calculation must be made:
1. Drop rate per minute.

For the total IV intake, the following solutions must be added:
1. Volume of loading dose.
2. Volume of secondary IV for 8 hours.
3. Volume of primary IV for 8 hours.

Secondary IV

1. $\dfrac{D}{H} \times V = \dfrac{40 \text{ g}}{5 \text{ g}} \times 10 \text{ mL} = 80$ mL of magnesium sulfate or 8 ampules
2. Concentration of solution:
$$40 \text{ g} = 40{,}000 \text{ mg}$$
$$40{,}000 \text{ mg} : 1000 \text{ mL} :: X : 1 \text{ mL}$$
$$1000 \, X = 40{,}000$$
$$X = 40 \text{ mg}$$
The concentration of solution is 40 mg/mL.
3. Volume of loading dose:
$$4 \text{ g} = 4000 \text{ mg}$$
$$40 \text{ mg} : 1 \text{ mL} :: 4000 \text{ mg} : X \text{ mL}$$
$$40 \, X = 4000$$
$$X = 100 \text{ mL}$$

Flow rate for the pump:

$$100 \text{ mL} \div \frac{20 \text{ min}}{60 \text{ min/hr}} = 100 \times \frac{\overset{3}{\cancel{60}}}{\underset{1}{\cancel{20}}} = 300 \text{ mL/hr}$$

The rate on the infusion pump for the 4-g infusion of magnesium sulfate over 20 minutes is 300 mL/hr. When the infusion rate is this high, it must be monitored closely, and the patient must be observed for response to drug therapy.

4. Infusion rate: volume per hour:

$$2 \text{ g} = 2000 \text{ mg}$$

$$\frac{\text{Concentration/hr}}{\text{Concentration of solution}} = \text{Volume/hr} \qquad \frac{2000 \text{ mg/hr}}{40 \text{ mg/mL}} = 50 \text{ mL/hr}$$

The rate on the pump for the 2-g/hr infusion is 50 mL/hr.

Primary IV

After the loading dose of magnesium sulfate, the primary IV will run at 75 mL/hr.

Total IV Intake Over 8 Hours

Volume of loading dose		100 mL
Volume of secondary IV	50 mL × 8 =	400 mL
Volume of primary IV	75 mL × 8 =	+ 600 mL
		1100 mL

Because fluid overload is a potential problem for patients with preeclampsia, all IV fluids must be calculated accurately and the use of infusion pumps is essential.

INTRAVENOUS FLUID BOLUS

An IV fluid *bolus* is a large volume, 500 to 1000 mL, of IV fluid infused over a short time (1 hour or less). A bolus may be given before administration of regional anesthesia or to a patient experiencing preterm labor.

In the next example, calculate the flow rate of an IV bolus from the primary IV followed by an infusion of a tocolytic drug given by titration. At the end of this example, calculate the patient's fluid intake for 8 hours.

EXAMPLES

1. Start 1000 mL LR at 300 mL/10 min, then reduce to 125 mL/hr.
2. Mix terbutaline 7.5 mg in 500 mL of NS; start at 2.5 mcg/min; increase 2.5 mcg/min every 20 min until contractions subside.

Available: Primary set:
    1000 mL LR
    IV set drop factor 20 gtt/mL
    infusion pump
  Secondary set:
    terbutaline 1 mg/mL
    500 mL NS
    IV set 20 gtt/mL
    infusion pump

For the *secondary* IV line, the following calculations must be made:
1. The dose of terbutaline in IV.
2. Concentration of solution.
3. Infusion rates: volume per minute and hour.
4. Titration factor for 2.5 mcg/mL.

For the *primary* IV line, determine the following:
1. Set pump to infuse 300 mL over 10 minutes and then 125 mL/hr.
2. Balance the primary IV with the secondary IV to achieve a rate of 125 mL/hr.
Total the IV fluids for 8 hours.

Secondary IV

1. $\dfrac{D}{H} \times V = \dfrac{7.5 \text{ mg}}{1 \text{ mg}} \times 1 \text{ mL} = 7.5 \text{ mL of terbutaline}$

2. Concentration of solution:

$$7.5 \text{ mg} = 7500 \text{ mcg}$$
$$7500 \text{ mcg} : 500 \text{ mL} :: X \text{ mcg} : 1 \text{ mL}$$
$$500 \text{ X} = 7500$$
$$X = 15 \text{ mcg}$$

The concentration of solution is 15 mcg/mL.
3. Infusion rates: volume per minute and volume per hour.

$$\dfrac{2.5 \text{ mcg/min}}{15 \text{ mcg/mL}} = 0.166 \text{ mL/min} \times 60 \text{ min/hr} = 9.96 \text{ mL/hr or 10 mL/hr}$$

4. Titration factor: To increase the concentration by increments of 2.5 mcg/min, the volume of the increment of change must be calculated per minute and per hour:

$$\dfrac{\text{Concentration/minute}}{\text{Concentration of solution}} = \text{mL/min} \qquad \dfrac{2.5 \text{ mcg/min}}{15 \text{ mcg/mL}} = 0.166 \text{ mL/min}$$
$$\text{Volume/min} \times 60 \text{ min/hr} = \text{Volume/hr}$$
$$0.166 \text{ mL/min} \times 60 \text{ min/hr} = 9.96 \text{ mL/hr or 10 mL}$$

The titration factor is 0.166 mL/min or 10 mL/hr. Increasing or decreasing the infusion rate by 2.5 mcg/min will correspond to an increase or decrease in volume by 0.166 mL/min or 10 mL/hr.

Primary IV

1. Set infusion pump at 300 mL over 10 minutes, then reduce rate to 125 mL/hr.

Total IV Intake Over 8 Hours

Volume of loading dose		300 mL
Volume of primary set	115 mL × 8 =	920 mL
Volume of secondary set	10 mL × 8 =	+ 80 mL
		1300 mL

Assume that an average of 10 mL/hr of terbutaline was given.

SUMMARY PRACTICE PROBLEMS

Answers can be found on pages 323 to 325.

1. Preeclamptic labor.

   a. Mix magnesium sulfate 20 g in 500 mL NS.

   b. Infuse 4 g over 30 minutes, then maintain at 2 g/hr.

   c. Start LR 1000 mL at 75 mL/hr after loading dose of magnesium sulfate.

   Available: Secondary set:
   magnesium sulfate 50% (5 g in 10 mL)
   1000 mL NS
   IV set 20 gtt/mL
   infusion pump
   Primary set:
   1000 mL LR
   IV set 20 gtt/mL

   Determine the following:

   a. Secondary IV:
   (1) Magnesium sulfate dosage.
   (2) Concentration of solution.
   (3) Volume of loading dose and infusion rate for pump.
   (4) Infusion rate per hour of magnesium sulfate.

   b. Primary IV: 75 mL/hr.

   c. Total fluid intake for 8 hours.

2. Oxytocin/Pitocin for augmentation of labor.

   a. Give LR 500 mL over 30 minutes, then infuse at 75 mL/hr.

   b. Mix 15 units of oxytocin/Pitocin in 250 mL NS.

   Start infusion at 2 milliunits/min, increase by 1 to 2 milliunits/min until labor pattern is established and contractions are 2 to 3 minutes apart. Notify physician before exceeding 40 milliunits/min.

   Available: Secondary set:
   oxytocin 10 units/mL
   250 mL NS
   IV set 20 gtt/mL
   infusion pump
   Primary set:
   1000 mL LR
   IV set 20 gtt/mL

   For secondary IV line, the following calculations must be made:
   (1) Dose of oxytocin for IV.
   (2) Concentration of solution.
   (3) Infusion rate: volume per minute and volume per hour.
   (4) Titration factor in milliunits per minute.

   For primary IV line, the following calculation must be made:
   (1) Infusion rate for 500 mL over 30 minutes.

3. Preterm labor.

   a. Mix terbutaline 5 mg in 250 mL NS.

   Begin infusion at 15 mcg/min; increase by 2 mcg/min until contractions subside. Do not exceed 80 mcg/min.

   b. Start NS 1 L at 100 mL/hr.

   Available: Secondary set:
      terbutaline 1 mg/1 mL ampule
      250 mL NS
      IV set 20 gtt/mL
   Primary set:
      1000 L NS
      IV set 20 gtt/mL

   For secondary IV line, the following calculations must be made:
      (1) Dose of terbutaline for IV.
      (2) Concentration of solution.
      (3) Infusion rate: volume per minute and volume per hour.
      (4) Titration factor in micrograms per minute and hour.

   For primary IV line, the following calculation must be made:

      (1) Infusion rate for 100 mL/hr.

4. Oxytocin/Pitocin for augmentation of labor.

   a. Mix 20 units of IV oxytocin in 1000 mL D_5W.

   Start infusion at 4 milliunits/min; increase by 3 milliunits/min until regular contractions begin.

   b. Give 1000 mL $D_5\frac{1}{2}NS$ over 2 hours.

   Available: Secondary set:
      oxytocin 10 units/mL
      1000 mL D_5W
      IV set 20 gtt/mL
      infusion pump
   Primary set:
      1000 mL $D_5\frac{1}{2}NS$
      IV set 20 gtt/mL

   For secondary IV line, the following calculations must be made:
      (1) Dose of oxytocin for IV.
      (2) Concentration of solution.
      (3) Infusion rate: volume per minute and volume per hour.
      (4) Titration factor in micrograms per minute.

   For primary IV line, the following calculation must be made:
      (1) Infusion rate for 1000 mL over 2 hours.

ANSWERS SUMMARY PRACTICE PROBLEMS

1. a. Secondary IV:
   (1) Magnesium sulfate dosage:

$$\frac{D}{H} \times V = \frac{20\ g}{5\ g} \times 10\ mL = 40\ mL \text{ or 4 ampules of magnesium sulfate}$$

   (2) Concentration of solution:

$$20\ g = 20,000\ mg$$
$$20,000\ mg : 500\ mL :: X\ mg : 1\ mL$$
$$500\ X = 20,000$$
$$X = 40\ mg$$

   The concentration of solution is 40 mg/mL.
   (3) Volume of loading dose:

$$4\ g = 4000\ mg$$
$$40\ mg : 1\ mL :: 4000\ mg : X\ mL$$
$$40\ X = 4000$$
$$X = 100\ mL$$

   Infusion rate for 30 minutes:

$$100\ mL \div \frac{30\ min}{60\ min/hr} = 100 \times \frac{\overset{2}{\cancel{60}}}{\underset{1}{\cancel{30}}} = 200\ mL/hr$$

   (4) Infusion rate: volume per hour:

$$2\ g = 2000\ mg$$
$$\frac{2000\ mg/hr}{40\ mg/mL} = 50\ mL/hr$$

b. Primary IV:
   After the loading dose: Set IV rate at 75 mL/hr.
c. Total IV intake over 8 hours:

Volume of loading dose		100 mL
Volume of secondary IV	50 mL × 8 =	400 mL
Volume of primary IV	75 mL × 8 =	+600 mL
		1100 mL

2. Augmentation of labor
   a. Secondary IV:

   (1) Oxytocin dosage: $\dfrac{D}{H} \times V = \dfrac{15\ units}{10\ units} \times 1\ mL = 1.5\ mL$

   Add 1.5 mL of oxytocin to 250 mL of NS.
   (2) Concentration of solution

$$15\ units = 15,000\ milliunits$$
$$15,000\ milliunits : 250\ mL = X\ milliunits : 1\ mL$$
$$250\ X = 15,000$$
$$X = 60\ milliunits/mL$$

   (3) Infusion rate: $\dfrac{\text{Concentration/minute}}{\text{Concentration of solution}} = \dfrac{2\ milliunits/min}{60\ milliunits/mL}$

$$= 0.033\ mL/min$$
$$= 19.8\ mL/hr$$

(4) Titration factor: $\dfrac{2 \text{ milliunits/min}}{60 \text{ milliunits/mL}} = 0.033 \text{ mL/min} \times 60 \text{ min/hr} = 1.9 \text{ mL/hr or } 2 \text{ mL/hr}$

$\dfrac{3 \text{ milliunits/min}}{60 \text{ milliunits/mL}} = 0.05 \text{ mL/min} \times 60 \text{ min/hr} = 3 \text{ mL/hr}$

$\dfrac{4 \text{ milliunits/min}}{60 \text{ milliunits/mL}} = 0.06 \text{ mL/min} \times 60 \text{ min/hr} = 3.6 \text{ mL/hr or } 4 \text{ mL/hr}$

$\dfrac{5 \text{ milliunits/min}}{60 \text{ milliunits/mL}} = 0.08 \text{ mL/min} \times 60 \text{ min/hr} = 4.8 \text{ mL/hr or } 5 \text{ mL/hr}$

Note: With this concentration of solution, there is a 1:1 relationship between milliunits/mL and mL/hr.

b. Primary IV: 500 mL LR $\div \dfrac{\text{Minutes to administer}}{60 \text{ min/hr}} = 500 \text{ mL} \div \dfrac{30 \text{ minutes}}{60 \text{ min/hr}}$

$= 500 \times \dfrac{60}{30}$

$= 1000 \text{ mL in 30 min}$

3. a. Secondary IV:
  (1) Terbutaline dosage:

$$\frac{D}{H} \times V = \frac{5 \text{ mg}}{1 \text{ mg}} \times 1 \text{ mL} = 5 \text{ mL or 5 ampules of terbutaline}$$

  Add 5 mL of terbutaline to 250 mL NS.
  (2) Concentration of solution:
$$5 \text{ mg} = 5000 \text{ mcg}$$
$$5000 \text{ mcg} : 250 \text{ mL} :: \text{X mcg} : 1 \text{ mL}$$
$$250\,\text{X} = 5000$$
$$\text{X} = 20 \text{ mcg/mL}$$

  (3) Infusion rate:

$$\frac{\text{Concentration/minute}}{\text{Concentration of solution}} = \frac{15 \text{ mcg/min}}{20 \text{ mcg/mL}}$$
$$= 0.75 \text{ mL/min}$$
$$= 0.75 \times 60 = 45 \text{ mL/hr}$$

  (4) Titration factor:

$$\frac{20 \text{ mcg/min}}{60 \text{ mcg/mL}} = 0.1 \text{ mL/min}$$
$$0.1 \text{ mL/min} \times 60 \text{ min/hr} = 6 \text{ mL/hr}$$

b. Primary IV: Set infusion pump to deliver 100 mL/hr.
4. a. Secondary IV:
  (1) Oxytocin dosage:

$$\frac{D}{H} \times V = \frac{20 \text{ units}}{10 \text{ units}} \times 1 \text{ mL} = 2 \text{ mL}$$

  Add 2 mL of oxytocin to 1000 mL of D_5W.

(2) Concentration of solution:

$$20 \text{ units} = 20,000 \text{ milliunits}$$
$$20,000 \text{ milliunits}: 1000 \text{ mL}::X \text{ milliunits}: 1 \text{ mL}$$
$$1000 \, X = 20,000$$
$$X = 20 \text{ milliunits/mL}$$

(3) Infusion rate:

$$\frac{\text{Concentration/minute}}{\text{Concentration of solution}} = \frac{4 \text{ milliunits/min}}{20 \text{ milliunits/mL}}$$
$$= 0.2 \text{ mL/min}$$
$$= 0.2 \times 60 = 12 \text{ mL/hr}$$

(4) Titration factor:

$$\frac{7 \text{ milliunits/min}}{20 \text{ milliunits/mL}} = 0.35 \text{ mL/min}$$

$$\frac{10 \text{ milliunits/min}}{20 \text{ milliunits/mL}} = 0.5 \text{ mL/min}$$

$$\frac{13 \text{ milliunits/min}}{20 \text{ milliunits/mL}} = 0.65 \text{ mL/min}$$

b. Primary IV: $1000 \text{ mL } D_5\frac{1}{2}NS \div \dfrac{\text{Minutes to administer}}{60 \text{ min/hr}} = 1000 \text{ mL} \div \dfrac{120 \text{ minutes}}{60 \text{ min/hr}}$

$$= 1000 \times \frac{60}{120}$$
$$= 500 \text{ mL/hr}$$

---

evolve   Additional practice problems are available in the Basic Calculations and Advanced Calculations sections of Drug Calculations Companion, version 5, on Evolve.

CHAPTER 16

Community

Although the metric system is widespread in the clinical area, the home setting generally does not have the devices of metric measure. This becomes a problem when liquid medication is prescribed in metric measure for the home patient. Measuring spoons and syringes with metric measurements are available in pharmacies, and families should be encouraged to purchase them. All pediatric liquid medication must be measured using a metric measuring device. If metric devices are not available, the community nurse should be able to assist the adult patient in converting metric to household measure.

Preparation of solutions in the home setting may involve conversion between the metric and household systems. Solutions used in the home setting can be used for oral fluid replacement, topical application, irrigation, or disinfection. Although the majority of the solutions are available in stores, solutions that can be prepared in the home can be effective and less costly than the commercially premixed items.

When commercially prepared drugs are too concentrated for the patient's use and must be diluted, it is necessary to calculate the strength of the solution to meet the therapeutic need as prescribed by the physician. Knowledge of solution preparation and of metric-household conversion can be useful skills for the community nurse.

METRIC TO HOUSEHOLD CONVERSION

When changing from metric to household measure, use the ounce from the apothecary system as an intermediary, because there is no clear conversion between the two systems.

The conversion factors for volume are:

Ounces to milliliters: multiply ounces $\times$ 29.57 or 30
Milliliters to ounces: multiply milliliters $\times$ 0.034

The conversion factors for weight are:

Ounces to grams: multiply ounces $\times$ 28.35
Grams to ounces: multiply grams $\times$ 0.035

Note that weight and volume measures differ in the metric system. The properties of crystals, powders, and other solids account for the differences more so than the liquids. Also, as liquid measures increase in volume, there are greater discrepancies between metric and standard household measure. Table 16-1 shows the current approximate equivalents. Deciliters and liters are also included with the volume measurements. These terms will be seen more commonly as the use of the metric system increases. Although conversion charts are helpful guides, a metric measuring device would be optimal for drug administration. Standard household measuring devices should be used instead of tableware if a metric device is not available.

NOTE

When a measuring device comes from the manufacturer with a drug, it should be used. If a liquid drug has no measuring device, one should be purchased from the pharmacy, and the pharmacist can help choose the correct device. If a measuring device cannot be obtained, then standard household measuring devices can be used.

TABLE 16-1 Household to Metric Conversions (Approximate)

Standard Household Measure	Apothecary	Metric Volume	Metric Weight
$1/8$ teaspoon	7-8 gtt or $1/48$ oz	0.6 mL	0.6 g
$1/4$ teaspoon	15 gtt or $1/24$ oz	1.25 mL	1.25 g
$1/2$ teaspoon	30 gtt or $1/12$ oz	2.5 mL	2.5 g
1 teaspoon	60 gtt or $1/6$ oz	5 mL	5 g
1 tablespoon or 3 teaspoons	$1/2$ oz	15 mL	15 g
2 tablespoons or 6 teaspoons	1 oz	$1/4$ dL or 30 mL	30 g
$1/4$ cup or 4 tablespoons	2 oz	$1/2$ dL or 60 mL	60 g
$1/3$ cup or 5 tablespoons	$2 1/2$ oz	$3/4$ dL or 75 mL	75 g
$1/2$ cup	4 oz	1 dL or 120 mL	120 g
1 cup	8 oz	$1/4$ L or 250 mL	230 g
1 pint	16 oz	$1/2$ L or 480-500 mL	
1 quart	32 oz	1 L or 1000 mL	
2 quarts or $1/2$ gallon	64 oz	2 L or 2000 mL	
1 gallon	128 oz	$3 3/4$ L or 3840-4000 mL	

PRACTICE PROBLEMS ▶ I METRIC TO HOUSEHOLD CONVERSION

Answers can be found on page 336.

Use Table 16-1 to convert metric to household measure.

1. Bismuth subsalicylate 15 mL every hour up to 120 mL in 24 hr.

   _____

2. Ceclor 5 mL four times per day.

   _____

3. Tylenol elixir 1.25 mL every 6 hours as necessary for temperature greater than 102° F.

   _____

4. Maalox 30 mL after meals and at bedtime.

   _____

5. Neo-Calglucon 7.5 mL three times per day.

   _____

6. Gani-Tuss NR liquid 10 mL, q6h, prn.

   _____

7. Castor oil 60 mL at bedtime.

   _____

Use Table 16-1 for conversions.

8. Metamucil 5 g in 1 glass of water every morning.

   _____

9. Dilantin-30 pediatric suspension 10 mL twice per day.

   _____

10. Homemade pediatric electrolyte solution:

    H_2O 1 L, boiled _____

    Sugar 30 g _____

    Salt 1.5 g _____

    Lite salt 2.5 g _____

    Baking soda 2.5 g _____

11. A nonalcoholic mouthwash:

    H_2O 500 mL boiled _____

    Table salt 5 g _____

    Baking soda 5 g _____

12. Magic mouthwash:

    Benadryl 50 mg/10 mL _____

    Maalox 10 mL _____

13. Gastrointestinal cocktail for gastric upset:

Belladonna/phenobarbital elixir, 10 mL _____

Maalox, 30 mL _____

Viscous lidocaine, 10 mL _____

PREPARING A SOLUTION OF A DESIRED CONCENTRATION

All solutions contain a solute (drug) and a solvent (liquid). Solutions can be mixed three different ways:
1. *Weight to weight:* Involves mixing the weight of a given solute with the weight of a given liquid.

EXAMPLE   5 g sugar with 100 g H_2O

This type of preparation is used in the pharmaceutical setting and is the *most accurate.* Scales for weight to weight preparation are not usually found in the home setting.
2. *Weight to volume:* Uses the weight of a given solute with the volume of an appropriate amount of solvent.

EXAMPLE   10 g of salt in 1 L of H_2O

or

$\frac{1}{3}$ oz of salt in 1 qt of H_2O

Again, a scale is needed for this preparation.
3. *Volume to volume:* Means that a given volume of solution is mixed with a given volume of solution.

EXAMPLE   30 mL of hydrogen peroxide 3% in 1 dL H_2O

or

2 T of hydrogen peroxide 3% in $\frac{1}{2}$ c H_2O

Preparation of solutions volume to volume is commonly used in both clinical and home settings. After a solution is prepared, the strength can be expressed numerically in three different ways:
1. A ratio—1:20 acetic acid
2. A fraction—5 g/100 mL acetic acid
3. A percentage—5% acetic acid

With a ratio, the first number is the solute and the second number is the solvent. In a fraction, the numerator is the solid and the denominator is the liquid. A solution labeled by percentage indicates the amount of solute in 100 mL of liquid. All pharmaceutically prepared solutions use the metric system, and the ratio, fraction, and percentages are interpreted in *grams per milliliter.*

Changing a Ratio to Fractions and Percentages

Change a ratio to a percentage or a fraction by setting up a proportion using the following variables:

Known drug : Known volume :: Desired drug : Desired volume

A proportion can also be set up like a fraction:

$$\frac{Known\ drug}{Known\ volume} = \frac{Desired\ drug}{Desired\ volume}$$

YOU MUST REMEMBER

Any variable in this formula can be found if the other three variables are known.

EXAMPLE Change acetic acid 1:20 to a percentage

$$1 \text{ g}:20 \text{ mL} = X \text{ g}:100 \text{ mL}$$
$$20 \text{ X} = 100$$
$$X = 5 \text{ g}$$
$$1 \text{ g}:20 \text{ mL} = 5 \text{ g}:100 \text{ mL}$$

Note: In percentage, the volume of liquid is 100 mL.

The ratio can be expressed as a fraction, 5 g/100 mL, or as a percentage, 5%. Another method of changing a ratio to a percentage involves finding a multiple of 100 for volume (denominator), then multiplying both terms by that multiple.

PRACTICE PROBLEMS ▶ **II PREPARING A SOLUTION OF A DESIRED CONCENTRATION**

Answers can be found on pages 336 and 337.

Change the following ratios to fractions and percentages.

1. 4:1

2. 2:1

3. 1:50

4. 1:3

5. 1:1000

6. 1:10,000

7. 1:4

8. 1:5000

9. 1:200

10. 1:10

In the previous problems, grams per milliliter is the unit of measure used for preparing solutions. Scales for measuring grams are rarely found in the clinical area or the home environment. Volume (in milliliters) is the common measurement of drugs for administration. Drugs that are powders, crystals, or liquids are measured in graduated measuring cups with metric, apothecary, or household units. The milliliter, although a volume measure, can be substituted for a gram, a measure of mass, because at 4° C, 1 mL of water weighs 1 g. Mass and volume differ with the type of substance; thus grams and milliliters are not exact equivalents in all instances, but they can be accepted as approximate values for preparation of solutions.

Calculating a Solution From a Ratio

To obtain a solution from a ratio, use the proportion or fraction method.

EXAMPLES **PROBLEM 1:** Prepare 500 mL of a 1:100 vinegar-water solution for a vaginal douche.

$$\text{Known drug}:\text{Known volume}::\text{Desired drug}:\text{Desired volume}$$
$$1 \text{ mL} \quad : \quad 100 \text{ mL} \quad :: \quad X \text{ mL} \quad : \quad 500 \text{ mL}$$
$$100 \text{ X} = 500$$
$$X = 5 \text{ mL}$$

or

$$\frac{\text{Known drug}}{\text{Known volume}} = \frac{\text{Desired drug}}{\text{Desired volume}}$$

$$\frac{1 \text{ mL}}{100 \text{ mL}} = \frac{X}{500 \text{ mL}}$$

$$100 \text{ X} = 500$$
$$X = 5 \text{ mL}$$

Answer: 5 mL of vinegar added to 500 mL of water is a 1:100 vinegar-water solution.
Note: Five milliliters did not increase the volume of the solution by a large amount. When volume and volume solutions are mixed, the total amount of *desired volume* should not be exceeded. Therefore it is important to determine the volume of desired drug first, then remove that volume from the appropriate amount of solvent (solution). When mixing the solution, begin with the desired drug and add the premeasured solvent. This process ensures that the solution has an accurate concentration.

PROBLEM 2: Prepare 100 mL of a 1:4 hydrogen peroxide 3% and normal saline mouthwash.

$$\text{Known drug : Known volume :: Desired drug : Desired volume}$$
$$1\text{ mL} \quad : \quad 4\text{ mL} \quad :: \quad X\text{ mL} \quad : \quad 100\text{ mL}$$
$$4\,X = 100\text{ mL}$$
$$X = 25\text{ mL}$$

25 mL of hydrogen peroxide 3% is the amount of desired drug. To calculate the amount of normal saline, use the following formula:

$$\text{Desired volume} - \text{Desired drug} = \text{Desired solvent}$$
$$100\text{ mL} \quad - \quad 25\text{ mL} \quad = \quad 75\text{ mL}$$

Answer: 75 mL of saline and 25 mL of hydrogen peroxide 3% make 100 mL of a 1:4 mouthwash.

Calculating a Solution From a Percentage

To obtain a solution from a percentage, use the same formula with either the proportion or fraction method.

EXAMPLE   Prepare 1000 mL of a 0.9% NaCl solution.

$$\text{Known drug : Known volume :: Desired drug : Desired volume}$$
$$0.9\text{ g} \quad : \quad 100\text{ mL} \quad :: \quad X\text{ g} \quad : \quad 1000\text{ mL}$$
$$100\,X = 900$$
$$X = 9\text{ g or 9 mL}$$

Answer: 9 g or 9 mL of NaCl in 1000 mL makes a 0.9% NaCl solution.

PREPARING A WEAKER SOLUTION FROM A STRONGER SOLUTION

When a situation requires the preparation of a weaker solution from a stronger solution, the amount of desired drug must be determined. The known variables are the desired solution, the available or on-hand solution, and the desired volume. The formula can be set up with the strength of the solutions expressed in either ratio or percentage. The proportion method or the fractional method can be used to solve the problem. The first ratio or fraction, the desired solution (weaker solution), is the numerator, and the available or on-hand solution (stronger solution) is the denominator.

$$\text{Desired solution : Available solution :: Desired drug : Desired volume}$$

or

$$\frac{\text{Desired solution}}{\text{Available solution}} = \frac{\text{Desired drug}}{\text{Desired volume}}$$

EXAMPLES Prepare 500 mL of a 2.5% aluminum acetate solution from a 5% aluminum acetate solution. Use water as the solvent.

$$2.5\% : 5\% :: X : 500 \text{ mL}$$
$$2.5 \text{ mL} : 5 \text{ mL} :: X : 500 \text{ mL}$$
$$5 X = 1250$$
$$X = 250 \text{ mL}$$

Answer: Use 250 mL of 5% aluminum acetate to make 500 mL of 2.5% aluminum acetate solution.

Determine the amount of water needed.

$$\text{Desired volume} - \text{Desired drug} = \text{Desired solvent}$$
$$500 \text{ mL} \quad - \quad 250 \text{ mL} \quad = \quad 250 \text{ mL}$$

or

Same problem using the fractional method:

$$\frac{2.5\%}{5\%} \times \frac{X}{500 \text{ mL}} =$$
$$5 X = 1250$$
$$X = 250 \text{ mL of 5\% aluminum acetate}$$

or

Same problem but stated as a ratio:

Prepare 500 mL of a 1:40 aluminum acetate solution from a 1:20 aluminum acetate solution with water as the solvent.

$$\frac{1}{40} : \frac{1}{20} :: X : 500 \text{ mL}$$

$$\frac{1}{20}X = \frac{500}{40}$$

$$X = \frac{500}{\underset{2}{40}} \times \frac{\overset{1}{20}}{1} = \frac{500}{2}$$

$$X = 250 \text{ mL of 5\% aluminum acetate solution}$$

Guidelines for Home Solutions

For solutions prepared by patients in the home, directions need to be very specific and in written form, if possible. People often think that more is better. Teach the patient that solutions can be dangerous if they are too concentrated. Higher concentrations of solutions can irritate tissues and prevent the desired effect. Recommend that standard measuring spoons and cups be used rather than tableware. Level measures rather than heaping measures of dry solutes should be used. Utensils and containers for solution preparation should be *clean or sterilized by boiling* if used for infants. Mixing acidic solutions in aluminum containers should be avoided, especially if the solution is for oral use. Although there is no evidence of toxicity, a metallic taste is noticeable. Glass, enamel, or plastic containers can be used. Solutions should be made fresh daily or just before use. Oral solutions, especially for infants, require refrigeration; topical solutions do not.

When preparing the solution, start with the desired drug and then add the solvent. This helps to disperse the drug and ensures that the desired volume of solution is not exceeded. If the volume of solvent is several liters, then it is not always practical to subtract a small volume of solute.

Solution problems are best calculated within the metric system. Fractional and percentage dosages are difficult to determine within the household system.

PRACTICE PROBLEMS ▸ III PREPARING A WEAKER SOLUTION FROM A STRONGER ONE

Answers can be found on pages 337 to 339.

Identify the known variables and choose the appropriate formula. Perform calculations needed to obtain the following solutions using the metric system. Use Table 16-1 to obtain the household equivalent.

1. Prepare 250 mL of a 0.9% NaCl and sterile water solution for nose drops.

   _____

2. Prepare 250 mL of a 5% glucose and sterile water solution for an infant feeding.

   _____

3. Prepare 1000 mL of a 25% Betadine solution with sterile saline for a foot soak.

   _____

4. Prepare 2 L of a 2% Lysol solution for cleaning a changing area.

   _____

5. Prepare 20 L of a 2% sodium bicarbonate solution for a bath.

   _____

6. Prepare 100 mL of a 50% hydrogen peroxide 3% and water solution for a mouthwash.

   _____

7. Prepare 500 mL of a modified Dakin's solution 0.5% from a 5% sodium hypochlorite solution with sterile water as the solvent.

   _____

8. Prepare 1500 mL of a 0.9% NaCl solution for an enema.

   _____

9. Prepare 2 L of a 1:1000 Neosporin bladder irrigation with sterile saline. (Omit the household conversion.)

   _____

10. Determine how much alcohol is needed for a 3:1 alcohol and white vinegar solution for an external ear irrigation. Vinegar 30 mL is used. Solve using the proportion method.

    _____

11. Prepare 1000 mL of a 1:10 sodium hypochlorite and water solution for cleaning.

    _____

12. Prepare 1000 mL of a 3% sodium hypochlorite and water solution.

    _____

13. Prepare 2000 L of a 1:9 Lysol solution to clean colorfast linens soiled with body fluids. (Omit the household conversion.)

_____

14. Prepare 6 L of a 1:1200 bleach bath solution, using household bleach and water, for eczema. Determine how much bleach is needed.

_____

15. Prepare a 0.12% bleach bath solution, using household bleach and 20 gallons of water, to reduce methicillin-resistant *Staphylococcus aureus* (MRSA) colonization. Determine how much bleach is needed.

_____

HYDRATION MANAGEMENT

Calculate Daily Fluid Intake for an Adult

Hydration problems normally increase with age as total body water is lost when muscle mass decreases. With aging, the sensation of thirst diminishes and the physiological response to dehydration is not sufficient to meet metabolic needs. Kidney function begins to decline in middle age, slowly decreasing the ability of the kidney to concentrate urine, resulting in increasing water loss. Add health care problems, such as dementia and diabetes, along with commonly used medication that increases fluid loss, such as diuretics and laxatives, and dehydration is a real risk.

Dehydration can exacerbate problems such as urinary tract and respiratory tract infections but can cause more subtle problems in the elderly, such as confusion, decreased cognitive function, incontinence, constipation, and falls. All elderly adults, especially those over 85 years old, should be assessed for dehydration on the basis of physical assessment, laboratory data, cognitive assessment, pattern of fluid intake, and medical condition. Once daily fluid intake is established, nursing measures can be taken to maintain an adequate hydration.

Standard Formula for Daily Fluid Intake*

100 mL/kg for the first 10 kg of weight
50 mL/kg for the next 10 kg of weight
15 mL/kg for the remaining kg

The standard formula includes fluid contained in foods. To determine how much liquid alone an adult needs to consume, multiply the daily fluid intake by 75%.

EXAMPLE Adult weight is 94 kg

$$
\begin{aligned}
&\underline{-10 \text{ kg}} \times 100 \text{ mL} = 1000 \text{ mL} \\
&84 \text{ kg} \\
&\underline{-10 \text{ kg}} \times 50 \text{ mL} = 500 \text{ mL} \\
&74 \text{ kg} \times 15 \text{ mL} = \underline{1110 \text{ mL}} \\
&\phantom{-10 \text{ kg} \times 100 \text{ mL} = 1}2610 \text{ mL}
\end{aligned}
$$

2610 mL × 75% = 2610 × 0.75 = 1957.5 or 1958 mL fluid/day

_____

*Adapted from Skipper, A. (Ed.) (1998). *Dietitian's handbook of enteral and parenteral nutrition.* Rockville, Maryland: Aspen Publishers.

Calculate Daily Fluid Intake for a Febrile Adult

When an adult is febrile, the need for fluids increases by 6% for each degree over normal temperature. For example, a 94-kg adult with an oral temperature of 100.8° F, 2° above normal, needs a 12% increase in fluid. To find the increase, multiply the fluid/day, 1958 mL, by the percent increase, 12%, and add that to the total fluid/day.

$$1958 \text{ mL} \times 12\% = 1958 \times 0.12 = 234.9 \text{ or } 235 \text{ mL}$$
$$1958 \text{ mL} + 235 \text{ mL} = 2193 \text{ mL}$$

PRACTICE PROBLEMS ▶ IV HYDRATION MANAGEMENT

Answers can be found on pages 339 and 340.

1. Calculate the standard formula, then the fluid need of an adult weighing 84 kg.

2. Calculate the standard formula, then the fluid need of an adult weighing 63 kg.

3. Calculate the standard formula, then the fluid need of an adult weighing 70 kg.

4. Calculate the standard formula, then the fluid need of an adult weighing 100 kg.

5. Calculate the standard formula, then the fluid need of an adult weighing 69 kg with a fever of 101° F.

BODY MASS INDEX (BMI)

The importance of weight for the determination of overall health status and drug therapy must be emphasized. The current international standard is "body mass index" for adults and children as the criteria for healthy weight, overweight, and obese persons.

Body mass index (BMI) is a weight-for-height index that takes the place of previously used height and weight tables. BMI is a part of health assessments and is used as an indicator of risk factors for chronic diseases.

Calculate Body Mass Index Using Two Formulas

a. BMI pounds and inches formula:

$$\frac{\text{Weight in pounds}}{(\text{Height in inches}) \, (\text{Height in inches})} \times 703$$

EXAMPLE A person who weighs 165 pounds and is 6 ft 1 inch (73 inches) has a BMI of:

$$\frac{165}{73 \times 73} \times 703 = 21.8 \text{ BMI}$$

b. BMI metric formula:

$$\frac{\text{Weight in kg}}{(\text{Height in meters}) \, (\text{Height in meters})}$$

EXAMPLE A person who weighs 165 pounds and is 6 ft 1 inch (73 inches) has a BMI of:

$$73 \text{ inches} \times 0.0254 \text{ meters} = 1.854 \text{ meters}$$
$$165 \text{ lb} \div 2.2 \text{ kg} = 75 \text{ kg}$$

$$\frac{75}{(1.854) \, (1.854)} = \frac{75}{3.437} = 21.8 \text{ BMI}$$

Answers can be found on page 340.

1. What is the BMI for a female weighing 208 lb and who is 5 ft 2?

2. What is the BMI for a male weighing 198 lb and who is 5 ft 11?

3. What is the BMI for a female weighing 112 lb and who is 5 ft 4 inches tall?

4. What is the BMI for a male weighing 165 lb and who is 6 ft 1 inch tall?

5. What is the BMI for a male weighing 60 lb with a height of 3 ft 10 inches?

ANSWERS

I Metric to Household Conversion

1. Bismuth subsalicylate 15 mL = 1 T; no more than 8 T in 24 hr
2. Ceclor 5 mL = 1 t
3. Tylenol elixir 1.25 mL = $^1/_4$ t
4. Maalox 30 mL = 2 T
5. Neo-Calglucon 7.5 mL = $1^1/_2$ t
6. Gani-Tuss NR 10 mL = 2 t
7. Castor oil 60 mL = 4 T or $^1/_4$ c
8. Metamucil 5 g = 1 t
9. Dilantin-30 pediatric suspension 10 mL = 2 t

10. H_2O 1 L = 1 qt
    Sugar 30 g = 2 T
    Salt 1.25 g = $^1/_4$ t
    Lite salt 2.5 g = $^1/_2$ t
    Baking soda 2.5 g = $^1/_2$ t
11. H_2O 500 mL = 1 pt
    Table salt 5 mL = 1 t
    Baking soda 5 mL = 1 t
12. Benadryl 50 mg/10 mL = 2 t
    Maalox 10 mL = 2 t
13. Belladonna/phenobarbital elixir, 10 mL = 2 t
    Maalox 30 mL = 2 T
    Viscous lidocaine 10 mL = 2 t

II Preparing a Solution of a Desired Concentration

1. 4:1 = X:100
   X = 400
   $\frac{400}{100}$, 400%
2. 2:1 = X:100
   X = 200
   $\frac{200}{100}$, 200%
3. 1:50 = X:100
   50 X = 100
   X = 2
   $\frac{2}{100}$, 2%

4. 1:3 = X:100
   3 X = 100
   X = 33.3
   $\frac{33.3}{100}$, 33.3%
5. 1:1000 = X:100
   1000 X = 100
   X = 0.1
   $\frac{0.1}{100}$, 0.1%
6. 1:10,000 = X:100
   10,000 X = 100
   X = 0.01
   $\frac{1}{10,000}$, 0.01%

7. $1:4 = X:100$
$\quad 4\,X = 100$
$\qquad X = 25$
$\quad \dfrac{25}{100}, 25\%$

8. $1:5000 = X:100$
$\quad 5000\,X = 100$
$\qquad X = 0.02$
$\quad \dfrac{0.02}{100}, 0.02\%$

9. $1:200 = X:100$
$\quad 200\,X = 100$
$\qquad X = 0.5$
$\quad \dfrac{0.5}{100}, 0.5\%$

10. $1:10 = X:100$
$\quad 10\,X = 100$
$\qquad X = 10$
$\quad \dfrac{10}{100}, 10\%$

III Preparing a Weaker Solution From a Stronger One

1. Known drug: 0.9% NaCl $0.9:100::X:250$
    Known volume: 100 mL $100\,X = 225$
    Desired drug: X $X = 2.25$ mL
    Desired volume: 250 mL

2.25 mL of NaCl in 250 mL of water yields a 0.9% NaCl solution. Household equivalents are approximately $\frac{1}{2}$ teaspoon salt and 1 cup sterile water.

2. Known drug: 5% glucose (sugar) $5:100::X:250$
    Known volume: 100 mL $100\,X = 1250$
    Desired drug: X $X = 12.5$ mL
    Desired volume: 250 mL

12.5 mL of sugar in 250 mL of water yields a 5% glucose solution. Household equivalents are approximately 1 tablespoon in 1 cup of sterile water.

3. Known drug: 25% Betadine $25:100::X:1000$
    Known volume: 100 mL $100\,X = 25{,}000$
    Desired drug: X $X = 250$ mL
    Desired volume: 1000 mL   1000 mL $-$ 250 mL $=$ 750 mL

250 mL of Betadine in 750 mL saline yields a 25% Betadine solution. Household equivalents are 1 cup Betadine in 3 cups sterile saline.

4. Known drug: 2% Lysol $2:100::X:2000$ mL
    Known volume: 100 mL $100\,X = 4000$
    Desired drug: X $X = 40$ mL
    Desired volume: 2 L = 2000 mL

40 mL of Lysol in 2 L of water yields a 2% Lysol solution. Household equivalents are 2 tablespoons and 2 teaspoons (40 mL) of Lysol to 2 quarts or $\frac{1}{2}$ gallon of water.

5. Known drug: 2% sodium bicarbonate $2:100::X:20{,}000$ mL
    Known volume: 100 mL $100\,X = 40{,}000$
    Desired drug: X $X = 400$ mL or 400 g
    Desired volume: 20,000 mL

400 mL or 400 g of sodium bicarbonate (baking soda) in 20,000 mL of water yields a 2% sodium bicarbonate solution. Household equivalents are $1\frac{1}{2}$ cups and 2 tablespoons baking soda in 5 gallons of water.

6. Known drug: 50% hydrogen peroxide   50:100::X:100
   Known volume: 100 mL   100 X = 5000
   Desired drug: X   X = 50 mL
   Desired volume: 100 mL   100 mL − 50 mL = 50 mL

   50 mL of hydrogen peroxide 3% in 50 mL water yields a 50% solution. Household equivalents are approximately 3 tablespoons of hydrogen peroxide 3% in 3 tablespoons of water.

7. Known drug: 0.5%   0.5:5::X:500
   Available solution: 5%   5 X = 250
   Desired drug: X   X = 50 mL
   Desired volume: 500 mL   500 mL − 50 mL = 450 mL

   50 mL of 5% sodium hypochlorite in 450 mL sterile water yields a 0.5% modified Dakin's solution. Household equivalents are 3 tablespoons and 1 teaspoon of Dakin's solution in 1 pint minus 3 tablespoons of water.

8. Known drug: 0.9%   0.9:100::X:1500
   Known volume: 100 mL   100 X = 1350
   Desired drug: X   X = 13.5 mL
   Desired volume: 1500 mL

   13.5 mL of NaCl in 1500 mL water yields a 0.9% NaCl solution. Household equivalents are $2\frac{1}{2}$ teaspoons of salt in $1\frac{1}{2}$ quarts of water.

9. Known drug: 1 mL   1:1000::X:2000
   Known volume: 1000 mL   1000 X = 2000
   Desired drug: X   X = 2 mL
   Desired volume: 2000 mL

   2 mL of Neosporin irrigant in 2000 mL of sterile saline yields a 1:1000 solution for continuous bladder irrigation. This treatment is done primarily in the clinical setting.

10. Use ratio and proportion to solve this problem.
    3:1::X:30 mL
      X = 90 mL

    Add 90 mL of alcohol to 30 mL of vinegar to yield a 3:1 solution for an external ear wash. Household equivalents are 6 tablespoons of alcohol and 2 tablespoons of vinegar.

11. Known drug: 1 mL   1:10::X:1000
    Known volume: 10 mL   10 X = 1000
    Desired drug: X   X = 100 mL
    Desired volume: 1000 mL   1000 mL − 100 mL = 900 mL

    100 mL of sodium hypochlorite (bleach) in 900 mL water yields a 1:10 sodium hypochlorite solution. Household equivalents are $\frac{1}{3}$ cup and 2 tablespoons sodium hypochlorite in approximately 1 quart minus $\frac{1}{3}$ cup and 2 tablespoons of water.

12. Known drug: 3 mL   3:100::X:1000
    Known volume: 100 mL   100 X = 3000
    Desired drug: X   X = 30 mL
    Desired volume: 1000 mL   1000 mL − 30 mL = 970 mL

    30 mL of sodium hypochlorite (bleach) in 970 mL water yields a 3% sodium hypochlorite solution. Household equivalents are 2 tablespoons in 1 quart minus 2 tablespoons of water.

13. Use ratio and proportion to solve this problem.

$$1:9::X:2000 \text{ mL}$$
$$9\,X = 2000 \text{ mL}$$
$$X = 222 \text{ mL}$$

Desired volume − Desired drug = Desired solvent
2000 mL − 222 mL   = 1778 mL

222 mL of Lysol in 1778 mL of water yields a 1:9 cleansing solution for colorfast linens soiled with body fluids.

14. Use ratio and proportion to solve this problem.

$$1:1200::X:6000 \text{ mL}$$
$$1200\,X = 6000$$
$$X = 5 \text{ mL}$$

5 mL of household bleach in 6 L of water yields a 1:1200 bleach bath solution for eczema.

15. Convert gallons to liters.

1 gallon = 4 liters
20 gallons × 4 liters/gallon = 80 liters

Use ratio and proportion to solve this problem.

$$0.12 \text{ mL}:0.1 \text{ L}::X:80 \text{ L}$$
$$0.1\,X = 9.6$$
$$X = 96 \text{ mL or } 3\frac{1}{4} \text{ ounces}$$

3¼ ounces of bleach in 20 gallons of water yields a 0.12% bleach bath solution for MRSA decolonization.

IV Hydration Management

1. Adult weight is 84 kg

−10 kg × 100 mL = 1000 mL
74 kg
−10 kg × 50 mL = 500 mL
64 kg × 15 mL = 960 mL
2460 mL
2460 mL × 75% = 2460 × 0.75 = 1845 mL

2. Adult weight is 63 kg

−10 kg × 100 mL = 1000 mL
53 kg
−10 kg × 50 mL = 500 mL
43 kg × 15 mL = 645 mL
2145 mL
2145 mL × 75% = 2145 × 0.75 = 1608.75 or 1609 mL

3. Adult weight is 70 kg

$$\begin{array}{r} -10\ kg \times 100\ mL = 1000\ mL \\ \hline 60\ kg \\ -10\ kg \times\ \ 50\ mL = \ \ 500\ mL \\ \hline 50\ kg \times\ \ 15\ mL = \ \ 750\ mL \\ \hline 2250\ mL \end{array}$$

2250 mL × 75% = 2250 × 0.75 = 1687.5 or 1688 mL

4. Adult weight is 100 kg

$$\begin{array}{r} -10\ kg \times 100\ mL = 1000\ mL \\ \hline 90\ kg \\ -10\ kg \times\ \ 50\ mL = \ \ 500\ mL \\ \hline 80\ kg \times\ \ 15\ mL = 1200\ mL \\ \hline 2700\ mL \end{array}$$

2700 mL × 75% = 2700 × 0.75 = 2025 mL

5. Adult weight is 69 kg

$$\begin{array}{r} -10\ kg \times 100\ mL = 1000\ mL \\ \hline 59\ kg \\ -10\ kg \times\ \ 50\ mL = \ \ 500\ mL \\ \hline 49\ kg \times\ \ 15\ mL = \ \ 735\ mL \\ \hline 2235\ mL \end{array}$$

2235 mL × 75% = 2235 × 0.75 = 1676 mL

6% × 3° = 18% for increased temperature.
1676 mL × 18% = 1676 × 0.18 = 301.6 or 302 mL
1676 mL + 302 mL = 1978 mL

V Body Mass Index

1. 5 feet 2 inches = 62 inches (12 × 5 = 60 inches + 2 inches = 62 inches)

$$\frac{208}{(62)\ \ (62)} \times 703 = \frac{208}{3844} \times 703 = 0.054 \times 703 = 38\ BMI$$

2. 5 feet 11 inches = 71 inches

$$\frac{198}{(71)\ \ (71)} \times 703 = \frac{198}{5041} \times 703 = 0.039 \times 703 = 27.4\ BMI$$

3. 5 feet 4 inches = 64 inches

$$\frac{112}{(64)\ \ (64)} \times 703 = \frac{112}{4096} \times 703 = 0.027 \times 703 = 19\ BMI$$

4. 6 feet 1 inch = 73 inches

$$\frac{165}{(73)\ \ (73)} \times 703 = \frac{165}{5329} \times 703 = 0.031 \times 703 = 21.8\ BMI$$

5. 3 feet 10 inches = 46 inches

$$\frac{60}{(46)\ \ (46)} \times 703 = \frac{60}{2116} \times 703 = 0.028 \times 703 = 19.7\ BMI$$

PART V

POST-TEST: ORAL PREPARATIONS, INJECTABLES, INTRAVENOUS, AND PEDIATRICS

The post-test is for testing the content of Part III, Oral Preparations, Injectables (subcutaneous and intramuscular), Insulin, Intravenous, and Chapter 14, Pediatric Critical Care. The test is divided into four sections. There are 65 drug problems, which should take 1 to 1½ hours to complete. You may use a conversion table as needed. The minimum passing score is 57 correct, or 88%. If you have more than two drug problems wrong in a section of the test, return to the chapter in the book for that test section and rework the practice problems.

ORAL PREPARATIONS

Answers can be found on pages 368 to 370.

1. **Order:** nifedipine (Adalat CC) 60 mg, po, daily for 1 week; then 90 mg, po, daily.
   Drug available:

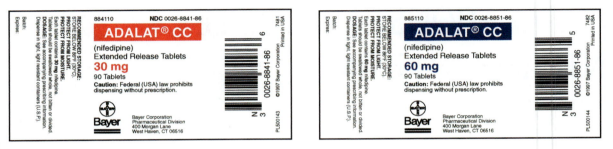

   a. Which Adalat CC container would you use for the first week? _____

   b. Explain how you would give 90 mg. _____

2. **Order:** Crestor (rosuvastatin calcium)
   10 mg, po, daily at bedtime.
   Drug available:

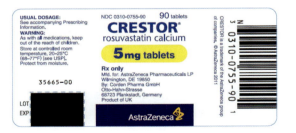

   a. How many tablet(s) would you give? _____

   b. When is/are the tablet(s) given? _____

3. Order: pravastatin sodium (Pravachol) 20 mg, po, at bedtime.

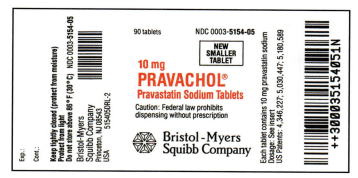

How many tablets of Pravachol should the patient receive? _____

4. Order: nitroglycerin (Nitrostat) gr 1/200, SL, STAT.
Drug available:

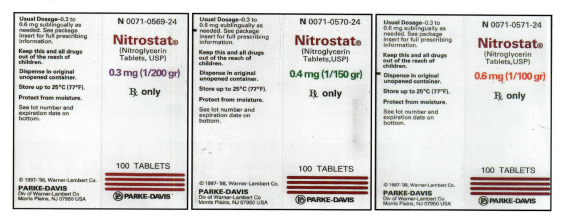

This drug dosage is ordered in the apothecary system, but the metric dosage is also on the drug label.

The drug is available in three different strengths. Which drug label would you select? Why?

_____

5. Order: clorazepate dipotassium (Tranxene) 7.5 mg in AM and 15 mg, po, at bedtime.
Drug available:

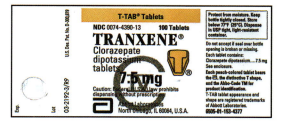

a. How many tablet(s) should the patient receive in the AM? _____.

b. How many tablets should the patient receive at bedtime? _____.

6. Order: clarithromycin (Biaxin) 0.5 g, bid × 10 days, po.
Drug available:

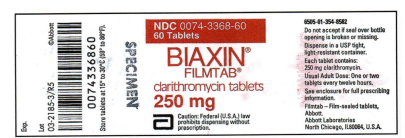

    a. 0.5 gram is equivalent to _____ milligrams.

    b. How many tablets would you give per dose? _____

7. Order: acetaminophen (Tylenol) 650 mg, po, prn, for headache.
Drug available:

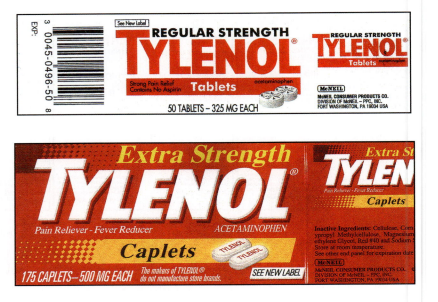

    a. Which Tylenol bottle would you select? _____

    b. How many tablets or caplets should the patient receive? _____

8. Order: allopurinol (Zyloprim) 0.2 g, po, bid.
   Drug available:

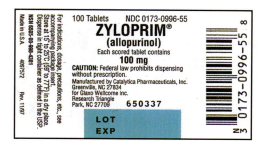

   a. 0.2 g is equivalent to _____ milligrams.

   b. The patient should receive how many tablets of allopurinol per dose? _____

9. Order: prochlorperazine (Compazine) 10 mg, po, tid.
   Drug available:

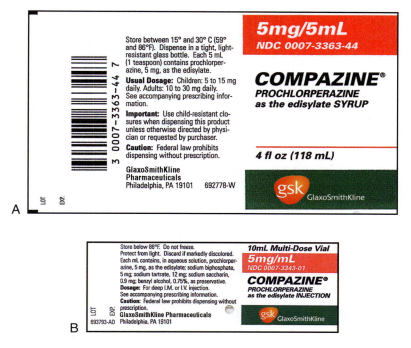

   a. Which Compazine bottle would you select? Why? _____

   b. How many milliliters would you give? _____

10. **Order:** olanzapine (Zyprexa) 10 mg, po, daily.
    Drug available:

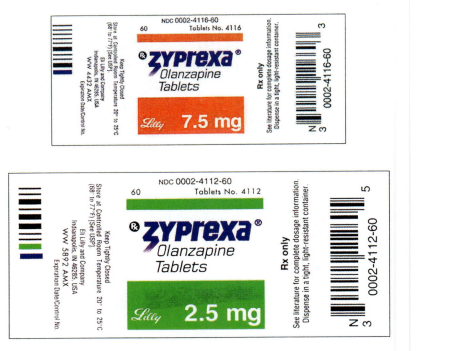

a. Which Zyprexa bottle would you select? Why? _____

b. How many tablet(s) would you give? _____

11. **Order:** Synthroid (levothyroxine) 0.0375 mg, po, daily.
    Drug available:

a. The micrograms for 0.0375 mg would be? _____

b. Which Synthroid bottle would you select? _____

c. How many tablet(s) would you give per day? _____

12. **Order:** cefuroxime axetil (Ceftin) 500 mg, po, q12h.
    Drug available:

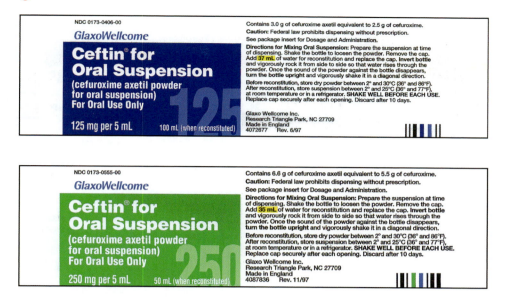

a. Which Ceftin bottle would you select? Explain. _____

b. The patient would receive how many grams _____ or milligrams _____ of Ceftin per day?

c. How many milliliters should the patient receive per dose? _____

13. Order: cefaclor (Ceclor) 250 mg, po, q8h.
Drug available:

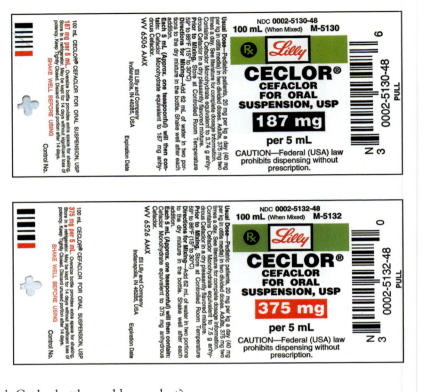

a. Which Ceclor bottle would you select? _____

b. How many milliliters should the patient receive per dose? _____

c. Is there another solution to this drug problem? _____

14. Order: simvastatin (Zocor) 40 mg, po, daily.
Drug available:

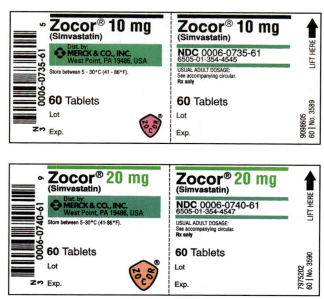

a. Which Zocor bottle would you select? Why? _____

b. How many tablets should the patient receive? _____

15. Order: ziprasidone (Geodon) 40 mg, po, bid.
After a week (7 days later) 60 mg, po, bid.
Drug available:

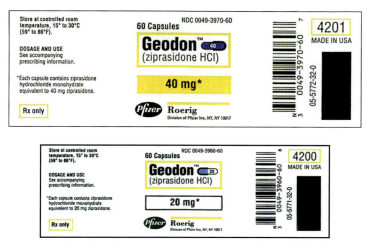

a. Which Geodon bottle(s) would you select to give 40 mg? _____

b. How many Geodon capsule(s) would you give for 40 mg per dose per day? _____

c. Which Geodon bottle(s) would you select to give 60 mg per dose? _____

d. How many Geodon capsule(s) from which bottle would you give per dose? _____

Per day? _____

16. Order: Amoxil (amoxicillin) 0.4 g, po, q8h.
Drug available:

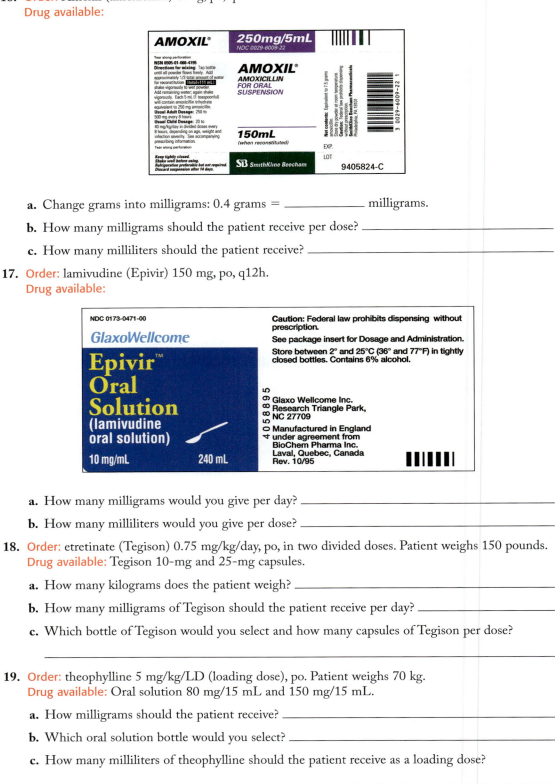

a. Change grams into milligrams: 0.4 grams = _____ milligrams.

b. How many milligrams should the patient receive per dose? _____

c. How many milliliters should the patient receive? _____

17. Order: lamivudine (Epivir) 150 mg, po, q12h.
Drug available:

a. How many milligrams would you give per day? _____

b. How many milliliters would you give per dose? _____

18. Order: etretinate (Tegison) 0.75 mg/kg/day, po, in two divided doses. Patient weighs 150 pounds.
Drug available: Tegison 10-mg and 25-mg capsules.

a. How many kilograms does the patient weigh? _____

b. How many milligrams of Tegison should the patient receive per day? _____

c. Which bottle of Tegison would you select and how many capsules of Tegison per dose?

_____

19. Order: theophylline 5 mg/kg/LD (loading dose), po. Patient weighs 70 kg.
Drug available: Oral solution 80 mg/15 mL and 150 mg/15 mL.

a. How milligrams should the patient receive? _____

b. Which oral solution bottle would you select? _____

c. How many milliliters of theophylline should the patient receive as a loading dose?

_____

20. Order: docusate sodium (Colace) 100 mg, po, bid per NG (nasogastric) tube.
Drug available: Colace 50 mg/5 mL. Osmolality of docusate sodium is 3900 mOsm. The desired osmolality is 500 mOsm.

    a. How many milliliters of Colace should the client receive? _____

    b. How much water dilution is needed to obtain the desired osmolality? _____

INJECTABLES

Answers can be found on pages 370 to 372.

21. Order: hydroxyzine (Vistaril) 25 mg, deep IM, STAT.
Drug available: (50 mg = 1 mL)

FOR INTRAMUSCULAR USE ONLY	**10 mL** NDC 0049-5460-74	Store below 86°F (30°C)
USUAL ADULT DOSE: Intramuscularly: 25 - 100 mg stat; repeat every 4 to 6 hours, as needed. See accompanying prescribing information.	**Vistaril®** (hydroxyzine hydrochloride)	PROTECT FROM FREEZING PATIENT: _____
Each mL contains **50 mg** of hydroxyzine hydrochloride, 0.9% benzyl alcohol and sodium hydroxide to adjust to optimum pH. To avoid discoloration, protect from prolonged exposure to light.	*Intramuscular Solution* 50 mg/mL	ROOM NO.: _____
CAUTION: Federal law prohibits dispensing without prescription.	*Pfizer* **Roerig** Division of Pfizer Inc, NY, NY 10017	05-1111-00-3 MADE IN USA **9249**

How many milliliters of Vistaril would you give? _____

22. Order: digoxin (Lanoxin) 0.25 mg, IM, daily.
Drug available:

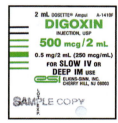

How many milliliters of digoxin would you give per dose? _____

23. Order: meperidine (Demerol) 40 mg and atropine sulfate 0.5 mg, IM, STAT.
Drug available:

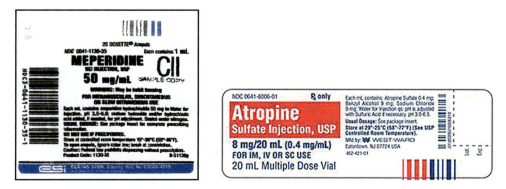

    a. How many milliliters of meperidine and how many milliliters of atropine would you

        administer? _____

    b. Explain how the two drugs would be mixed. _____

24. **Order:** heparin 2500 units, subcut, q6h.
Drug available:

Each mL contains heparin sodium 5000 USP units, sodium chloride 7 mg and benzyl alcohol 0.01 mL in Water for Injection. pH 5.0-7.5; sodium hydroxide and/or hydrochloric acid added, if needed, for pH adjustment.

DERIVED FROM PORCINE INTESTINES

Caution: Federal law prohibits dispensing without prescription. SAMPLE COPY

esi
10 mL
MULTIPLE DOSE Vial
NDC 0641-2460-41
HEPARIN
SODIUM INJECTION, USP
5000 USP units **/ 1** mL
FOR INTRAVENOUS OR SUBCUTANEOUS USE
esi ELKINS-SINN Cherry Hill, NJ 08003

Each mL contains heparin sodium 10,000 USP units, sodium chloride 6 mg and benzyl alcohol 0.01 mL in Water for Injection. pH 5.0-7.5; sodium hydroxide and/or hydrochloric acid added, if needed, for pH adjustment.

DERIVED FROM PORCINE INTESTINES

Caution: Federal law prohibits dispensing without prescription. SAMPLE COPY

esi
4 mL
MULTIPLE DOSE Vial
NDC 0641-2470-41
HEPARIN
SODIUM INJECTION, USP
10,000 USP units **/ 1** mL
FOR INTRAVENOUS OR SUBCUTANEOUS USE
esi ELKINS-SINN Cherry Hill, NJ 08003

a. Which heparin would you use? _____

b. How many milliliters of heparin should the patient receive? _____

25. **Order:** Lovenox (enovaparin sodium) 20 mg, subcut, q12h.
Drug available:

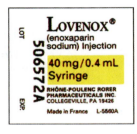

LOVENOX®
(enoxaparin sodium) Injection
40 mg/0.4 mL Syringe
RHÔNE-POULENC RORER PHARMACEUTICALS INC.
COLLEGEVILLE, PA 19426
Made in France   L-5560A
LOT 506572A   EXP:

How many milliliters would you give? _____

26. **Order:** naloxone (Narcan) 0.5 mg, IM, STAT.
Drug available:

Each mL contains naloxone hydrochloride 400 mcg, sodium chloride 8.6 mg, methylparaben 1.8 mg and propylparaben 0.2 mg in Water for Injection. pH 3.0-4.5; hydrochloric acid and/or sodium hydroxide added, if needed, for pH adjustment. Sealed under nitrogen. USUAL DOSAGE: See package insert for complete prescribing information.

10 mL Multiple Dose Vial
NDC 0641-2521-41
NALOXONE
HCl INJECTION, USP
400 mcg/mL
(0.4 mg/mL)
FOR INTRAMUSCULAR, SUBCUTANEOUS OR INTRAVENOUS USE

Store at controlled room temperature 15°-30°C (59°-86°F). Avoid freezing. PROTECT FROM LIGHT: Keep covered in carton for duration of use. Caution: Federal law prohibits dispensing without prescription. Product Code 2521b A-2521b
LOT   EXP   SAMPLE COPY

esi ELKINS-SINN, INC. Cherry Hill, NJ 08003
A subsidiary of A. H. Robins Company

How many milliliters of naloxone should the patient receive? _____

27. Order: Humulin 70/30 insulin 35 units, subcut, in AM.
    Drug available:

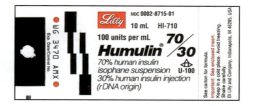

Indicate on the unit-100 insulin syringe how many units of 70/30 insulin should be given.

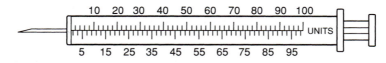

28. Order: Humulin N insulin 45 units and Humulin R (regular) 10 units.

    a. Explain the method for mixing the two insulins.

    _____

    b. Mark on the unit-100 insulin syringe how much Humulin R insulin and Humulin N insulin should be withdrawn.

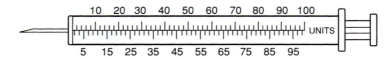

29. Order: vitamin B_{12} 500 mcg, IM, 3 times a week.
    Drug available:

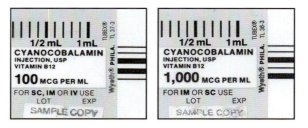

    a. Which cyanocobalamin would you select? Why?

    _____

    b. How many milliliters would you give? _____

30. **Order:** morphine 8 mg IM, STAT.
   Drug available:

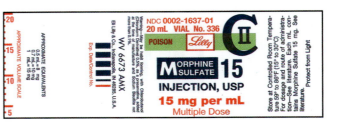

How many milliliters of morphine would you administer? _____

31. **Order:** phytonadione (AquaMEPHYTON) 5 mg, IM, STAT.
   Drug available:

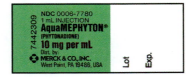

How many milliliters of AquaMEPHYTON would you administer? _____

32. **Order:** ranitidine HCl (Zantac) 35 mg, IM, q8h.
   Drug available:

NDC 0173-0363-01
GlaxoWellcome
Zantac®
(ranitidine hydrochloride) Injection
25 mg/mL*
Sterile
6-mL Multidose Vial

Caution: Federal law prohibits dispensing without prescription.
* Each mL contains ranitidine 25 mg (as the hydrochloride) in a buffered aqueous solution with phenol 5 mg as preservative.
Usual Adult Dosage: 50 mg (2 mL) every 6 to 8 hours or 150 mg (6 mL) over 24 hours.
For IV or IM injection, or IV infusion.
See package insert for full prescribing information.
Store between 4° and 30°C (39° and 86°F). Protect from light.
Zantac® Injection tends to exhibit a yellow color that may intensify over time without adversely affecting potency.
U.S. Patent No. 4,585,790

Glaxo Wellcome Inc.
Research Triangle Park,
NC 27709
Made in England
Rev. 4/97

4 0 7 6 7 8 8

How many milliliters of Zantac should the patient receive per dose? _____

33. Order: tobramycin (Nebcin) 3 mg/kg/day, IM, in three divided doses.
Patient weighs 145 pounds.
Drug available: (80 mg = 2 mL)

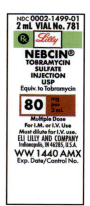

a. How many kilograms does the patient weigh? _____

b. How many milligrams of Nebcin should the patient receive per day? _____

c. How many milligrams of Nebcin should the patient receive per dose? _____

d. How many milliliters of Nebcin would you administer per dose? _____

34. Order: bethanechol chloride (Urecholine) 2.5 mg, subcut, STAT and may repeat in 1 hour.
Drug available: (Note: 5.15 mg = 5 mg or 5.15 mg = 5.2 mg [tenths])

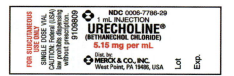

How many milliliters of Urecholine would you give? _____

35. Order: methotrexate 20 mg, IM, every other week.
Drug available:

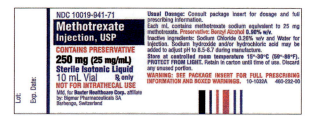

How many milliliters should the nurse administer? _____

36. Order: Tazidime (ceftazidime) 250 mg, IM, q8h.
Drug available:

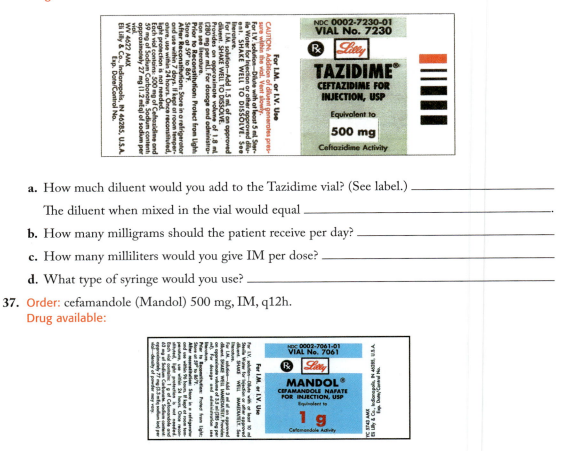

a. How much diluent would you add to the Tazidime vial? (See label.) _____

The diluent when mixed in the vial would equal _____.

b. How many milligrams should the patient receive per day? _____

c. How many milliliters would you give IM per dose? _____

d. What type of syringe would you use? _____

37. Order: cefamandole (Mandol) 500 mg, IM, q12h.
Drug available:

a. How much diluent would you mix with the Mandol powder? (See label for mixing.)

_____

b. How many milliliters should be given per dose? _____

38. Order: cefazolin (Ancef) 0.25 g, IM, q12h.
Mixing: Add 2.0 mL of diluent = 2.2 mL of drug solution.
Drug available:

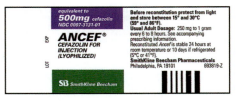

a. Change grams in order to milligrams; drug label is in milligrams. _____

b. How many milliliters of Ancef should the patient receive per dose? _____

39. Order: Rocephin (ceftriaxone) 500 mg, IM, q12h. Suggested dose: 1-2 g/day.
Drug available:

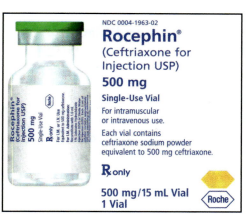

    a. Is the dose per day within the suggested drug parameters? _____

       Explain _____

    b. How many milliliters of sterile water should be injected into the Rocephin 1-g vial? _____

    c. After reconstitution, 1 mL of Rocephin solution would yield _____.

    d. How many mL of the Rocephin solution would you give per dose? _____

40. Order: ceftazidime (Fortaz) 750 mg, IM, q12h.
Add 2.5 mL of diluent = 3 mL of drug solution.
Drug available:

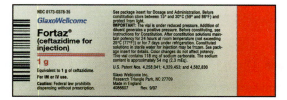

How many milliliters of ceftazidime would you administer per dose? _____

41. Order: gentamicin sulfate 4 mg/kg/day, IM, in three divided doses.
Patient weighs 165 pounds.
Drug available: gentamicin 10 mg/mL and 40 mg/mL.

    a. How many kilograms does the patient weigh? _____

    b. How many milligrams of gentamicin per day should the patient receive? _____

    c. How many milligrams of gentamicin per dose? _____

    d. Which gentamicin bottle would you select? Explain.

    _____

    e. How many milliliters of gentamicin per dose should the patient receive? _____

DIRECT IV ADMINISTRATION

Answers can be found on page 372.

42. Order: furosemide (Lasix) 30 mg, IV direct, STAT.
Drug available:

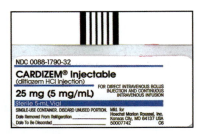

Instruction: Direct IV infusion not to exceed 10 mg/min.

a. How many milliliters should the patient receive? _____

b. Number of minutes to administer? _____

43. Order: diltiazem (Cardizem) 15 mg, IV direct, STAT.
Drug available:

Instruction: Direct IV infusion. Initial dose: 0.25 mg/kg over 2 minutes. Patient weights 60 kg.

a. How many milligrams should the patient receive? _____

b. Is the Cardizem dose ordered within the drug parameter? _____

c. Give the number of milliliters and number of minutes to administer.

_____

INTRAVENOUS

Answers can be found on page 373 to 374.

44. Order: 1000 mL of 5% dextrose/0.45% NaCl in 8 hours.
Available: 1 liter of 5% D/½ NS; IV set labeled 10 gtt/mL.
How many drops per minute should the patient receive?

_____

45. Order: 500 mL of D_5W in 2 hours.
Available: 500 mL of D_5W; IV set labeled 15 gtt/mL.
How many drops per minute should the patient receive?

_____

46. Order: potassium chloride 20 mEq in 1000 mL in D_5W to run 8 hours.
Drug available:

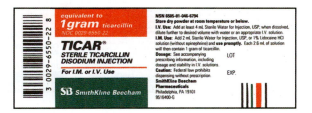

   a. How many milliliters should be mixed in 1000 mL of 5% dextrose in water to be given IV over 8 hours? _____

   b. How many drops per minute should the patient receive using a macrodrip IV set (10 gtt/mL)?
_____

47. Order: ticarcillin disodium (Ticar) 600 mg, IV, q6h.
Available: Calibrated cylinder (Buretrol) set with drop factor 60 gtt/mL; 500 mL D_5W.
Drug available: add 2 mL of diluent = 2.6 mL drug solution

Instruction: Dilute drug in 60 mL of D_5W and infuse in 30 minutes.

  a. *Drug calculation:*

_____

  b. *Flow rate calculation:*

_____

48. Order: cefazolin (Kefzol) 500 mg, IV, q6h.
Available: Secondary set: drop factor 15 gtt/mL; 100 mL D$_5$W.
Add 2.5 mL of diluent to yield 3 mL of drug solution.
Drug available:

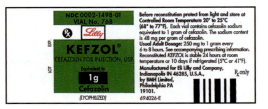

Instruction: Dilute drug in 100 mL D$_5$W and infuse in 45 minutes.

a. *Drug calculation:*

_____

b. *Flow rate calculation:*

_____

49. Order: chlorpromazine HCl (Thorazine) 50 mg, IV, to run for 4 hours.
Available: Secondary set: drop factor 15 gtt/mL; 500 mL of NS (normal saline solution).
Drug available:

Instruction: Dilute Thorazine 50 mg in 500 mL of 0.9% NaCl (NS) to run for 4 hours.

a. *Drug calculation:*

_____

b. *Flow rate calculation:*

_____

50. Order: cefoxitin (Mefoxin) 1 g, IV, q6h.
Drug available: ADD-Vantage vial

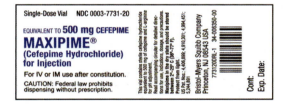

Set and solution: 50 mL of IV diluent bag for ADD-Vantage; Mefoxin 1 g vial for ADD-Vantage.
Instruction: Dilute Mefoxin in 50 mL of NaCl bag and infuse in 30 minutes.

a. How would you prepare Mefoxin 1 g powdered vial using the diluent bag? (See page 225.)

_____

b. Infusion pump rate (mL/hr): _____

51. Order: cefepime HCl (Maxipime) 0.5 g, IV, q12h.
Available: Infusion pump.
Add 2.0 mL diluent = 2.5 mL.
Drug available:

Instruction: Dilute in 50 mL of D₅W and infuse over 20 minutes.

a. *Drug calculation:*

_____

b. *Infusion pump rate:*

_____

52. Order: diltiazem (Cardizem) 10 mg/hr, IV for 5 hours.
Available: Infusion pump; 500 mL of D_5W.
Drug available:

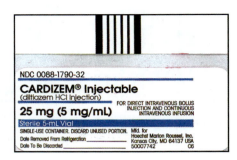

Instruction: Infuse diltiazem 10 mg/hr over 5 hours.
Drug parameter: 5–15 mg/hr for 24 hours.

  a. *Drug calculation:* How many milligrams of Cardizem should the patient receive over 5 hours?

  _____

  b. How many milliliters of Cardizem should be mixed in the 500 mL of D_5W? _____

  c. *Infusion pump rate:*

  _____

53. Order: ciprofloxacin (Cipro) 100 mg, IV, q6h.
Drug available:

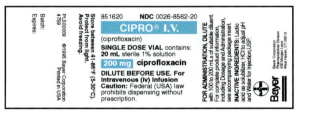

Set and solution: Secondary set with drop factor 15 gtt/mL; 100 mL of D_5W.
Instruction: Dilute drug in 100 mL of D_5W and infuse in 30 minutes; also calculate rate for infusion pump.

  a. *Drug calculation:* _____

  b. *Flow rate calculation* with secondary set (gtt/min): _____

  c. *Infusion pump rate* (mL/hr): _____

54. Order: ifosfamide (Ifex) 1.2 g/m²/day for 5 consecutive days.
    Patient: Weight: 150 pounds; height: 70 inches = 1.98 m².
    Available: Infusion pump; 5% dextrose solution.
    Add 20 mL of diluent to 1 g of Ifex.
    Drug available:

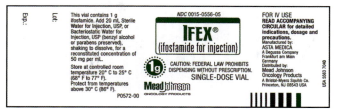

Instruction: Dilute Ifex in 50 mL of D₅W; infuse over 30 minutes.

   a. *Drug calculation:*

_____

How many grams or milligrams of Ifex should the patient receive?

_____

   b. How much diluent would you add to 2.4 g of Ifex? _____

   c. *Infusion pump rate:*

_____

PEDIATRICS

Answers can be found on pages 374 to 376.

55. Child with cardiac disorder.
    Order: Lanoxin pediatric elixir 0.4 mg, po, daily.
    Drug available:

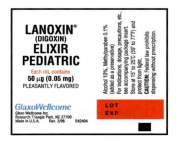

Child's age and weight: 3 years, 12 kg.
Pediatric dose range: 0.03–0.04 mg/kg.

   a. Is this drug dose within the safe range? _____

   b. How many milliliters would you administer? _____

56. Child with high fever.
Order: ibuprofen (Motrin) 0.1 g, prn temperature greater than 102° F.
Child's age and weight: 3 years, 15 kg.
Pediatric dose range: 100 mg, q6-8h, not to exceed 400 mg/day.
Drug available: (100 mg = 5 mL)

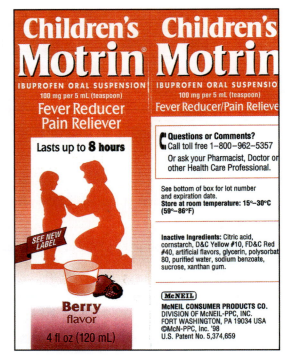

a. Is this drug dose within the safe range? _____

b. How many milliliters should the child receive per dose? _____

57. Child with strep throat.
Order: penicillin V potassium (Veetids) 400,000 units, po, q6h.
Child's age and weight: 8 years, 53 pounds.
Pediatric dose range: 25,000–90,000 units/kg/day in three to six divided doses.
Drug available:

a. Is the drug dose within the safe range? _____

b. How many milliliters of penicillin V would you give? _____

58. Child with otitis media.

Order: amoxicillin (Amoxil) 250 mg, po, q6h.

Child's age and weight: 5 years, 19 kg.

Pediatric dose range: 20-40 mg/kg/day in three divided doses.

Drug available:

a. Is the drug dose within the safe range? _____

b. How many milliliters would you give? _____

59. Child with pruritus.

Order: diphenhydramine HCl (Benadryl) 25 mg, po, tid.

Child's age and weight: 2 years, 16 kg.

Pediatric dose: 5 mg/kg/day.

Drug available: Benadryl 12.5 mg/5 mL.

a. Is the drug dose within the safe range? _____

b. How many milliliters would you give? _____

60. Child with severe bacterial infection.
    Order: clindamycin (Cleocin) 150 mg, po, q8h for 7 days.
    Child's weight: 45 pounds.
    Pediatric dose range: 20-40 mg/kg/day in three divided doses.
    Drug available:

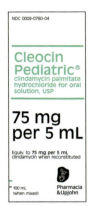

a. How many kilograms does the child weigh? _____

b. What are the dosage parameters? _____

c. Is the dosage within drug parameters? _____

d. How many milligrams should the child receive per day? _____

e. How many milliliters should the child receive per dose? _____

61. Child with a lower respiratory tract infection.
    Order: cefaclor (Ceclor) 100 mg, q8h.
    Child's age and weight: 4 years, 44 pounds.
    Pediatric dose range: 20-40 mg/kg/day in three divided doses.
    Drug available:

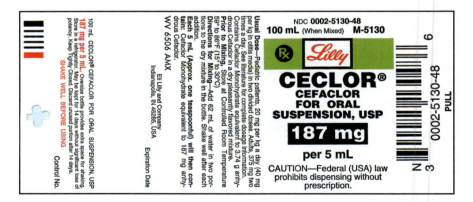

a. How many kilograms does the child weigh? _____

b. Is the drug dose within the safe range? _____

c. How many milliliters should the child receive? _____

62. Child with severe systemic infection.
    Order: tobramycin (Nebcin) 15 mg, IV, q8h.
    Child's age and weight: 18 months, 10 kg.
    Pediatric dose range: 3-5 mg/kg/day in three divided doses.
    Drug available:

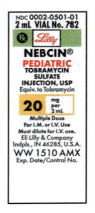

    a. Is the drug dose within the safe range? _____

    b. How many milliliters of tobramycin would you give per dose? _____

63. Child with a severe central nervous system (CNS) infection.
    Order: ceftazidime (Fortaz) 250 mg, IV, q6h.
    Child's age and weight: 6 years, 27 kg.
    Pediatric dose range: 30-50 mg/kg/day in three divided doses.
    Add 2.0 mL of diluent = 2.4 mL of drug solution.
    Drug available:

    a. Is the drug dose within the safe range? _____

    b. How many milliliters of Fortaz would be given? _____

64. Order: Cefazolin (Ancef) 400 mg, IV, q8h.
Child weight: 49 pounds.
Parameters: 50-100 mg/kg/day in three divided doses.
Drug available:

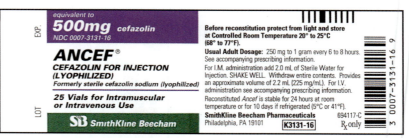

Instruction: Mix Ancef with 1.8 mL to equal 2.0 mL = 500 mg. Buretrol: Dilute drug in 50 mL of IV diluent; infuse in 30 minutes.

a. How many kg does the child weigh? _____

b. Is the drug dose within drug parameters? _____

c. How many mL of Ancef should be withdrawn from the vial? _____

d. Flow rate calculation (gtt/min): _____

65. Child with a severe respiratory tract infection.
Order: kanamycin (Kantrex) 60 mg, IV, q8h.
Child's age and weight: 1 year, 26 pounds.
Pediatric dose range: 15 mg/kg/day, q8-12h.
Drug available:

a. How many milligrams of kanamycin will the child receive per day? Per dose? _____

b. How many milliliters of kanamycin will the child receive per dose? _____

c. Is the drug dose within the safe range? _____

ANSWERS

Oral Preparations

1. a. The Adalat CC, 60-mg tablet container
   b. For 90 mg, remove 1 tablet from the 30-mg tablet container and 1 tablet from the 60-mg tablet container.
2. (a) 2 tablets; (b) in the evening or bedtime
3. 2 tablets of Pravachol
4. Nitrostat 0.3 mg (use conversion table as needed)
5. a. 1 tablet in the AM
   b. 2 tablets at bedtime

6. **a.** 0.5 gram = 500 mg
   b. 2 tablets
7. **a.** 325-mg bottle
   b. 2 tablets from the 325-mg bottle
8. **a.** 0.2 g = 200 mg
   b. 2 tablets
9. **a.** Compazine 5 mg/5 mL; Compazine 5 mg/mL is for injection.
   b. 10 mL
10. **a.** Select Zyprexa 2.5-mg tablets. The nurse could give 1 tablet of Zyprexa 7.5 mg and 1 tablet of Zyprexa 2.5 mg = 10 mg. If the nurse does not have the 2 strengths of Zyprexa, then the nurse should use the 2.5-mg tablets.

   b. BF: $\dfrac{D}{H} \times V = \dfrac{10 \text{ mg}}{2.5 \text{ mg}} \times 1 \text{ tab} = 4 \text{ tablets}$

   or
   RP: H : V ::   D :X
         2.5 mg:1 tab :: 10 mg:X
                    2.5 X = 10
                        X = 4 tablets

11. **a.** 37.5 mcg = 0.0375 mg
    b. 0.025-mg or 25-mcg bottle

    c. BF: $\dfrac{D}{H} \times V = \dfrac{0.0375}{0.025} \times 1 =$

    $1\frac{1}{2}$ tablets

    or
    RP: H   : V ::   D   : X
        0.025 mg:1 tab :: 0.0375 mg:X tab
                    0.025 X = 0.0375
                          X = $1\frac{1}{2}$ tablets

    or
    FE: $\dfrac{H}{V} = \dfrac{D}{X} = \dfrac{25 \text{ mcg}}{1 \text{ tab}} = \dfrac{37.5 \text{ mcg}}{X} =$
    (Cross multiply) 25 X = 37.5
                        X = $1\frac{1}{2}$ tablets

    or
    DA: tab $= \dfrac{1 \text{ tab} \quad \times 0.0375 \text{ mg}}{0.025 \text{ mg} \times \quad 1} = 1\frac{1}{2}$ tablets

12. **a.** Select 250-mg/5-mL bottle. However, either bottle could be used; 125 mg/5 mL = 20 mL.
    b. 1 gram; 1000 mg
    c. 500 mg = 10 mL of Ceftin 250 mg/5 mL
13. **a.** Either 187 mg/5 mL or 375 mg/5 mL.
    b. With (preferred) 187-mg/5-mL bottle:

    $\dfrac{250 \text{ mg}}{187 \text{ mg}} \times 5 \text{ mL} = \dfrac{1250}{187} = 6.68 \text{ or } 7 \text{ mL per dose}$

    c. With the 375 mg/5 mL, 3.3 mL per dose.
14. **a.** Zocor 20-mg bottle. Either bottle; however, with the 10-mg Zocor bottle, more tablets would be taken (Zocor 10-mg bottle = 4 tablets).
    b. 2 tablets (Zocor 20-mg bottle)
15. **a.** Select Geodon 40-mg bottle.
    b. 1 capsule of Geodon 40 mg per dose; 2 capsules per day.
    c. Select both Geodon 40 mg and Geodon 20 mg to equal 60 mg.
    d. Per dose, give 1 capsule from the 40-mg bottle and 1 capsule from the 20-mg bottle to equal 60 mg. You can NOT cut a capsule in half, so both bottles of Geodon would be needed. Per day, give 2 capsules from Geodon 40-mg bottle and 2 capsules from the Geodon 20-mg bottle.

16. a. Change 0.4 grams to milligrams = 400 mg
   b. 400 mg per dose.

c. BF: $\dfrac{D}{H} \times V = \dfrac{400 \text{ mg}}{250 \text{ mg}} \times 5 \text{ mL} =$
        8 mL of amoxicillin

or
RP: H : V :: D : X
     250 mg : 5 mL :: 400 mg : X mL
            250 X = 2000
                 X = 8 mL

or
FE: $\dfrac{H}{V} = \dfrac{D}{X} = \dfrac{250}{5} = \dfrac{400}{X} =$

(Cross multiply) 250 X = 2000
              X = 8 mL of amoxicillin

or
DA: mL $= \dfrac{5 \text{ mL} \times \overset{4}{\cancel{1000 \text{ mg}}} \times 0.4 \text{ \cancel{g}}}{\underset{1}{\cancel{250 \text{ mg}}} \times 1 \text{ \cancel{g}} \times 1} = 8 \text{ mL}$

17. a. 300 mg per day

b. BF: $\dfrac{D}{H} \times V = \dfrac{150 \text{ mg}}{10 \text{ mg}} \times 1 \text{ mL} =$

$\dfrac{150}{10} = 15 \text{ mL}$

or
DA: mL $= \dfrac{1 \text{ mL} \times \overset{15}{\cancel{150 \text{ mg}}}}{\cancel{10 \text{ mg}} \times 1} = 15 \text{ mL}$

18. a. 150 pounds = 68 kg
   b. 0.75 × 68 = 51 mg or 50 mg per day
   c. Select 25-mg capsule bottle. One capsule per dose.
19. a. 5 mg × 70 kg = 350-mg loading dose
   b. Select the 150-mg/15-mL bottle.

c. BF: $\dfrac{D}{H} \times V = \dfrac{\overset{7}{\cancel{350 \text{ mg}}}}{\underset{3}{\cancel{150 \text{ mg}}}} \times 15 \text{ mL} = \dfrac{105}{3} = 35 \text{ mL theophylline}$

or
DA: mL $= \dfrac{15 \text{ mL} \times \overset{7}{\cancel{350 \text{ mg}}}}{\underset{3}{\cancel{150 \text{ mg}}} \times 1} = \dfrac{105}{3} = 35 \text{ mL theophylline}$

20. a. 10 mL = 100 mg Colace

b. $\dfrac{Known \ mOsm \ (3900) \times \text{Volume of drug (10 mL)}}{\text{desired mOsm (500)}} = \dfrac{39,000}{500} = 78 \text{ mL drug solution and water}$

78 mL of drug solution and water − 10 mL of drug solution = 68 mL of water to dilute the osmolality of the drug

Injectables

21. ½ mL or 0.5 mL

BF: $\dfrac{D}{H} \times V = \dfrac{\overset{1}{\cancel{25 \text{ mg}}}}{\underset{2}{\cancel{50 \text{ mg}}}} \times 1 \text{ mL} = \frac{1}{2} \text{ mL}$

or
RP: H : V :: D : X
     50 mg : 1 mL :: 25 mg : X
          50 X = 25
             X =   ½ mL or 0.5 mL

or
DA: no conversion factor needed

mL $= \dfrac{1 \text{ mL} \times \overset{1}{\cancel{25 \text{ mg}}}}{\underset{2}{\cancel{50 \text{ mg}}} \times 1} = \frac{1}{2} \text{ mL or 0.5 mL}$

22. 1 mL
23. a. Meperidine 0.8 mL; atropine 1.25 mL or 1.3 mL
   b. (1) Draw 1.25 mL of air and insert into the atropine bottle.
      (2) Withdraw 1.25 mL of atropine and 0.8 mL of meperidine from the ampule.
24. a. Could use either vial, units 5000/mL or units 10,000/mL.
   b. 0.5 mL from the units 5000 vial or 0.25 mL from the units 10,000 vial.
25. 0.2 mL of Lovenox
26. 1.25 mL of Naloxone
27. Withdraw 35 units of Humulin 70/30.

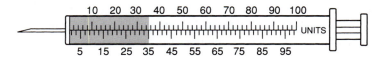

28. a. Withdraw the regular Humulin R insulin first and then the Humulin N insulin.

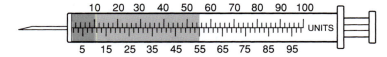

   b. Total of 55 units of Humulin R and Humulin N insulin (10 units regular, 45 units Humulin N).
29. a. Select 1000 mcg/mL. If you chose the 100-mcg/mL cartridge, you would need 5 cartridges to give 500 mcg.
   b. ½ mL or 0.5 mL
30. RP: H : V :: D : X
         15 mg : 1 mL :: 8 mg : X
               15 X = 8
                  X = 0.533 or 0.5 mL of morphine (round off to tenths)

or
DA: mL = $\dfrac{1 \text{ mL } \times 8 \text{ mg}}{15 \text{ mg } \times \quad 1} = \dfrac{8}{15}$ = 0.533 or 0.5 mL of morphine (round off to tenths)

31. ½ mL or 0.5 mL
32. 1.4 mL
33. a. 145 ÷ 2.2 = 65.9 kg or 66 kg
   b. 3 mg × 66 kg = 198 mg/day
   c. 198 ÷ 3 = 66 mg per dose

   d. BF: $\dfrac{66 \text{ mg}}{80} \times 2 \text{ mL} = \dfrac{132}{80}$ = 1.65 or 1.7 mL per dose (round off to tenths)

   or
   DA: mL = $\dfrac{2 \text{ mL } \times 66 \text{ mg}}{80 \text{ mg } \times \quad 1} = \dfrac{132}{80}$ = 1.7 mL per dose

34. 0.5 mL or 0.48 mL = 0.5 mL (tenths)
35. RP: H : V :: D : X   **or**
            25 mg : 1 mL :: 20 mg : X   DA: mL = $\dfrac{1 \text{ mL } \times 20 \text{ mg}}{25 \text{ mg } \times \quad 1} = \dfrac{20}{25}$ = 0.8 mL
               25 X = 20
                  X = 0.8 mL of methotrexate
      Give 0.8 mL of methotrexate.

36. **a.** Add 1.5 mL of diluent: 1.8 mL total
   b. 750 mg per day

   c. BF: $\dfrac{D}{H} \times V = \dfrac{250 \text{ mg}}{500 \text{ mg}} \times 1.8 \text{ mL} = 0.9 \text{ mL of Tazidime}$

   or
   RP: H : V :: D : X
       500 mg : 1.8 mL :: 250 mg : X mL
                 500 X = 450
                     X = 0.9 mL of Tazidime

   d. 3-mL syringe for mixing and administering; unable to mix the drug and diluent with a tuberculin syringe.
37. **a.** Add 3 mL diluent = 3.5 mL of drug solution; 1 g = 1000 mg.

   b. BF: $\dfrac{500 \text{ mg}}{1000 \text{ mg}} \times 3.5 \text{ mL} = \dfrac{1750}{1000} = 1.75 \text{ mL or } 1.8 \text{ mL per dose (round off to tenths)}$

38. **a.** 0.25 g = 250 mg

   b. BF: $\dfrac{250 \text{ mg}}{500} \times 2.2 \text{ mL} = \dfrac{550}{500} = 1.1 \text{ mL per dose}$ **or** 1 mL

   or
   RP: H : V :: D : X
       500 mg : 2.2 = 250 : X
            500 X = 550

            X = $\dfrac{550}{500}$ = 1.1 mL or 1 mL

   or
   DA: mL = $\dfrac{2.2 \text{ mL} \times 250 \text{ mg}}{500 \text{ mg} \times \quad 1} = 1.1 \text{ mL or 1 mL of Ancef}$

39. **a.** Yes, the total dose is 1000 mg daily (1 g = 1000 mg).
   b. Inject 2.1 mL of sterile water into the vial.
   c. After reconstitution, 1 mL of Rocephin solution would yield 350 mg.

   d. BF: $\dfrac{D}{H} \times V = \dfrac{500 \text{ mg}}{350 \text{ mg}} \times 1 \text{ mL} = 1.4 \text{ mL of Rocephin}$

40. 2.25 mL Fortaz
41. **a.** 165 lb ÷ 2.2 = 75 kg
   b. 4 mg × 75 kg = 300 mg/day
   c. 100 mg per dose
   d. Select 40-mg/mL bottle of gentamicin sulfate. (Normally less than 3 mL IM should be given at one site.)
   e. 2.5 mL of gentamicin per dose

Direct IV Administration

42. **a.** 3 mL
   b. Known drug : Known minutes :: Desired drug : Desired minutes
        10 mg   :   1 min   ::   30 mg   :   X
                            X = 3 min to administer 3 mg
43. **a.** 0.25 mg × 60 kg = 15 mg according to drug parameters of Cardizem IV direct (bolus) over 2 minutes
   b. Yes, dose is within drug parameters.
   c. Administer 3 mL of IV Cardizem over 2 minutes.

Intravenous

44. 125 mL per hour

$$\frac{125 \text{ mL} \times 10 \text{ gtt/min}}{60 \text{ min/hr}} = \frac{1250}{60} = 20.8 \text{ gtt/min or } 21 \text{ gtt/min}$$

45. $\dfrac{250 \text{ mL/hr} \times \overset{1}{\cancel{15}} \text{ gtt/mL}}{\underset{4}{\cancel{60}} \text{ min}} = \dfrac{250}{4} = 62.5 \text{ or } 63 \text{ gtt/min}$

46. a. BF: $\dfrac{D}{H} \times V = \dfrac{\overset{2}{\cancel{20}} \text{ mEq}}{\underset{3}{\cancel{30}} \text{ mEq}} \times 15 \text{ mL} = \dfrac{30}{3} = 10 \text{ mL of KCl}$

Inject 10 mL of potassium chloride in 1000 mL D$_5$W. The KCl should be injected into the IV bag and mixed well before the IV is hung.

b. 1000 ÷ 8 = 125 mL

$$\frac{125 \text{ mL} \times 10 \text{ gtt}}{60 \text{ min/hr}} = \frac{1250}{60} = 21 \text{ gtt/min}$$

47. Add 2.0 mL diluent = 2.6 mL of drug solution; 1 g = 1000 mg.

a. $\dfrac{\cancel{600} \text{ mg}}{\cancel{1000} \text{ mg}} \times 2.6 \text{ mL} = \dfrac{15.6}{10} = 1.56 \text{ mL or } 1.6 \text{ mL Ticar per dose (round off to tenths)}$

b. $\dfrac{\text{Amount of solution} \times \text{gtt/mL}}{\text{Minutes}} = \dfrac{60 \text{ mL} \times \overset{2}{\cancel{60}} \text{ gtt/mL}}{\underset{1}{\cancel{30}} \text{ min}} = 120 \text{ gtt/min}$

48. a. 1.5 mL

b. $\dfrac{100 \text{ mL} \times \overset{1}{\cancel{15}} \text{ gtt/mL}}{\underset{3}{\cancel{45}} \text{ min}} = \dfrac{100}{3} = 33.3 \text{ or } 33 \text{ gtt/min}$

49. a. Add 2 mL Thorazine to 500 mL. For 4 hours: 500 mL ÷ 4 = 125 mL/hr.

b. $\dfrac{125 \text{ mL} \times \overset{1}{\cancel{15}} \text{ gtt/mL}}{\underset{4}{\cancel{60}} \text{ min/1 hr}} = \dfrac{125}{4} = 31 \text{ gtt/min for 4 hours}$

50. a. Use the Mefoxin 1-g vial for ADD-Vantage and mix drug in the 50 mL IV bag for ADD-Vantage.

b. Amount of sol ÷ $\dfrac{\text{Minutes to admin}}{60 \text{ min/hr}}$ = mL/hr

$50 \text{ mL} \div \dfrac{30 \text{ min}}{60 \text{ min}} = 50 \text{ mL} \times \dfrac{\overset{2}{\cancel{60}} \text{ min}}{\underset{1}{\cancel{30}} \text{ min}} = 100 \text{ mL/hr}$

51. a. 0.5 g = 500 mg; add 2.0 mL of diluent = 2.5 mL of drug solution; 500 mg = 2.5 mL

b. Amount of solution ÷ $\dfrac{\text{Min to admin}}{60 \text{ min/hr}}$ = mL/hr

$2.5 \text{ mL drug} + 50 \text{ mL} \div \dfrac{20 \text{ min}}{60 \text{ min/hr}} = 52.5 \text{ mL} \times \dfrac{\overset{3}{\cancel{60}}}{\underset{1}{\cancel{20}}} = 157.5 \text{ mL/hr or } 158 \text{ mL/hr}$

Set pump to deliver in 20 minutes.

52. a. 10 mg/hr $\times$ 5 hr = 50 mg Cardizem

    b. $\dfrac{50 \text{ mg}}{5} \times 1 \text{ mL} = 10 \text{ mL}$ Cardizem to add to 500 mL

    c. 10 mL drug solution + 500 mL $\div \dfrac{300 \text{ min (5 hr)}}{60 \text{ min/hr}} = 510 \text{ mL} \times \dfrac{\overset{1}{60} \text{ min}}{\underset{5}{300} \text{ min (5 hr)}} = \dfrac{510}{5} = 102$ mL/hr

53. a. *Drug calculation:*

    BF: $\dfrac{D}{H} \times V = \dfrac{100 \text{ mg}}{200 \text{ mg}} \times 20 \text{ mL} = 10 \text{ mL}$ **or**   RP: H   :   V   ::   D   :   X
                                                               200 mg : 20 mL :: 100 mg : X mL
                                                                  200 X = 2000
                                                                     X = 10 mL

    or
    FE: $\dfrac{H}{V} = \dfrac{D}{X} = \dfrac{200}{20} = \dfrac{100}{X} =$ **or**
                                                   DA: mL $= \dfrac{20 \text{ mL} \times \overset{1}{100} \text{ mg}}{\underset{2}{200} \text{ mg} \times 1} = 10 \text{ mL}$

    (Cross multiply) 200X = 2000
                               X = 10 mL

    b. *Flow rate calculation* (secondary set):

    $\dfrac{110 \text{ mL } (100 + 10) \times \overset{1}{15} \text{ gtt/mL (set)}}{\underset{2}{30} \text{ min}} = 55 \text{ gtt/min}$

    c. *Infusion pump rate:*

    $110 \text{ mL} \div \dfrac{30 \text{ min to admin}}{60 \text{ min/hr}} = 110 \times \dfrac{\overset{2}{60}}{\underset{1}{30}} = 220 \text{ mL/hr}$

54. a. 1.2 g $\times$ 1.98 m^2 = 2.37 g or 2.4 g or 2400 mg
    b. 2.4 g $\times$ 20 mL = 48 mL diluent added to Ifex vials

    c. (48 mL of drug solution + 50 mL) $\div \dfrac{30 \text{ min}}{60 \text{ min}} = 98 \text{ mL} \times \dfrac{\overset{2}{60} \text{ min}}{\underset{1}{30} \text{ min}} = 196 \text{ mL/hr}$

    Set pump to deliver in 30 minutes.

Pediatrics

55. a. Drug dose is within safe range.
    0.03 mg $\times$ 12 kg = 0.36 mg
    0.04 mg $\times$ 12 kg = 0.48 mg
    b. BF: $\dfrac{D}{H} \times V = \dfrac{0.4 \text{ mg}}{0.05 \text{ mg}} \times 1 = 8 \text{ mL}$ of digoxin (Lanoxin)

    DA: mL $= \dfrac{1 \text{ mL} \times 0.4 \text{ mg}}{0.05 \text{ mg} \times 1} = \dfrac{0.4 \text{ mg}}{0.05 \text{ mg}} = 8 \text{ mL}$ of digoxin

56. a. Drug dose is within safe range.
    b. 5 mL

57. a. Drug dose is within safe range; 53 pounds ÷ 2.2 = 24 kg. 25,000 × 24 = 600,000 units; 90,000 × 24 = 2,160,000 units/day. Child receives 400,000 units × 4 (q6h) = 1,600,000 units/day.

   b. RP: H   :   V   ::   D   :X

              200,000 units : 5 mL :: 400,000 units : X

                      200,000 X = 2,000,000

                              X = 10 mL of penicillin

   400,000 units = 10 mL per dose

58. a. No; the drug dose is *NOT* within safe range. Do *NOT* give. Contact the physician or health care provider.
   Dosage parameters: 380 to 760 mg/day
   Order 250 mg × 4 (q6h) = 1000 mg/day; *not safe; exceeds parameters*

   b. Would not give medication.

59. a. Drug dose is within safe range.
   5 mg × 16 kg = 80 mg; child receives 25 mg × 3 (tid) = 75 mg; *SAFE*

   b. 10 mL

60. a. Child's weight: 45 lb ÷ 2.2 = 20.45 or 20.5 kg.

   b. Dosage parameters:
   20 mg × 20.5 kg/day = 410 mg/day.
   40 mg × 20.5 kg/day = 820 mg/day.

   c. Drug dose is safe, within the parameters.

   d. 150 mg × 3 doses = 450 mg.
   The child should receive 450 mg of Cleocin per day.

   e. BF: $\dfrac{D}{H} \times V = \dfrac{\overset{2}{\cancel{150}}}{\underset{1}{\cancel{75}}} \times 5 \text{ mL} = 10 \text{ mL per dose}$ **or**   DA: mL $= \dfrac{5 \text{ mL} \times \overset{2}{\cancel{150}} \text{ mg}}{\underset{1}{\cancel{75}} \text{ mg} \times 1} = 10 \text{ mL per dose}$

61. a. 44 lb ÷ 2.2 = 20 kg

   b. Drug dose is less than pediatric drug range.
   Check with the health care provider.
   20 mg × 20 kg = 400 mg/day; 40 mg × 20 kg = 800 mg/day.
   Child to receive 100 mg × 3 (q8h) = 300 mg/day; less than 400-800 mg/day.

   c. BF: $\dfrac{D}{H} \times V = \dfrac{100 \text{ mg}}{187 \text{ mg}} \times 5 \text{ mL} = \dfrac{500}{187} = 2.67$ or 2.7 mL of Ceclor (round off to tenths)

62. a. Drug dose is within safe range.
   3 mg × 10 kg = 30 mg/day; 5 mg × 10 kg = 50 mg/day.
   Child to receive 15 mg × 3 (q8h) = 45 mg/day.

   b. 1.5 mL per dose

63. a. Drug dose is within the safe range.
   30 mg × 27 kg = 810 mg/day; 50 mg × 27 kg = 1350 mg/day.
   Child to receive 250 mg × 4 (q6h) = 1000 mg/day.

   b. DA: mL $= \dfrac{2.4 \text{ mL} \times \overset{1}{\cancel{250}} \text{ mg}}{\underset{2}{\cancel{500}} \text{ mg} \times 1} = 1.2 \text{ mL of Fortaz}$

64. **a.** 22 kg (child's weight in kg); 49 lb ÷ 2.2 = 22.2 or 22 kg
    b. Yes, the daily dose is within the parameters; 50 × 22 = 1100 mg/day and 100 × 22 = 2200 mg/day.
    c. *Drug calculation:* Child is to receive 400 mg × 3 = 1200 mg/day or 400 mg q8h.

$$BF: \frac{D}{H} \times V = \frac{400 \text{ mg}}{500 \text{ mg}} \times 2 \text{ mL} = \frac{8}{5} = 1.6 \text{ mL}$$

$$DA: mL = \frac{2 \text{ mL} \times \overset{4}{\cancel{400 \text{ mg}}}}{\underset{5}{\cancel{500 \text{ mg}}} \times 1} = \frac{8}{5} = 1.6 \text{ mL}$$

   d. *Flow rate calculation:* $\dfrac{50 \text{ mL} \times \overset{2}{\cancel{60}} \text{ gtt/mL}}{\underset{1}{\cancel{30}} \text{ min}} = 100 \text{ gtt/min}$

65. **a.** 180 mg/day; 60 mg/dose
    b. $BF: \dfrac{60}{75} \times 2 \text{ mL} = \dfrac{120}{75} = 1.6 \text{ mL per dose}$

$$FE: \frac{H}{V} = \frac{D}{X} = \frac{75 \text{ mg}}{2 \text{ mL}} = \frac{60 \text{ mg}}{X}$$

   (Cross multiply) 75 X = 120
   $\qquad\qquad\qquad$ X = 1.6 mL of Kantrex
    c. Drug dose is within safe range.
    Child's weight: 26 lb ÷ 2.2 = 11.8 or 12 kg
    15 mg × 12 kg = 180 mg/day; child to receive 180 mg/day or 60 mg per dose.

---

evolve $\qquad$ Additional practice problems are available in the Comprehensive Post-Test section of Drug Calculations Companion, version 5, on Evolve.

APPENDIX A

Guidelines for Administration of Medications

Outline **GENERAL DRUG ADMINISTRATION**
ORAL MEDICATIONS
INJECTABLE MEDICATIONS
INTRAVENOUS FLUID AND MEDICATIONS

GENERAL DRUG ADMINISTRATION

1. Wash hands and don gloves before preparing **all** medications.
2. All medication should be prepared in a clean, distraction-free environment.
3. Check medication order against physician's orders in the MAR (medication administration record) or eMAR (electronic medication administration record). Check for medication administration parameters, such as heart rate, respiration, and blood pressure.
4. Check label of drug container against medication order and physician's order. Verify 5 "rights": that you have the right patient, medication, dose, route of administration, and time of administration. If something is amiss, ask another nurse to verify the medication reconciliation with you.
5. Check all drug labels for an expiration date. Notify the pharmacy of outdated drugs, and return expired medication.
6. If a drug order is unclear, do not guess. Verify order with charge nurse, physician, and/or pharmacist.
7. Nurses are patient advocates and have the right to question and clarify drug orders. Physicians are responsible for medication orders. Nurses are responsible for administering medications correctly and safely.
8. Do not give medications that are poured or drawn up by someone else unless you witness the drug preparation. Dosages should be verified before administering them.
9. Do not leave medication sitting out unsupervised or out of your sight.
10. Identify patients by using their identification bracelets (ID bands) and by asking each patient to state his or her name and birth date.
11. Check if patient has any allergies to the drug or drug class. Patient should be wearing an allergy bracelet.
12. Explain to the patient what medication he or she is receiving and why.
13. Assist patient as necessary with taking medication (i.e., positioning or providing water). You must stay with the patient to make sure the medication is taken. Manage time by giving medications last to patients who need more assistance.

14. Promptly document in patient's MAR or eMAR that medication was given (especially STAT medications). If patient did not receive medication, document why in MAR or eMAR.
15. Record the amount of fluid taken orally or intravascularly with each medication if client's intake (I) and output (O) are being recorded.
16. Immediately report any medication errors to the physician and charge nurse. Document incident per your institution's policy. Evaluate the patient's condition immediately.
17. Nurses have a window of 30 minutes before and after the scheduled time to administer ordered medications. Check hospital policy because some facilities vary on time allowed before and after the scheduled administration time.
18. Patients have the right to refuse medications. Provide education for these patients. Notify physician of patient's refusal. Document refusal on patient's MAR or eMAR.

ORAL MEDICATIONS

1. Wash hands and don gloves before preparing oral medications.
2. Pour tablet or capsule into medicine cup (not your hand or into another medication container). Drugs prepared for unit dose can be opened at the time of administration in the patient's room. Discard drugs that are dropped on the floor and dispose of them per institutional policy.
3. Pour liquids into a container or cup placed on a flat surface and read measurement at eye level. Pour liquid medication from the opposite side of the bottle's label to avoid spilling on the label.
4. Do not mix liquid medications or tablets and liquid medications together. Ideally, medications should be given one at a time. Patient may take more than one tablet or capsule at a time (except oral narcotics, digoxin, and STAT medications) if they are comfortable doing so.
5. Evaluate patients' swallowing abilities by first having them take a sip of water. For a larger pill (e.g., potassium), ask patients if they feel comfortable swallowing it. Instant coughing after swallowing water may indicate that the patient is aspirating.
6. For the patient who has difficulty swallowing tablets and thin liquids, contact the physician and pharmacy to evaluate whether the medication can be crushed and given in applesauce.
7. Do not return poured medication to its container. Discard poured medication if unused.
8. Dilute liquid medication that irritates gastric mucosa (e.g., potassium products) or that could discolor or damage tooth enamel (e.g., saturated solution of potassium iodide). Evaluate whether these medications can be taken with meals.
9. Offer ice chips before administering bad-tasting medications to help numb patient's taste buds.
10. Assist patient into an upright position when administering oral medications. Stay with patient until medication is taken.
11. Give 50 to 100 mL of oral fluids with medications unless the patient has a fluid restriction.
12. Patients who have a nasogastric or gastric tube should receive their oral medications via this route. Tablets should be thoroughly crushed and diluted in sterile water or normal saline (NS). Medications should be given one at a time and flushed with sterile water or NS between each medication. Some medications cannot be crushed; therefore the form would need to be changed. Refer to your institution's policy. (See Chapter 8 for additional information.)
13. For drugs given by oral syringe, direct the syringe across the tongue and toward the side of the mouth.
14. If a patient spits out all of the liquid medication, repeat the dose. If the patient spits out half of the medication, repeat half of the dose. Notify the physician if there is a question regarding repeated doses. The physician may need to select another route of administration.

INJECTABLE MEDICATIONS

1. Wash hands and don gloves before preparing injectable medications.
2. Check medication order and medication label to determine method(s) for drug administration (e.g., intramuscular [IM] or subcutaneous [subcut]).
3. Check for drug compatibility before mixing drugs in the same syringe. Check institution's policy before mixing compatible drugs in a syringe to administer.
4. Do not give medications that are cloudy, discolored, or that have precipitated.
5. Select the proper syringe and needle size for the route and type of medication to be administered.
6. Select the injection site according to the drug, patient's age, and disease process.
7. Medication in ampules should be drawn up using a 15-micron filtered needle or filter straw. Once opened, the ampule cannot be used again and the unused solution should be discarded.
8. Do not reuse vials, needles, or syringes between patients.
9. Avoid the use of multiple-dose vials. If multiple-dose vials must be used, each patient should have his or her own vial, labeled with the date it was opened and stored according to manufacturer's directions.
10. Know alternative sites of administration. Do not administer injections into inflamed, edematous, or infected tissue. Lesions (moles, birthmarks, and scar tissue) and surgical sites should also be avoided.
11. When administering IM medications, aspirate the plunger before injecting the medication. If blood is aspirated, do not administer. Withdraw the needle and prepare a new solution. Check your institution's policy about aspirate when giving IM injections.
12. Do not massage the injection site when using the Z-track method, intradermal injections, or any anticoagulant solution.
13. Recognize that patients experiencing edema, shock, or poor circulation will have a slower tissue absorption rate with IM injections.
14. The site of injection on the patient's skin should be cleansed with an alcohol swab before injection.
15. Do not administer IM medications subcutaneously. Poor medication absorption and sloughing of the skin could occur.
16. Specific medications (e.g., narcotics) need to be discarded with a colleague and documented per your institution's policy.
17. Discard medication per your institution's policy. Discard needles into the proper sharps container.

INTRAVENOUS FLUID AND MEDICATIONS

1. Wash hands and don gloves before preparing and priming IV drugs or fluids.
2. Use aseptic technique when inserting IV catheters, administering medications, and changing IV tubing and fluids.
3. All products and medications for IV infusion should be clearly labeled with trade and generic names, along with the dosage and concentration of the drug or fluid, route of administration, expiration date, frequency, infusion rate, and sterility state.
4. Recognize signs of catheter-related infection, such as erythema, edema, induration or drainage at vascular access site, fever, and chills. These changes should be reported immediately to the charge nurse and physician.
5. Use peripheral access over central access when appropriate. Avoid placing an IV in areas of inflammation, bruises, breakdown, or infection; in the lower extremities; at surgical sites; or in extremities with neuromuscular or motor deficits.
6. IV tubing and fluid bags should be labeled with date, time, and initials of nurse. When multiple catheters or lumens are being used, all lines should be labeled (at the sites where they connect to the patient) with the name of the medication or fluid that is infusing.

7. Check patency of IV catheter before using by flushing the IV catheter with 2 mL of normal saline (NS). To clear IV tubing of a medication's solution, flush tubing with 15 mL of NS.

8. Do not forcefully irrigate IV catheters. The IV catheter could be kinked, infiltrated, or the force could dislodge a clot from the catheter site, leading to an embolus.

9. IV sites that are saline locked should be flushed at intervals that adhere to your institution's protocols.

10. Check for air bubbles in tubing. Remove air from tubing by repriming the tubing or by clamping below the air bubble and removing the air by aspirating with a syringe. Use the method that is indicated by unit policy.

11. Monitor all IV flow rates hourly or as needed. IV flow rates can be easily altered by the patient's position or by kinked tubing. Promptly address pump alarms.

12. Assess for signs of an allergic reaction to the IV drug. If signs of a reaction are noted, stop the administration of the drug and notify the prescriber immediately.

13. Use an infusion pump for any high-risk medications with a narrow therapeutic range to prevent medication errors. Every precaution should be taken to prevent "free flow" incidence of IV fluids. Check that the pump is infusing accurately.

14. Check compatibility of IV medications before infusing them together. Stop infusion immediately if precipitation is noted in the tubing.

15. Assess IV sites for signs of infiltration: swelling, coolness, leakage, and pain at insertion site. If these symptoms are found, remove IV and elevate arm. Use an infiltration scale to grade severity of the infiltration when documenting (see following page).

16. Monitor IV sites for signs of phlebitis, which is an inflammation of the vein, causing erythema and pain along the vessel. Remove the IV catheter if signs are present. A phlebitis scale should be used when documenting this site (see following page).

17. IV sites should be secured with tape or stat lock and stabilized to prevent the loss of IV access.

18. Change IV site dressing when soiled and per institution's policy. Ensure that IV sites are labeled with date and time of insertion, gauge size, and initials.

19. Change IV tubing every 24 to 48 hours. This includes all add-on devices, such as filters, extensions, ports, stopcocks, access caps, and needleless systems. Change IV fluid every 24 hours. Follow institution's policy.

20. Vascular access sites should be flushed at intervals according to institutional policies and procedures and manufacturer's recommendations.

21. Choose the flow-control device that best meets the clinical application for patients. Base this choice on factors such as severity of illness, type of therapy, clinical setting, age, and mobility.

Infiltration Scale

Grade	Clinical Criteria
0	No symptoms
1	Skin blanched
	Edema less than 1 inch in any direction
	Cool to touch
	With or without pain
2	Skin blanched
	Edema 1–6 inches in any direction
	Cool to touch
	With or without pain
3	Skin blanched, translucent
	Gross edema greater than 6 inches in any direction
	Cool to touch
	Mild to moderate pain
	Possible numbness
4	Skin blanched, translucent
	Skin tight, leaking
	Skin discolored, bruised, swollen
	Gross edema greater than 6 inches in any direction
	Deep pitting tissue edema
	Circulatory impairment
	Moderate to severe pain
	Infiltration of any amount of blood product, irritant, or vesicant

From *Infusion Nursing Standards of Practice.* (2006). New York: Infusion Nurses Society, p. S60.

Phlebitis Scale

Grade	Clinical Criteria
0	No symptoms
1	Erythema at access site with or without pain
2	Pain at access site with erythema and/or edema
3	Pain at access site with erythema and/or edema
	Streak formation
	Palpable venous cord
4	Pain at access site with erythema and/or edema
	Streak formation
	Palpable venous cord greater than 1 inch in length
	Purulent drainage

From *Infusion Nursing Standards of Practice.* (2006). New York: Infusion Nurses Society, p. S59.

APPENDIX B

Nomograms

HEIGHT
BODY SURFACE AREA (BSA)
WEIGHT

```
cm 200 —┬ 79 inch          ┬ 2.80 m²         kg 150 ┬ 330 lb
        ├ 78                                   145 ─┤ 320
  195 ─┤ 77                 ┤ 2.70            140 ─┤ 310
        ├ 76                                   135 ─┤ 300
  190 ─┤ 75                 ┤ 2.60            130 ─┤ 290
        ├ 74                                   125 ─┤ 280
  185 ─┤ 73                 ┤ 2.50            120 ─┤ 270
        ├ 72                 ┤ 2.40                 ┤ 260
  180 ─┤ 71                 ┤ 2.30            115 ─┤ 250
        ├ 70
  175 ─┤ 69                 ┤ 2.20            110 ─┤ 240
        ├ 68                                   105 ─┤ 230
  170 ─┤ 67                 ┤ 2.10            100 ─┤ 220
        ├ 66
  165 ─┤ 65                 ┤ 2.00             95 ─┤ 210
        ├ 64                 ┤ 1.95                 ┤
  160 ─┤ 63                 ┤ 1.90             90 ─┤ 200
        ├ 62                 ┤ 1.85             85 ─┤ 190
  155 ─┤ 61                 ┤ 1.80
        ├ 60                 ┤ 1.75             80 ─┤ 180
  150 ─┤ 59                 ┤ 1.70                 ┤ 170
        ├ 58                 ┤ 1.65             75 ─┤
  145 ─┤ 57                 ┤ 1.60                 ┤ 160
        ├ 56                 ┤ 1.55             70 ─┤ 150
  140 ─┤ 55                 ┤ 1.50
        ├ 54                 ┤ 1.45             65 ─┤ 140
  135 ─┤ 53                 ┤ 1.40             60 ─┤ 130
        ├ 52                 ┤ 1.35
  130 ─┤ 51                 ┤ 1.30             55 ─┤ 120
        ├ 50                 ┤ 1.25
  125 ─┤ 49                 ┤ 1.20             50 ─┤ 110
        ├ 48                 ┤ 1.15                 ┤ 105
  120 ─┤ 47                                     45 ─┤ 100
        ├ 46                 ┤ 1.10                 ┤ 95
  115 ─┤ 45                 ┤ 1.05             40 ─┤ 90
        ├ 44                 ┤ 1.00                 ┤ 85
  110 ─┤ 43                                         ┤ 80
        ├ 42                 ┤ 0.95             35 ─┤ 75
  105 ─┤ 41                 ┤ 0.90                 ┤ 70
        ├ 40
cm 100 ─┴ 39 in             ┴ 0.86 m²         kg 30 ┴ 66 lb
```

Body surface area (BSA) nomogram for adults. *Directions:* (1) Find height; (2) find weight; (3) draw a straight line connecting the height and weight. Where the line intersects on the BSA column is the body surface area (m²). (From Deglin, J.H., Vallerand, A.H., & Russin, M.M. [1991]. *Davis's Drug Guide for Nurses* [2nd ed.]. Philadelphia: F.A. Davis, p. 1218. Used with permission from Lentner C. [Ed.]. [1981]. *Geigy Scientific Tables.* [8th ed.] Vol. 1. Basel, Switzerland: Ciba-Geigy, pp. 226-227.)

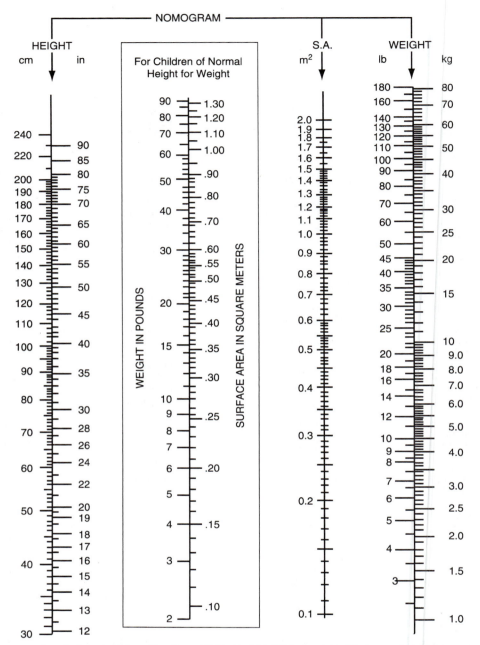

West nomogram for infants and children. *Directions: (1) Find height; (2) find weight; (3) draw a straight line connecting the height and weight. Where the line intersects on the S.A. (surface area) column is the body surface area in square meters (m²).* (Modified from data by E. Boyd & C. D. West. In Kliegman, R. M., Stanton, B. F., St. Geme, J. W., et al [2011]: *Nelson textbook of pediatrics,* ed. 19, Philadelphia: Saunders.)

REFERENCES

Adachi, W., & Lodolce, A. E. (2005). Use of failure mode and effects analysis in improving the safety of I.V. drug administration [electronic version]. *American Journal of Health-Systems Pharmacy, 62*(9):917-920.

ALARIS Medical Systems. (1999). *Volumetric infusion pump manual.*

Beckwith, C.M., Feddema, S.S., Barton, R.G., & Graves, C. (2004). A guide to drug therapy in patients with enteral feedingtubes: dosage form selection and administration methods. *Hospital Pharmacy, 39*:231.

Briars, G.L., & Bailey, B.J. (1994). Surface area estimation: pocket calculator vs. nomogram. *Archives of Disease in Childhood, 70*:246-247.

Brunton L., & Chabner, B. (2011). *Goodman & Gilman's the pharmacological basis of therapeutics* (12th ed.). New York: McGraw-Hill.

Bryn Mawr Hospital. (2005). Perinatal units: policy and procedural manual. Bryn Mawr, Pa: Auhor.

Burz, S. (2006). *Smart pumps get smarter.* Retrieved from www.nursezone. com/job/technologyreport.asp?article ID_15520.

Carayon, P., Wetterneck, T.B., Schoofs Hundt, A., et al. (2008). Observing nurse interaction with infusion pump technologies [electronic version]. *Advances in Patient Safety: From Research to Implementation, 2*:349-364.

CNA Medical. (n.d.). *Refurbished infusion pumps.* Retrieved from www. cnamedical.com/infusionpumps.htm.

Conklin, S. (2004). *UW Hospital and clinics install "smart" intravenous pumps.* Retrieved from www.wistechnology.com/article. php?id_1186.

Cowan, D. (2009). "Mission zero" with smart pumps [electronic version]. *Pharmacy Solutions,* a supplement of *Nursing Management, 40*(11): 1-2.

Crass, R. (2001). *Improving intravenous (IV) medication safety at the point of care.* Boston: ALARIS.

Dennison, R.D. (2006). High alert drugs: Strategies for safe I.V. infusions. *American Nurse Today, 1*(2).

Department of Veterans Affairs, Veterans Health Administration. (2002). *Bar code medication administration, version 2, training manual.* Washington, D.C.: Authors.

Food and Drug Administration. (n.d.). *Dailymed.* Retrieved from http://dailymed.nlm.nih.gov/dailymed/.

Foster, J. (2006). *Intravenous in-line filters for preventing morbidity and mortality in neonates.* Retrieved from www.nichd.nih.gov/cochrane/ foster2FOSTER.HTM.

Gahart, B., & Nazarento, A. (2015). *Intravenous medications* (31st ed.). St. Louis: Mosby.

Gardner, S.L., & Carter, B.S. (2011). *Merenstein & Gardner's handbook of neonatal intensive care* (7th ed). St. Louis: Mosby.

Gin, T., Chan, M.T., Chan, K.L., & Yen, P.M. (2002). Prolonged neuromuscular block after rocuronium in postpartum patient. *Anesthesia-Analgesia, 94*(3):686-689.

Green, B. (2004). *What is the best size descriptor to use for pharmacokinetic studies in the obese?* Retrieved from www.ncbi.nlm.nih.gov/entrez/ query.fegi?cmd.

Gurney, H. (1996). Dose calculation of anticancer drugs: a review of current practice and introduction of an alternative. *Journal of Clinical Oncology, 14*(9):590-611.

Gurney, H.P., Ackland, S., Gebski, V., & Farrell, G. (1998). Factors affecting epirubicin pharmacokinetics and toxicity: evidence against using body-surface areas for dose calculation. *Journal of Clinical Oncology, 16*:2299-2304.

Han, P.Y., Coombes, I.D., & Green, B. (October 4, 2004). *Factors predictive of intravenous fluid administration errors in Australian surgical care wards.* Retrieved from www.qhc.bmjjournals.com/cgi/content/ full/14/3/179.

Hasler, R.A. (2004). *Administration of blood products.* ALARIS. Retrieved from www.cardinalhealth.com/alaris/support/clinical/ pdfs/wp836.asp.

Hegenbarth, M.A., & American Academy of Pediatarics Committee on Drugs. (2008). Preparing for pediatric emergencies: Drugs to consider, *Pediatrics 121*(2):433-443.

Hockenberry, M.J., & Wilson, D. (2011). *Wong's Nursing care of infants* (9th ed). St. Louis: Elsevier/Mosby.

Hodgson, B., & Kizior, R. (2006). *Mosby's 2006 drug consult for nurses.* St. Louis: Elsevier.

Husch, M., Sullivan, C., & Rooney, D. (2005). Insights from the sharp end of intravenous medication errors: Implications for infusion pump technology, *Quality & Safety in Health Care, 14*(2):80-86.

Infusion Nurses Society. (2011). *Infusion nursing: Standards of practice,* vol. 34. Philadelphia: Lippincott Williams & Wilkins.

Institute for Safe Medication Practices. (2005). *Preventing magnesium toxicity in obstetrics.* Retrieved from www.ismp.org/newsletters/ acutecare/articles/20051020.asp

Institute for Safe Medication Practices. (2010). *ISMP's guidelines for standard order sets.* Retrieved from http://www.ismp.org/Tools/ guidelines/StandardOrderSets.asp.

Institute for Safe Medication Practices. (2013). *ISMP's list of error-prone abbreviations, symbols, and dose designations.* Retrieved from www. ismp.org.

Joanna Briggs Institute. (2001). *Maintaining oral hydration in older people,* vol 5. Retrieved from www.joannabriggs.edu.au/best_practice/ BPIShyd.php.

Johnson, N.L., Huang, J.T., & Chang, T. (1996) Control of a multichannel drug infusion pump using a pharmacokinetic model. United States. Abbott Laboratories (Abbott Park, IL). Retrieved from http://www.freepatentsonline.com/5522798.html.

The Joint Commission. (2000). *Infusion pumps: Preventing future adverse effects* (15th ed.). Retrieved from www.jointcommission.org/ SentinelEvents/SentinelEventAlert/sea_15.htm.

The Joint Commission. (2001). *Sentinel event alert: Medication errors related to potentially dangerous abbreviations.* Retrieved from www. jointcommission.org.

Kaboli, P.J., Glasgow, J.M., Jaipaul, C.K., et al. (2010). Identifying medication misadventures: Poor agreement among medical record, physician, nurse, and patient reports [electronic version]. *Pharmacotherapy, 30*(5):529-538.

Kalyn, A., Blatz, S., & Pinelli, M. (2000). A comparison of continuous infusion and intermittent flushing methods in peripheral intravenous catheters in neonates. *Journal of Intravenous Nursing, 23*(3):146-153.

Kazemi, A., Fors, U.G.F., Tofighi, S., et al. (2010). Physician order entry or nurse order entry? Comparison of two implementation strategies for a computerized order entry system aimed at reducing dosing mediation errors. *Journal of Medical Internet Research, 12*(1):e5.

Kee, J.L., Hayes, E.R., & McCuistion, L. (2012). *Pharmacology: A nursing process approach* (7th ed.). Philadelphia: Saunders.

Kee, J.L., Paulanka, J.B., & Polek, C. (2010). *Fluids and electrolytes with clinical applications* (8th ed.). Albany, NY: Delmar Publishers.

Krupp, K., & Heximer, B. (1998). The flow. *Nursing '98, 4*:54-55.

Kuczmarski, R.J., & Flegal, K.M., (2000). Criteria for definition of overweight in transition: Background and recommendations for the United States. *American Society for Clinical Nutrition, 72*:1074-1081.

Kuschel, C. (2004). *Newborn services drug protocol.* Retrieved from http://www.adhb.govt.nz/newborn/DrugProtocols/Default.htm

Lack, J.A., & Stuart-Taylor, M.E. (1997). Calculation of drug dosage and body surface area of children. *British Journal of Anaesthesia, 78*:601-605.

Lacy, C. (1990-2000). *Drug information handbook* (7th ed.). Cleveland: Lexi-Corp, Inc.

Leahy-Patano, M. (2008). Safety at the pump [electronic version]. *Acuity Care Technology.*

Leidel, B.A., Kirchhoff, C., Bogner, V., et al. (2012). Comparison of intraosseous versus central venous vascular access in adults under resuscitation in the emergency department with in accessible peripheral veins. *Resuscitation 83*(1):40-45.

Lilley, L.L., & Guanci, R. (1994). Getting back to basics. *American Journal of Nursing, 9:*15-16.

Lu, M., & Okeke, C. (2005). *Requirements for compounding sterile preparations: Evolution of USP's chapter.* Retrieved from http://www.usp.org/hqi/practitioner-Programs/newsletters/capsLink/

Macklin, D., Chernecky, C., & Infortuna, M.H. (2011). *Math for clinical practice* (2nd ed.) St. Louis: Elsevier/Mosby.

Maddox, R.R., Danello, S., Williams, C.K., & Fields, M. (2008). Intravenous infusion safety initiative: Collaboration, evidence-based best practices, and "smart" technology help avert high-risk adverse drug events and improve patient outcomes [electronic version]. *Advances in Patient Safety: New Directions and Alternative Approaches, 1*(4):1-14.

Magnuson, V., Clifford, T.M., Hoskins, L.A., Bernard, A.C. (2005). Enteral nutrition and drug administration, interactions, and complications. *Nutrition in Clinical Practice, 20*(6):618-624. Retrieved from www.ncp.aspenjournals.org/cgi/content/full/20/6/618.

McKinley Medical. (2001). *Ambulatory infusion pump.* Retrieved from www.mckinleymed.com.

McKinley Medical. (2001). *High tech IVs raise issues—intravenous infusion systems.* Retrieved from www.mckinleymed.com.

McKinley Medical. (n.d.). *Intravenous therapy.* Retrieved from www.mckinleymed.com/intravenous-therapy.shtml.

McKinley Medical. (n.d.). *Infusion pumps.* Retrieved from www.mckinleymed.com/infusion-pump-systems.shtml.

Medscape. (2006). *ASHP National Survey of pharmacy practice.* Retrieved from www.medscape.com/viewarticle/523005.

Mentes, J.C. (2004). *Hydration management evidence based-practice guidelines.* Iowa City: University of Iowa.

Mentes, J.C. (2006). Oral hydration in older adults. *American Journal of Nursing, 106*(6):40-48.

MMWR. (2005). *Immunization management issues,* CDC. Retrieved from www.cdc.gov/mmwr/preview/mmwrhtml/rr5416a3.htm.

Morris, D.G. (2010). Calculate with confidence (5th ed). St. Louis: Elsevier/Mosby.

Mulholland, J.M. (2011). *The nurse, the math, the meds* (2nd ed). St. Louis: Elsevier/Mosby.

Murray, M.D. (n.d.). *Unit-dose drug distribution systems.* Retrieved from www.ahrq.gov/clinic/ptsafety/chap10.htm.

National Coordinating Council for Medication Error Reporting and Prevention. (2005). *Council recommendation.* Retrieved from www.nccmerp.org/council/council1996-09-04.html.

National Institute of Health (NIH). (1998). *First federal obesity clinical guidelines released.* Retrieved from www.nhlbi.nih.gov/new/press/ober14f.htm.

Neville, K., Galinkin J.I., Green, T.P., et al. (2015). Metric units and the preferred dosing of orally administered liquid medications. [electronic Version]. *Pediatrics, 1359*(4):784-787.

Niemi, K., Geary, S., Larrabee, M., & Brown, K.R. (2005). Standardized vasoactive medications: a unified system for every patient, everywhere. *Hospital Pharmacy, 40*(11): 984-993.

Ogden, S.J. (2012). Calculation of drug dosages (9th ed.). St. Louis: Elsevier/Mosby.

Okeke, C. (2005). Pharmaceutical calculations in prescription compounding [electronic version]. *Pharmacopeial Forum, 31*(3):846.

Owen, D., Jew, R., Kaufman, D., & Balmer, D. (1997). Osmolality of commonly used medications and formulas in the neonatal intensive care unit. *Nutrition Clinics, 12*(4).

Oyama, A. (2000). Intravenous line management and prevention of catheter-related infections in America. *Journal of Intravenous Nursing, 23*(3):170-175.

PALL Medical. (n.d.). *Posidyne ELD intravenous filter set.* Retrieved from www.pall.com.

Partners Healthcare System, Inc. (2003). *Project 4: safe intravenous infusion systems.* Retrieved from www.coesafety.bwh.harvard.edu/linkPages/projectsPages/project4.htm.

PatientPlus. (n.d.). *Prescribing in children.* Retrieved from www.patient.co/uk/showdoc/40024942.

Physicians' Desk Reference. (69th ed.). Montvale, NJ: PDR Network, LLC.

Pinkney, S., Trbovich, P., Rothwell, S., et al. (2009). Smart medication delivery system: Infusion pumps. *Healthcare Human Factors Group.* Retrieved from http://www.ehealthinnovation.org/?q_smartpumps.

Ratain, M.J. (1998). Body-surface area as a basis for dosing of anticancer agents: science, myth, or habit? *Journal of Clinical Oncology, 16*(7):2297-2298.

Rothschild, J.M. (2003). *Intelligent intravenous infusion pumps to improve medical administration safety.* AMIA Annual Symposium Process. Retrieved from www.pubmedcentral.nih.gov.articlerender.fegi?artid_1480207.

Savinetti-Rose, B., & Bolmer, L. (1997). Understanding continuous subcutaneous insulin infusion therapy. *American Journal of Nursing, 97:*42-49.

Skokal, W. (1997). Infusion pump update. *RN, 60:*35-38.

Spratto, G., & Woods, A. (2003). *PDR Nurse's drug handbook.* Albany, NY: Delmar Publishers.

Taxis, K. (2005). *Safety infusion devices.* Grogingen: BMJ Publishing Group. Retrieved from www.qhc.bmjjournals.com/cgi/content/ful/14/2/76.

Terry, J., Baranowski, L., Lonsway, R., & Hedrick, C. (1995). *Intravenous therapy: Clinical principles and practice.* Philadelphia: W.B. Saunders.

Tessella Support Services. (2005). *Software that saves your life.* ALARIS. Retrieved from www.tessella.com/literature/articles/tessarchive/alaris.htm.

Thimbleby, H., & Williams, D. (2013).Using nomograms to reduce harm from clinical calculations. *Proceedings of IEEE International Conference on Healthcare Informatics,* 461-470.

Toedter Williams, N. (2009). Medical administration through enteral feeding tubes [electronic version]. *American Journal of Health-Systems Pharmacy, 65*(24):2347-2357.

Truax Group (The). (2010). *Infusion pump safety.* Retrieved from http://www.patientsafetysolutions.com/docs/April_27_2010_Infusion_Pump_Safety.htm.

Vanderveen, T. (2002). *Impact of intravenous (IV) infusion medication errors.* Retrieved from www.cardinalhealth.com/alaris/support/clinical/pdfs/wpguardrails.asp.

Vanderveen, T. (2005). *Medication safety: averting high-risk errors is first priority.* Patient Safety & Quality Healthcare. Retrieved from www.psqh.com/mayjun05/averting.html.

Wideman, M.V., Whittler, M.E., & Anderson, T.M. (n.d.). *Barcode medication administration: lessons learned from an intensive card unit implementation.* Columbia, Mo: Agency for Healthcare Research and Quality.

Wyeth Laboratories. (1988). *Intramuscular injections.* Philadelphia: Wyeth Laboratories.

Youngberg Webb, P., & Chilamkurti, R. (2009). Formulations: RTU drug products, the keys to RTU parenterals [electronic version]. *Pharmaceutical Formulation & Quality.*

INDEX

Page references with f indicate figures; those with t, tables.